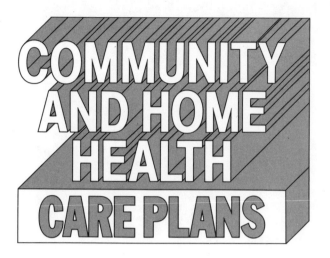

COMMUNITY AND HOME HEALTH CARE PLANS

Marion B. Dolan, RN

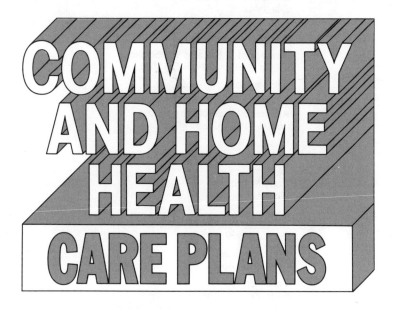

COMMUNITY AND HOME HEALTH CARE PLANS

Marion B. Dolan, RN

Springhouse Corporation
Springhouse, Pennsylvania

Staff

Executive Director, Editorial
Stanley Loeb

Executive Director, Creative Services
Jean Robinson

Director of Trade and Textbooks
Minnie B. Rose, RN, BSN, MEd

Art Director
John Hubbard

Associate Acquisitions Editor
Bernadette M. Glenn

Editors
Kevin Law (editorial manager), David
Moreau

Copy Editor
Elizabeth Kiselev

Designers
Stephanie Peters (associate art director),
Donna Giannola

Art Production
Donna Giannola

Typography
David Kosten (director), Diane Paluba
(assistant manager), Elizabeth Bergman,
Joyce Rossi Biletz, Robin Rantz, Valerie
Rosenberger

Manufacturing
Deborah Meiris (manager), T.A. Landis,
Jennifer Suter

Production Coordination
Aline S. Miller (manager), Colleen Hayman

CHCP-021090

Library of Congress Cataloging-in-Publication Data
Dolan, Marion B.
  Community and home health care plans / Marion B. Dolan.
    p. cm.
  Includes bibliographical references.
  1. Nursing care plans.   2. Community health nursing.   3. Home nursing.   4. Nursing. I. Title
    [DNLM: 1. Community Health Nursing.
2. Home Care Services.   3. Patient Care Planning.
WY 115 D659c]
RT49.D65 1989
362.1′4—dc20
DNLM/DLC   89-21823
ISBN 0-87434-225-2   CIP

For information about our audio products, write us at:
Newbridge Book Clubs, 3000 Cindel Drive, Delran, NJ 08370

Contents

Acknowledgments

The author wishes to thank the following people for their contributions:

Bernadette Glenn, Acquisitions Editor, Springhouse, for her support and guidance in helping the idea of a book on home health become a reality.

Kevin Law, Editorial Manager, Springhouse, for his wisdom and humor in helping to mold the material on home care planning into the fruition of a book.

Linda Maines, Administrative Assistant, Heritage, for her dedication and loyalty to the care plan project.

My dad, Stanley Muchewicz, for believing in home health, hospice, and especially me.

DEDICATION

To Louise and Veronica, who by their deaths at home, and Alyssa Lyn and Matthew, who by their births, have taught me that the only thing that truly matters is how we spend the time in between the two events.

Contributors and Consultants

Contributors

Shirley Avellino, RN
Hospice Coordinator
Heritage Home Health
Heritage Hospice
Bristol, N.H.
(Pain)

Sondra Bergman Baird, RN, MEd, MSN
Nursing Instructor
Abington (Pa.) Memorial Hospital
(Cellulitis)

Nancy Barton, RN, MSN
Gerontology Clinical Specialist
Northeast Georgia Medical Center
Gainesville
(Angina Pectoris)

Linda M. Benton, RN
ABC Home Health Services Inc.
Commerce, Ga.
(Hepatitis)

Carole Bloom, RN
Southern New Jersey Visiting
Nurses Association (SNJVNA)
Woodbury
Community Health and Nursing
Services (CHANS)
Collingswood, N.J.
(Breast Cancer)

Marcia Gilbert Bower, RN,C MSN
Instructor
Abington (Pa.) Memorial Hospital
(Osteomyelitis, Total Parenteral Nutrition)

Diane M. Breckenridge, RN, MSN
Independent Renal Nurse Consultant
and Nursing Instructor
Abington (Pa.) Memorial Hospital
(Neurogenic Bladder)

Elizabeth A. Burtt, RN, BS, MS, MPH
Coordinator
Tuberculosis Control Program and
Tuberculosis Control Officer (Retired, 1988)
Bureau of Disease Control
New Hampshire Division of Public Health Services
Concord
(Tuberculosis)

Joyce Cameron, RN, MSN
Instructor
Capstone College of Nursing
University of Alabama
Tuscaloosa
(Amputation)

Cristol Ward Cannon, RN
Administrator
ABC Home Health Services Inc.
Dublin, Ga.
(Osteoporosis)

Sister Alberta Carey, SC, RN, MA
Associate Director
Director of Training
Office of Substance Abuse
Ministry
Archdiocese of New York
(Substance Abuse)

Katherine Kerins Carr, MS, ARNP
Assistant Professor of Nursing
St. Anselm College
Manchester, N.H.
"Homeless Project"
Adult Nurse Practitioner
Manchester (N.H.) Visiting Nurse Association
(Chronic Congestive Heart Failure)

Patricia Carr, RN
Quality Assurance Coordinator
Florida Home Health Services
Sarasota, Inc.
Sarasota
(Brain Tumors, Cerebrovascular Accident, Cirrhosis,
Colostomy, Diabetes Mellitus, Lung Cancer, Total
Hip Replacement, Total Knee Replacement,
Uterine Cancer)

Barbara A. Davis, RN, BS, MS
Clinical Instructor
Watts School of Nursing
Durham County Hospital Corp.
Home Health Services RN
Medical Personnel Pool
Durham, N.C.
(Gastrointestinal Cancer)

Ellen Thomas Eggland, RN, MN
Vice President
Healthcare Personnel, Inc.
Naples, Fla.
(Osteoarthritis)

Joann Kelly Erb, RN,C, MSN
Nursing Instructor
Abington (Pa.) Memorial Hospital
School of Nursing
(Chronic Bronchitis)

Helen Flaherty, RN, MEd
Level Coordinator
Medical-Surgical Instructor
Abington (Pa.) Memorial Hospital
(Hiatal Hernia)

Janet Carol Fox, RN,C, BSN, MSN
Instructor
Abington (Pa.) Memorial Hospital
School of Nursing
(Esophagitis, Gastroenteritis)

Diane Broadbent Friedman, RN, MSN, CS
Formerly, Clinical Nurse Specialist,
Epilepsy and Sleep Disorders
Department of Neurology
Cleveland (Ohio) Clinic Foundation
(Seizure Disorders, Sleep Disorders)

Teresa Byron Fuller, RN
Discharge Planning Nurse
Mary Hitchcock Memorial Hospital
Hanover, N.H.
(Prostate Cancer)

Linda Garner, RN, MSN
Rehabilitation Specialist
Rehabilitation Management Services
Birmingham, Ala.
(Hypertension)

Susan W. Gaskins, RN, MPH
Instructor
Capstone College of Nursing
The University of Alabama
Tuscaloosa
(Indwelling Catheter Care)

Claire J. Gordon, ARNP
Ob-Gyn Nurse Practitioner
Dartmouth Hitchcock Clinic
Bedford, N.H.
(Sexually Transmitted Diseases)

P. Allen Gray, Jr., RN, PhD
Assistant Professor and Director
RN ACCESS Program
School of Nursing
University of North Carolina
at Wilmington
(Sex and Sexuality)

Beulah Barnard Hall, RN, EdD
Director
B.S. Nursing Program
Hahnemann University
Philadelphia
(Manic-Depressive Illness, Schizophrenia)

Barbara S. Harrison, RN,C, EdS
Assistant Professor
School of Nursing
Hampton (Va.) University
(Psoriasis)

Beth H. Hensley, RN, BSN
Consultant-Owner
Advance Health Care Consultants
New Richmond, Ohio
(Thrombophlebitis)

Ann B. Howard
Executive Director
American Federation of Home Health Agencies
Silver Spring, Md.
(Perspectives and Trends)

Susan Montgomery Hunter, RN, BSN, MSN
Assistant Professor
Adult Health Nursing
College of Nursing
University of North Dakota
Grand Forks
(Pneumonia)

Donna Ignatavicius, RN, MS
Di Associates
Baltimore
(Fractured Hip)

Cynthia Lange Ingham, RN, BSN
Public Health Nursing Specialist
Vermont Department of Health
Burlington
(Developmental Disabilities)

Sheryl A. Innerarity, RN, PhD
Assistant Professor
Midwestern State University
Program of Nursing
Wichita Falls, Tex.
(Kidney Transplant)

Susan Keady, RN
Public Health Nurse
Bureau of Disease Control
Division of Public Health Services
Concord, N.H.
(Acquired Immunodeficiency Syndrome)

E. Juanita Lee, RN, EdD
Associate Professor
University of Southern California
Los Angeles
(Parkinson's Disease)

Helen D. Loiselle, RN
Clinical Coordinator
TPN Healthcare Services
Laconia, N.H.
(Smoking Cessation)

Preface

Although doctors rarely make house calls, legions of home health nurses are called upon to provide quality care for patients at home every day. Unfortunately, care plan guides written specifically for the home health nurse are scarce—and either maddeningly superficial or too detailed or too poorly organized to benefit the nurse and the patient. Without a comprehensive, practical resource for hands-on care planning in the home, many home health nurses still refer to hospital-oriented medical-surgical texts, which overlook the patient's home and community as factors influencing health.

In writing this book, I collaborated with more than 50 experts in community and home health nursing to provide current and vital information on community-based care planning in an easy-to-use format. My primary goals were the special needs of the patient being cared for at home and the challenges confronting the home health nurse. Because the patient's community plays a significant role during care, each of the 65 care plans includes information relevant to nurses working in various community settings, such as senior centers, neighborhood health centers, clinics, mental health centers, and community outreach locations. Nursing instructors and nursing students seeking a care planning model for community health nursing also will find the book a valuable reference.

We live in a time when more and more nurses are treating greater numbers of patients in the home and community rather than in a hospital. To provide quality care for these patients, the nurse must have a reliable resource of nursing diagnoses, interventions, and rationales appropriate to those settings. I hope this book proves to be such a resource.

—Marion B. Dolan

Section I

Introduction

Perspectives and Trends

Home care is on the cutting edge of change in nursing and health care. In a time of increasing concern over federal health care expenditures, home care represents a humane, sensible, cost-effective alternative to institutionalized health care for an increasing number of Americans. It also offers other benefits, including eliminating the risk of nosocomial infection, maintaining patients' and families' social and cultural patterns, and promoting patients' self-esteem, independence, and personal involvement in care.

Ongoing expansion of home health agencies, gradually increasing federal and private reimbursement for home care services, and growing consumer demand for home care demonstrate the increasing importance of home health care. Today, many diverse and often conflicting forces are influencing the direction of home health care. These forces include cost containment pressures and other financial trends, an increasing elderly population, increasing consumer demand for quality health care services, and increasing competition for health care dollars.

FINANCIAL TRENDS

The Medicare program provides a reliable predictor of changes in the health care delivery system. Because it finances a large percentage of the medical and nursing services provided in the United States, any changes in Medicare influence the entire system.

Medicare and home care

The establishment of the Medicare program in the mid-1960s transformed the home health delivery system. Before Medicare, most home care was provided by voluntary visiting nurse associations (VNAs), and most home care clients were elderly persons with chronic (but usually not critical) illnesses who required basic nursing care and homemaking assistance. Payment for these services came from social welfare agencies, charities, or personal funds.

The advent of Medicare changed not only the payment source, but also the very nature of home care. Under federal direction, doctors became involved in managing home care delivery, and the emphasis of home care shifted from a nursing-based to a medical-based model. Home care came to be viewed as a less-costly substitute for extended hospitalization or as an extension of hospital and nursing home care. Medicare focused on covering the costs of treating acute illnesses of relatively short duration in institutions; it reimbursed for home care only until the patient recovered from the acute phase of illness. A patient's eligibility for Medicare reimbursement for home health services was based on the patient's acute care needs and certain criteria—the patient must be homebound, in need of skilled care (defined as medically directed care provided by a

nurse or other health care professional), and under the care of a doctor, who must plan, review, and certify all treatment.

This shift to a medical-based emphasis largely overlooked the need for the preventive and health-promoting care provided by nurses, as well as for support services. Although VNAs and other agencies continued to provide this care and these services, Medicare provided minimal reimbursement. The new medical emphasis also resulted in more stringent requirements for home health agencies' certification for Medicare reimbursement. As a result of these changes, the number of voluntary home care agencies declined dramatically, and public, proprietary, and hospital-based home care agencies grew.

Overall, Medicare has achieved its original purpose. Although some important areas remain uncovered, the program does provide much-needed help with the costs of acute care for elderly and other eligible persons. However, in the decades since Medicare was enacted, the health needs of these persons have changed dramatically. Medicare has not addressed many of these needs—especially those related to long-term care.

Today, most elderly persons survive the acute phase of illness and face relatively long periods of chronic illness marked by ongoing debilitation. Home care is tailor-made for these persons. Unfortunately, because of the way in which Medicare is structured, many elderly Americans who cannot meet increasingly restrictive Medicare home health reimbursement requirements face a tough choice: seek institutionalized care to remain eligible for reimbursement or go without services. This situation has contributed to a startling increase in Medicare outlays, which in turn has spurred measures designed to curtail expenditures, coming from Congress and the Health Care Financing Administration (HCFA), which administers the Medicare program.

The next several decades will see a dramatic increase in the Medicare-eligible population. From approximately 31.5 million Americans ages 65 and over, demographers predict that by the year 2030, the number will rise to 55 million, nearly a quarter of our population. The 85-and-older population, those most in need of home care services, is predicted to double by 2030.

Although the demographics ensure that the demand for home care will increase, the shape of the home health benefit of the future is not clear. The national economy, actions of Congress and the HCFA, and the quality of care needed and delivered will all have an impact on this benefit.

Cost containment

For the foreseeable future, federal budget deficits will drive national health care policy. Political pressure to reduce the deficit is spurring congressional and executive branch action to control costs throughout the government. Existing and proposed programs will continue to be reviewed carefully for cost-effectiveness.

Although many critics point out that the federal deficit could be trimmed by raising taxes and by curtailing defense and domestic programs, politicians perceive the American public as resoundingly opposed to tax increases. At a time when support for reductions in defense spending is considered politically risky, deficit reduction pressures have fallen disproportionately on domestic programs. For most of this decade, the only major exception to applying significant limitations solely on the social service side has been the Gramm-Rudman-Hollings deficit reduction legislation, which includes defense spending in across-the-board cuts mandated if deficit reduction targets are not met. Such cuts have been imposed twice and remain a threat if Congress does not meet targets through program reductions and tax increases.

In federal health programs, budgetary pressures have led to demands for setting new priorities. In a sense, a triage system is developing as competition for limited federal dollars grows stiffer. Although considerable congressional support exists for expanding the home health benefit to address the needs of chronically ill Medicare beneficiaries, even some of home care's strongest congressional supporters believe that other concerns are more pressing—for example, health coverage for the nation's uninsured, a population that includes millions of children.

In any expansion of home health services, federal policymakers fear a perceived "woodwork effect": beneficiaries who now are making do with the assistance of family support, expenditure of their own financial resources, or even going without care would "come out of the woodwork" to claim services, thus straining federal resources even further. This argument does not address the issue of whether the current lack of such services places an unbearable strain on family and financial resources or whether services currently forgone are nevertheless needed.

While Congress has debated health care priorities, the executive branch has targeted home health for cuts that go well beyond congressional intent to provide a limited benefit or concerns about cost control. The HCFA's rationale for making home health a target appears to be that, on a percentage basis, home health care has grown faster than most other Medicare components in recent years. The HCFA's own statistics demonstrate that the growth of the benefit is due primarily to the increasing number of eligible beneficiaries, not to the overutilization of the benefit by patients or abuse by home health agencies and doctors. Nevertheless, over the last several years, the HCFA has curtailed the availability of home health services through restrictive regulations and directives to its fiscal intermediaries who review home health claims for the HCFA.

Recently, the HCFA has issued restrictive changes so rapidly that home health agencies can hardly adjust to one before several more are imposed. Many agencies have been unable to bear the cumulative effect, especially with the additional cash flow problems created for home health agencies, as cost-reimbursed providers, under reductions mandated by Gramm-Rudman-Hollings, the 1-year imposition of per discipline cost limits, and the lowering of these cost limits. Even while reducing reimbursement, the HCFA has continued to impose time-consuming policies and procedures that drive up costs—for example, the requirement for provision of "minimum data elements" on Forms 485, 486, and 487. Professionals must complete these forms, reducing highly skilled personnel to "paper pushers." These forms demonstrate the tendency of Medicare funds to flow toward additional regulatory burdens rather than toward actual patient care.

The HCFA apparently has attempted to create a climate of uncertainty for home health agencies in the hope that, rather than risk disallowances, agencies would arbitrarily cut back on the delivery of services—even when good medical practice would suggest that the visits should be made. The 1980s has brought a significant increase in the denial of home health claims (although the denial rate has leveled off in recent years). The pressure to increase claims denials came in part from the HCFA's mandate to fiscal intermediaries to produce specific dollar returns for every dollar expended for medical and utilization review. Not until Congress finally intervened did the HCFA suspend fiscal intermediary denial quotas for home health for the end of 1987 and all of 1988.

Catastrophic health insurance

The federal budget–driven curtailment of Medicare home health and other services throughout the 1980s has required congressional intervention time and again. Fortunately, beneficiaries and care providers have succeeded not only in stopping some of the most egregious HCFA practices restricting provision of services but also got across the message of the deficiencies of Medicare coverage itself. Thus, 1988 saw the first major expansion of the Medicare program, through passage of legislation addressing catastrophic health insurance coverage.

The Medicare Catastrophic Coverage Act, signed into law on July 1, 1988, is intended to provide protection for beneficiaries against the cost of catastrophic illness through:
• expansion of the home health and skilled nursing home benefit
• provision of unlimited hospital days
• implementation of an outpatient prescription drug benefit
• a cap on out-of-pocket beneficiary expenses.

Specific home health provisions, effective as of January 1, 1990, include:

• daily skilled nursing and home health aide services for up to 38 consecutive days, with *daily* defined as 7 days per week (Congress also intended additional daily care beyond the 38 days as necessary, with a doctor's certification of exceptional circumstances.)
• a limited in-home respite care benefit for chronically dependent persons—up to 80 hours over a 12-month period
• home I.V. therapy items and services, including fluids (antibiotic, chemotherapy, immunosupressive), medical supplies, equipment, and nursing care for I.V. delivery.

As with existing benefits, availability of the expanded program will depend largely on whether the administration elected in 1988 is serious about ensuring that beneficiaries receive the services to which they are entitled and on the tone set for fiscal intermediaries by the HCFA.

Catastrophic health insurance coverage has a major deficiency, however—it does not address costs associated with chronic long-term home health and nursing home care. In June 1988, Congress rejected one solution to the problem of lack of home care services for the chronically ill when the House of Representatives, on a procedural vote, turned aside Congressman Claude Pepper's Medicare Long-Term Home Care Catastrophic Protection Act. This legislation was designed to provide the six presently covered services, plus supplies and durable medical equipment, to chronically ill elderly and disabled people and to technology-dependent children unable to perform at least two activities of daily living. Even as the House took this action, powerful congressional opponents of the Pepper bill made commitments to move forward with consideration of long-term care legislation in the 101st Congress.

Even though it was defeated, the Pepper legislation represented the beginning of serious congressional debate on long-term care. Final passage of a long-term care bill could occur within a year or could be several years away.

Future legislative possibilities
The debate on the Pepper bill in the House of Representatives reflected the concern of many members of Congress that the legislation was not a comprehensive solution to the long-term care problem. A final package could take the form of the Pepper bill or it may well be a combination of several approaches, including both chronic long-term home health and nursing home care and encouragement of private sector initiatives. Many long-term care bills have been introduced in the Senate and House of Representatives incorporating various benefits and funding mechanisms. We should expect emergence of a compromise approach that appeals to all segments of the political spectrum.

Look for a basic chronic home health and nursing home benefit applying to Medicare-eligible Americans as well as for provisions to encourage private insurers to offer long-term care policies supplementing the basic benefit and to encourage employers to offer long-term care insurance as an employee benefit.

Any expansion of the Medicare home health benefit undoubtedly will be accompanied by various provisions for limiting use and controlling costs. These provisions may include:
• cost sharing, with care recipients paying an increasing percentage of health care charges
• case management and care management
• benefit eligibility restrictions
• limitations on types of services offered
• regulation of the number and frequency of home care visits.

A major Congressional concern in debate on the Pepper bill was cost. The program funding mechanism involves eliminating the $45,000 cap on the portion of individual income subject to the Medicare tax. Partial or complete lifting of the cap is a feature of nearly all of the long-term care bills under development.

This raises the question of how a president adamantly pledged to no tax increases would react to creation of a program financed by a hike in Medicare taxes. For the foreseeable future, cost will continue to be a major consideration in all federal programs and proposed legislation.

Nevertheless, long-term care is popular with American voters, making it a potentially potent issue with Republican and Democrat, conservative and liberal politicians. Voters strongly favor pro-long-term care candidates, according to a nationwide poll of 1,000 potential voters done by RL Associates for Long-Term Care '88. The poll found that 50% of the respondents are more likely to vote for a candidate who supports long-term care, and only 4% are less likely to support such a candidate. Various other national polls have indicated that long-term care for elderly Americans is a top priority of all voting age-groups.

We should expect any expanded home care services funded by the American taxpayers to be accompanied by an intensified scrutiny of the quality of care provided. Already, Congress has mandated:
• professional review organization (PRO) review of home health care agencies
• enumeration of patients' rights
• training requirements for home health aides
• creation of state toll-free hot lines and investigative units
• implementation of sanctions against home health care agencies found deficient.

OTHER TRENDS
Besides financial trends, various other trends are affecting the current nature and future direction of home care.

Changes in the health care delivery system
As an increasingly important segment of the American health care delivery system, home care has been and will continue to be affected by changes in this system. Over the next decade, an increasing number of regional intensive care units and surgical/trauma centers will force many smaller hospitals to close because of econ-

omic problems. As a result, more medical care will be delivered in the home setting, and more surviving hospitals will develop home care agencies. However, because of their enormous administrative overhead, many hospital-based home health agencies will find it difficult to cost-compete with non-hospital-based agencies. Look for partnerships between home care agencies and hospitals to provide patient care, with patient information shared between the hospital and the home care agency to prevent costly and perhaps dangerous duplication of tests and procedures and help minimize gaps in patient care.

Staffing trends

As its importance grows, home care will call for an increasing scope of nursing practice, requiring nurses working in home care settings to move from being generalists to specialists and requiring more nurses on agency staffs. More clinical nurse specialists and nurse practitioners will expand their primary practices into home care settings. Also, look for an increasing number of nurse-owned and -operated home health agencies.

Increasing numbers of other health care professionals, such as respiratory therapists, psychologists, and nutritionists, also will join home care agency staffs.

Another change will be the addition of doctors to home care agency staffs. Currently, 70% of doctors under age 35 are employed by a hospital, health maintenance organization (HMO), or other type of agency. By the year 2010, virtually all doctors in the United States will be employed by a hospital or agency—many by home care agencies. Having a doctor on staff will facilitate timely medical orders, revision of care plans, and recertifications for the home health agency.

Technological advances

Rapid technological advancement will continue to influence home care and home health nursing. Care of more acutely ill patients in the home will require increasingly sophisticated equipment and techniques. I.V. therapy, total parenteral nutrition, and dialysis are now commonplace in the home. In the near future, look for more medical equipment, such as respirators, and procedures, such as blood transfusions, in the home setting. These technological advancements will require that home health nurses develop not only increased knowledge and expertise, but also good teaching skills to instruct the patient and family on using sophisticated equipment and performing special procedures.

Paperwork reduction

The HCFA is finally starting to take steps to reduce the amount of paperwork required to document home care visits and secure reimbursement from Medicare for services provided. Currently, the cost of a home care visit averages $375—only $65 of which is attributable to nursing and other home care services. The remaining $310 derives from administrative costs for home health agencies, fiscal intermediaries, and the HCFA—costs that should be directed instead to patient services.

In an effort to reduce their paperwork and thus lower administrative costs, some home care agencies are using HCFA Forms 485, 486, and 487 not only as reimbursement and recertification forms, but also as patient care plan forms. This saves the home health nurse valuable time, which can be spent providing hands-on nursing care in the home.

Geriatric day care

Another trend in home care is toward geriatric day care. More than 1,500 geriatric day-care centers now serve about 60,000 elderly persons in the United States, and these numbers are growing rapidly. By setting up such a center, an agency can help keep its patients at home and out of the hospital.

Payment for this type of care still comes only from the private sector; however, within the next 10 years, look for geriatric day care to be funded on the federal and state levels.

Pediatric home care

Public perception traditionally has seen home health care as focusing on adults, particularly elderly adults. But with an increasing number of ill children being discharged from hospitals to home, pediatric home care is evolving as a distinct and important segment of home health care.

Usually, an ill child does much better in the home environment. Parents typically are highly motivated and dedicated caregivers, especially when support services are available from a home health agency. Home care enables the child to maintain emotional and physical closeness to the family, minimizing disruption of family patterns, and also helps the child maintain social contacts outside the family, contributing to continued normal social development.

Personal services

Recognizing the need to expand existing services to meet patient demands and to broaden their fiscal base, home care agencies are implementing various programs and services beyond traditional health care services. Popular services and programs include wellness clinics, shared housing, pet therapy, hospice care, and even transportation services that go beyond illness-related needs, such as doctor visits, to offer home care patients transportation for social events, shopping trips, and other personal needs.

Case management and care management

Perhaps the most important trend in home health care involves case management and care management. Although the two terms often are used interchangeably, case management and care management differ in terms of the caregiver or agencies involved and the services provided.

Case management may be defined as a system of assessing patient needs, planning and coordinating services, and making referrals to meet the multiple needs of home care patients. Home-health agencies, hospitals, insurance companies, and private entrepreneurs act as case managers. Reimbursed by fiscal intermediaries or care recipients, case managers offer referral services for financial, health, housing, and personal concerns. They may or may not offer nursing or health-care services.

Care management, on the other hand, focuses mainly on patients' health care concerns. Care management involves controlling, monitoring, reviewing, and directing health care in the most effective manner as well as recommending the most appropriate treatment in the most efficient environment. Care managers offer home care in the form of nurses, home health aides, homemakers, therapists, and rehabilitative services.

Despite their differences, both case management and care management grow logically from the basic precepts of nursing. They provide a guide for necessary items needed for health—housing, nutrition, sanitation, and human support. As the case and care management concepts evolve, home care will take on a more individualized, personalized approach encompassing not only skilled nursing services, but also every other service required by home care patients.

Case management and care management are valuable tools for home care agencies to help prevent patients from "falling through the cracks" in today's health care delivery system. They are needed most by elderly patients and other vulnerable members of society. However, the case or care management approach is not appropriate for every patient. A patient and family who are capable of managing their own care should be encouraged to do so to help them maintain their usual functional patterns and independence.

Ann B. Howard
Executive Director
American Federation of Home Health Agencies

Marion B. Dolan, RN
President
Heritage Home Health and Hospice and People-Match

Using the Care Plans

These care plans are designed to give the reader a maximum amount of information in a minimum number of pages. They are intended not as a substitute for more detailed nursing reference works, but rather as a guide for providing "hands on" nursing care for patients in the home setting.

Each care plan is formatted similarly, with various sections presenting specific information. Becoming familiar with the basic format will enable the nurse to use the plans more effectively. Explanations of each section follow, along with specific recommendations for using the care plans in practice.

Description and time focus

This section begins with a brief discussion of the disorder, procedure, or problem on which the care plan focuses. Information may include etiology and precipitating factors, incidence, possible treatments, potential complications, and morbidity and mortality statistics.

The section continues with the focus of care planning for a patient with the identified condition. Except for the Hospice Care entry (which focuses on preparing the patient and family for the patient's imminent death), each care plan focuses on nursing interventions that will enhance the patient's health, functional ability, and independence.

The section ends with information on typical home health care length of service and visit frequency, based on average duration and frequency of home health nursing care for the identified condition. Remember, these are average figures that can change if the patient meets his goals sooner than expected or if complications develop. Length of service also depends on the patient meeting the criteria for skilled care. The fiscal intermediary pays for skilled services; thus, as long as care meets the definition of skilled service, this care may continue. Skilled nursing care is a covered home health service under Medicare when services are ordered by a doctor and include a plan of treatment established by the doctor for the patient. For home care services to qualify, the services must be performed on an intermittent basis and be deemed reasonable and necessary; the patient also must be homebound and have a medical need for nursing care.

Health history findings, physical findings, and diagnostic studies

Next are three assessment sections that present findings common to most patients with the identified condition. The intent is to provide a vivid clinical picture of the typical patient presentation in a given condition.

The first section, "Health history findings," lists typical subjective assessment findings, including patient complaints (symptoms) and other factors (such as family history of disease) that may be linked to the condition's development or possible complications. The emphasis is on definitive or common findings for the identified condition, not on every possible finding the patient may report.

The next section, "Physical findings," lists typical objective assessment findings for a patient presenting with the identified condition. These findings are grouped by body system, beginning with the body system most closely linked to the condition and continuing in the order in which the body system–grouped care plans are presented within the book.

The final section, "Diagnostic studies," presents information on laboratory and diagnostic tests typically performed for a patient in the home setting after the patient has received a thorough diagnostic workup in a hospital or outpatient clinic. For example, a patient with diabetes will continue to measure blood glucose levels at home, and a patient recovering from acute myocardial infarction will have blood samples drawn periodically for measurement of prothrombin time and other hematologic values. For each test listed, information is given on its purpose (and sometimes usual findings) and its frequency. Not all tests listed may be performed on a particular patient; which tests are ordered depends on individual factors. However, this section helps the nurse be aware of the significance of tests that may pertain to the patient's condition.

Nursing diagnoses, interventions, and rationales

This section contains the main body of the care plan: the major problems typically associated with the identified condition, classified by specific nursing diagnoses. All of the nursing diagnoses in this book are derived from the latest NANDA taxonomy of nursing diagnoses (see Appendix 1).

According to nursing diagnoses, all problems are actual or potential. An actual problem is one that is present and usually can be identified by clinical signs and symptoms. A potential problem is one that the patient may develop—even though signs and symptoms are not present—based on the nurse's identification of risk factors in the patient's health history.

Each nursing diagnosis is followed by one or more nursing goals, which specify the focus of the nursing interventions that follow.

The interventions and rationales, presented in a two-column format, represent the "how to" section of the care plans. Simply stated, the interventions explain what to do and the rationales explain why. Interventions are based on clinical experience and nursing literature and thus represent a blend of practice and theory.

Keep in mind that all listed interventions may not apply to each patient with the identified condition. Of course, certain basic care practices—such as sterile dressing changes, proper hand-washing techniques, and proper disposal of contaminated medical waste—apply to all patients. But many others do not. The nurse must personalize care for each patient. The home is a unique environment in which to practice nursing. Each home health nurse soon becomes aware that, unlike a large hospital, which has specific written policies and procedures, each home has its own unwritten policies and procedures that the nurse must learn and respect.

The home health nurse, acting as case manager, must select the appropriate interventions to enable goal achievement. The home health nurse also must be astute enough to apply these interventions in a way that the patient and family will accept, taking into account personal characteristics and preferences. A home health nurse could be asked to leave and the service cancelled if the patient or family feels that the case is not being handled appropriately.

Associated care plans

Following the final nursing diagnosis and its interventions and rationales is a section listing other care plans in the book that the nurse may refer to for more information on the patient's condition and additional applicable nursing diagnoses and interventions. For example, Mrs. Smith, who is receiving home health care related to treatment for uterine cancer, has questions about sexual activity during treatment. Besides the Uterine Cancer care plan, the Sex and Sexuality care plan also will help the nurse plan care for this patient.

Networking of services

Meals On Wheels, Lifeline and other emergency response systems, fuel assistance programs, senior centers, retired senior volunteer programs, religious groups, the Women, Infants, and Children (WIC) free food program, and the Council on Aging are some of the resources offered in most communities for patients receiving home health care. This section lists appropriate services to help the home health nurse round out care planning. For example, Mr. Jones, who lives alone, has been discharged home to complete recovery from a hip fracture. Meals On Wheels can help compensate for his inability to shop for food and prepare meals, and a religious group may send a visitor regularly to help combat feelings of isolation and loneliness.

Care team involved

This section lists the health care team members who may be involved in providing home health care for a patient with the identified condition. Besides the nurse and the patient and family—who are always included—this list includes other professionals who can provide necessary services, such as a doctor, physical therapist, occupational therapist, speech therapist, home health aide, and medical social worker. This information allows the nurse to seek doctor's orders for all necessary and appropriate services.

Implications for home care

This section lists important factors for the nurse to consider when assessing the patient's home for suitability as a care setting. Often, the home must be adapted to accommodate changes in the patient's abilities. For example, a patient with a spinal cord injury may require several changes in the home's functional features, such as replacing stairs with ramps to ease access to the home, widening doorways to allow passage of a wheelchair, and installing grab bars in the bathroom to ease transfer to the toilet and bathtub. By identifying and arranging for necessary adaptations, the nurse can greatly enhance the effectiveness of home health care. Another important consideration is telephone service. Patients must communicate with health care providers about emergency and routine concerns, as well as with family and friends to help minimize feelings of loneliness and isolation. A telephone also allows the home health care agency to check on the patient without arranging for a nursing visit.

Patient education tools

This section lists various educational resources, such as brochures and pamphlets, that give the patient and family more information about a disorder, procedure, or problem. Sources may include drug and medical equipment manufacturers, the American Cancer Society, the Arthritis Foundation, the American Heart Association, the American Lung Association, the Easter Seal Foundation, and Planned Parenthood.

Discharge plan from home health care

This section presents criteria for the nurse to use in evaluating a patient's readiness for discontinuation of home health care and the patient's and family's ability to continue home care after the agency is no longer involved. These criteria can range from actual physiologic parameters (such as the ability to perform self-care adequately) to patient demonstrations of appropriate knowledge of treatments and other care procedures (such as proper use of prescribed medication) to evidence of plans for necessary follow-up care (such as telephone numbers of the home health care agency and doctor on hand and dates and times of scheduled appointments marked on a calendar). This list helps the nurse coordinate care and also provides the patient, home health care agency, doctor, and fiscal intermediary with a checklist of the care provided.

Selected references

Concluding each care plan is a list of selected references, which may prove helpful to the nurse seeking more information.

Organization of the book

This book presents three basic types of care plans. Section II presents clinical care plans that focus on a disorder or procedure and that are grouped by the body system most closely linked to the disorder or procedure. Section III contains general care plans that provide the nurse with information on common problems and procedures (such as pain, grief and grieving, and intermittent I.V. therapy) applicable to any patient. Section IV presents community-based care plans—including sexually transmitted diseases, acquired immunodeficiency syndrome (AIDS), and substance abuse—that have an impact not only on the patient and family, but also on the community as a whole.

Section II

Clinical Care Plans

Acute Myocardial Infarction

DESCRIPTION AND TIME FOCUS

Myocardial infarction (MI), or the necrosis of myocardial tissue, usually is caused by coronary artery occlusion or spasm. Post-acute myocardial infarction (AMI) care must focus on health maintenance so that the myocardium can heal. The patient's home provides an excellent environment for the home health nurse to monitor for complications (such as congestive heart failure) and to conduct patient teaching.

This clinical plan focuses on the patient discharged home from an acute-care hospital after diagnosis, management, and treatment of an AMI.

■ Typical home health care length of service for a patient with uncomplicated recovery from AMI: 4 weeks

■ Typical visit frequency: once weekly

HEALTH HISTORY FINDINGS

In a health history interview, the patient may report many of these findings:
• chest pain
• palpitations
• intermittent claudication
• dyspnea and shortness of breath on exertion
• recurrent nausea
• recurrent vomiting
• indigestion
• fatigue
• anxiety
• sedentary life-style
• emotional stress
• tobacco use
• high dietary fat intake
• occasional vertigo
• history of hypertension
• history of diabetes
• history of cardiac dysfunction
• family history of cardiac disease

PHYSICAL FINDINGS

In a physical examination, the nurse may detect many of these findings:

Cardiovascular
• tachycardia or bradycardia
• hypertension or hypotension
• dependent edema (pedal, presacral, pretibial)

Respiratory
• shallow, rapid respirations
• crackles

Gastrointestinal
• hepatomegaly

Integumentary
• xanthelasma (caused by hyperlipidemia)
• cyanosis (caused by hypoxia)
• diaphoresis

General
• obesity
• restlessness

DIAGNOSTIC STUDIES

The following studies may be performed to evaluate the patient's health status:
• stress test—2 to 4 weeks after AMI, to evaluate cardiac function during activity
• plasma lipid tests—monthly until normal range is reached
• electrocardiography (ECG)—monthly for the first 2 months post-AMI, then every 3 months for the next 6 months
• prothrombin time (for a patient receiving anticoagulant therapy)—usually twice weekly for 2 weeks, then monthly for the next 3 months

---

Nursing diagnosis: *Activity intolerance related to imbalance between oxygen supply and demand*

GOAL: To improve the patient's activity tolerance

Interventions

1. Plan adequate rest periods for the patient during waking hours. Encourage the patient to nap between 2 p.m. and 4 p.m. daily.

Rationales

1. Adequate rest helps the patient increase endurance and thus improves activity tolerance.

2. Evaluate the patient's past and present nocturnal sleep patterns, and explain their significance to him.

2. Poor sleep patterns can contribute to patient fatigue. Adequate sleep helps reduce stress, thus decreasing blood pressure and heart rate.

3. Obtain the results of baseline diagnostic studies from the patient's hospital records, and record the data on the patient's chart.

3. This information serves as comparison data if the patient's clinical status changes (for example, if his pulse rate rises 20 beats/minute above the baseline) or if he develops complications that would alter activity tolerance.

4. Assess the patient's understanding of the relationship between activity intolerance and stress, and fill in knowledge gaps as necessary.

4. The patient must understand that stress reduces activity tolerance and must recognize and report signs and symptoms of stress (such as sighing, nausea, anorexia, sweating, and hives or rashes) before he can adopt behaviors to reduce stress and increase his energy level.

5. Monitor and document the patient's pulse rate during periods of activity, rest, and sleep. Report any pulse rates over 120 beats/minute to the patient's doctor.

5. A patient's pulse rate provides insight into his activity tolerance. A pulse rate over 120 beats/minute accompanied by other signs and symptoms of cardiac dysfunction indicates that the heart is unable to meet the increased demands of exercise.

6. Monitor and document the patient's respiratory rate during periods of activity, rest, and sleep. Observe for stress-related signs and symptoms, such as apprehension, uncertainty, restlessness, hand tremors, and facial tension.

6. The respiratory rate is a reliable indicator of the patient's clinical status and helps to measure activity tolerance.

7. To obtain an accurate profile, monitor the patient's blood pressure with the patient in three positions: lying down, sitting, and standing.

7. Blood pressure readings help measure the patient's activity tolerance.

8. Encourage the patient to follow prescribed diet and medication regimens designed to combat hypertension.

8. Compliance with such diet and medication regimens helps to keep the patient normotensive, thus increasing endurance.

9. Monitor the patient for signs and symptoms of increased fatigue, such as cold, clammy skin; dizziness; and dyspnea.

9. Fatigue increases myocardial oxygen demands and impairs healing of cardiac tissue.

10. Instruct the patient to report all episodes of dyspnea to you or the doctor.

10. Patient reports of little or no dyspnea on exertion indicate that normal function is returning.

11. Teach the patient relaxation techniques, such as alternate nostril breathing, guided imagery, pet therapy, and music therapy.

11. Noninvasive relaxation techniques help reduce stress and promote feelings of calm and well-being.

Nursing diagnosis: *Sexual dysfunction related to physical limitations resulting from AMI and medication use*

GOAL: To help the patient understand and cope with any sexual limitations imposed by his condition

Interventions

1. Record the patient's sexual history. Include the patient's age, sex, sexual partner or partners, past and present sexual patterns, and any problems with erection, ejaculation, or orgasm.

Rationales

1. Assessing the patient's past and present sexual functioning establishes norms and helps the nurse plan future care.

2. Encourage the patient and partner to discuss fears and anxieties regarding any sexual problems and resumption of sexual activity. Remain warm, caring, honest, and reassuring throughout the discussion.

3. Evaluate the patient's medication regimen for drugs that may cause decreased libido or impotence. Such drugs include antihypertensives (such as reserpine, guanabenz, and methyldopa), diuretics (such as spironolactone), and beta blockers (such as propranolol and nadolol). If necessary, encourage the patient to speak with the doctor about altering the medication or dosage to eliminate or minimize adverse reactions.

4. Provide the patient and partner with information about AMI recovery and resumption of sexual activity. In general, a patient can safely resume normal sexual activity when he can climb two flights of stairs comfortably. (Sexual intercourse and climbing two flights of stairs involve approximately the same myocardial oxygen requirement.)

5. Instruct the patient to notify the doctor if the following symptoms occur during foreplay or intercourse: chest pain, increased heart rate and respirations persisting for more than 10 minutes after sexual activity, or extreme fatigue the day after sexual activity.

6. As appropriate, discuss alternatives to sexual intercourse that require less energy expenditure, such as hugging, kissing, cuddling, massage, and masturbation. Help the patient focus on the quality of the relationship rather than solely on the sex act.

7. Explain the value of lubricants and position changes during sexual intercourse.

8. Assess the patient's and partner's need for sex counseling and make appropriate referrals.

2. Such discussion can help the patient cope with his adjustment more effectively and help the nurse understand how the patient views his current situation—both of which are vital factors in the therapeutic regimen.

3. An alteration in medication regimen may eliminate or minimize the patient's sexual dysfunction, and the patient's awareness that his sexual dysfunction may result from medication effects can help decrease his anxiety.

4. Accurate information can help allay the patient's and partner's fears about resuming sexual activity too soon after AMI. (Fear of death during intercourse is common in post-AMI patients.)

5. These symptoms indicate that the activity is too strenuous and that the increased myocardial oxygen demand is not being met.

6. Emotional closeness is essential, particularly when the AMI patient first returns home. The patient may need guidance in exploring various methods of sexual expression. Masturbation, one method often not considered, is seen by sex therapists as a stress reducer.

7. Supplemental water-based lubricants can ease discomfort and increase the pleasure of sex acts. Certain sexual positions require less myocardial work than others; for example, the female-superior position for a male patient.

8. Sex therapy can help allay the patient's and partner's fears and foster emotional healing.

Nursing diagnosis: *Impaired home maintenance management related to recovery from AMI*

GOAL: To enhance the patient's self-care and home maintenance management abilities

Interventions

1. Assess the patient's home for safety and convenience. Count the number of stairs, and determine whether the patient must use stairs to reach the bathroom or answer the telephone.

2. Evaluate the patient's need for support systems, such as Meals On Wheels and Lifeline.

3. Determine the patient's need for durable medical equipment, such as a commode, cane, or shower chair, and arrange for provision of necessary equipment.

Rationales

1. Climbing and descending stairs can strain the endurance of the AMI patient. The nurse must evaluate how often the patient can safely walk between floors daily.

2. Appropriate support systems can alleviate many patient concerns, from emergency care to meal preparation.

3. Appropriate equipment promotes safety for the patient at home.

4. Evaluate the patient's ability to handle the financial burden of illness and recovery. Refer to social services as necessary.

5. Provide the patient and family with a list of service organizations, such as the American Heart Association (AHA), that can provide information and support.

4. The patient may be unaware of available resources. Referral may help the patient locate financial assistance.

5. Such organizations can provide the patient with information about AMI and rehabilitation, which can clear up any misunderstandings and help decrease anxiety.

ASSOCIATED CARE PLANS
• Angina Pectoris
• Chronic Congestive Heart Failure
• Grief and Grieving
• Hypertension
• Ineffective Coping
• Pain
• Sex and Sexuality

NETWORKING OF SERVICES
• Lifeline
• Meals On Wheels
• durable medical equipment (DME) supplier
• cardiac rehabilitation program
• respiratory therapy (for a patient requiring supplemental oxygen)

CARE TEAM INVOLVED
• nurse
• doctor
• patient and family
• medical social worker
• exercise physiologist
• massage therapist

IMPLICATIONS FOR HOME CARE
• functional features of the home (such as stairs and location of bathroom)
• telephone (communication)
• oxygen safety (if supplemental oxygen therapy is ordered)

PATIENT EDUCATION TOOLS
• list of normal readings for pulse, blood pressure, and respiratory rate
• written guidelines for oxygen use and safety measures (if supplemental oxygen is ordered)
• literature on each medication ordered, including dosage schedule and adverse effects
• AHA literature
• information about sexuality and alternative means of sexual expression

DISCHARGE PLAN FROM HOME HEALTH CARE
Before discharge from home health care, the patient should:
• know the medication regimen, dosage, desired effect, and adverse reactions

• state the prescribed diet regimen and discuss plans for compliance
• begin participating in a smoking cessation program (if a smoker)
• begin participating in a cardiac rehabilitation program
• be enrolled in a weight-reduction program (if necessary)
• be aware of stressors in his life and begin taking steps to eliminate or minimize them
• know the signs and symptoms of coronary problems
• understand that *heart attack* and *myocardial infarction* are synonymous
• be aware that he may require surgery after a second or third AMI
• have the telephone number of the home health agency for follow-up care
• know when he can resume sexual activity
• know the dates of doctor and laboratory appointments
• have Lifeline response in place
• have telephone numbers for the ambulance service and emergency department
• know the value of all family members learning cardiopulmonary resuscitation.

SELECTED REFERENCES
Conover, M. *Understanding Electrocardiography*, 5th ed. St. Louis: C.V. Mosby Co., 1988.
Diagnostics, 2nd ed. Nurse's Reference Library. Springhouse, Pa.: Springhouse Corp., 1987.
Guyton, A. *Textbook of Medical Physiology*, 7th ed. Philadelphia: W.B. Saunders Co., 1986.
Porth, C. *Pathophysiology*, 2nd ed. Philadelphia: J.B. Lippincott Co., 1986.
Weeks, L., ed. *Advanced Cardiovascular Nursing*. Boston: Blackwell Scientific Publications, 1986.

CARDIOVASCULAR SYSTEM

Chronic Congestive Heart Failure

DESCRIPTION AND TIME FOCUS

Congestive heart failure (CHF) is a complex clinical syndrome in which the heart fails to pump sufficient blood to meet the body's oxygen and nutritional needs. Decreased myocardial contractility is the primary dysfunction. Abnormalities in preload (blood volume in the ventricles after diastole) and afterload (how hard the heart must pump to circulate blood) also can contribute to CHF.

Chronic CHF typically involves both sides of the heart. Because both ventricles must function properly for the heart to pump efficiently, sustained failure of one ventricle almost always results in failure of the other. Left ventricular failure usually causes pulmonary congestion. Right ventricular failure causes congestion in peripheral tissues and viscera.

CHF onset is a symptom of an underlying problem, such as myocardial infarction, hypertension, fluid overload, coronary artery disease, dysrhythmias (especially tachycardia above 180 beats/minute or bradycardia below 30 beats/minute), or valvular heart disease. In all cases, pump failure results in hypoperfused tissue and pulmonary and systemic venous congestion, which starts a chain reaction of serious complications.

This clinical plan focuses on home care for the patient with chronic CHF. Key elements include ensuring that the patient and family understand and adhere to measures that improve the heart's performance. These measures can help the patient avoid secondary problems resulting from inadequate organ perfusion to such vital areas as the neurologic, renal, respiratory, and GI systems.

■ Typical home health care length of service for a patient with chronic CHF: 6 weeks

■ Typical visit frequency: twice weekly or until the patient becomes stable

HEALTH HISTORY FINDINGS

In a health history interview, the patient may report many of these findings:
• reduced exercise tolerance
• dyspnea on exertion
• orthopnea
• paroxysmal nocturnal dyspnea
• anorexia
• emotional stress
• pregnancy
• history of anemia
• history of respiratory acidosis
• history of pulmonary edema
• history of cardiopulmonary infection
• history of diabetes
• history of angina pectoris
• history of hyperkalemia
• history of hypothyroidism
• history of hypertension
• history of dysrhythmias
• history of fluid overload
• history of thiamin deficiency

PHYSICAL FINDINGS

In a physical examination, the nurse may detect many of these findings:

Cardiovascular
• tachycardia or other dysrhythmias
• third and fourth heart sounds (S_3 and S_4)
• pulsus alternans
• jugular vein distention
• peripheral and dependent edema
• elevated central venous pressure
• decreased capillary refill time

Respiratory
• rapid, shallow respirations
• Cheyne-Stokes respirations
• dry, hacking cough or frothy cough
• crackles, wheezes, rhonchi

Neurologic
• confusion
• impaired concentration

Gastrointestinal
• nausea and vomiting
• abdominal distention
• hepatomegaly
• ascites

Integumentary
• cool, clammy, or dry skin
• dusky nail beds

Renal and urinary
• oliguria
• fluid retention and edema
• dark amber urine

General
• restlessness
• lethargy
• fatigue
• somnolence or insomnia
• weight gain

DIAGNOSTIC STUDIES
The following studies may be performed to evaluate the patient's health status:
• electrolyte studies—monthly for 3 months, to reveal hyponatremia, hypokalemia, or hypochloremia
• blood chemistry profile—monthly for 3 months, to reveal increased blood urea nitrogen (BUN) and creatinine levels; mildly increased aspartate aminotransferase (AST, formerly serum glutamic-oxaloacetic transaminase or SGOT), bilirubin, and alkaline phosphatase levels
• electrocardiography (ECG)—monthly to detect ventricular hypertrophy, atrial hypertrophy, or tachycardia or other dysrhythmias

Nursing diagnosis: *Altered cardiac output: decreased, related to decreased myocardial contractility, altered cardiac rhythm, fluid volume overload, or increased cardiac afterload*

GOAL: To maintain optimal cardiac output within limits imposed by the patient's condition

Interventions

1. Monitor the patient's heart rate and rhythm, blood pressure, pulse pressure, and presence or absence of peripheral pulses. Compare findings against baseline assessment data and report any abnormalities to the doctor.

2. Auscultate for abnormal heart sounds.

3. Assess breath sounds for signs of pulmonary congestion, such as crackles, decreased breath sounds, and bronchial breath sounds.

4. Monitor and record fluid intake and output.

5. Administer medications (such as inotropes, diuretics, or anticoagulants) as ordered, and monitor the patient's response. Restrict sodium and fluid intake, as ordered.

6. Administer vasodilators as ordered, and monitor the patient's response.

7. Ensure that the patient gets adequate rest.

8. Teach the patient relaxation techniques to reduce his anxiety.

Rationales

1. Increased heart rate is one of the earliest signs of decreasing cardiac output. Decreased cardiac output also may be reflected by cardiac dysrhythmias, decreased blood pressure, and diminished pulse pressure or peripheral pulses.

2. A new S_3 sound or a systolic murmur may indicate increased fluid volume and decreasing cardiac output.

3. These signs may indicate pulmonary vascular congestion and pulmonary edema resulting from decreased cardiac output.

4. Decreased urine output may reflect fluid retention resulting from decreased cardiac output.

5. These actions help reduce preload, which strains myocardial fibers, reducing fiber contractility and cardiac output.

6. Vasodilators, such as hydralazine, reduce afterload but may lower blood pressure to such an extent as to impair organ perfusion.

7. Rest reduces myocardial oxygen consumption and improves cardiac output.

8. Anxiety can lead to increased catecholamine production, which increases afterload.

Nursing diagnosis: *Fluid volume excess related to decreased cardiac output*

GOAL: To maintain optimal fluid and electrolyte balance

Interventions

1. Instruct the patient to weigh himself at the same time each day, using the same scale, and to record the results. Check the patient's weight record each visit.

Rationales

1. Rapid weight gain of 1 to 2 lb/day indicates fluid retention, which may occur with decreased renal perfusion secondary to decreased cardiac output.

2. Maintain an accurate intake and output record.

2. Accurate intake and output records can alert the nurse to fluid overload early in the process.

3. As ordered, restrict the patient's fluid and sodium intake.

3. Fluid and sodium retention may result from decreased renal perfusion related to decreased cardiac output. A low-sodium diet helps decrease fluid retention, which can reduce cardiac preload and improve cardiac output.

4. Administer diuretics, as ordered, scheduling doses to permit uninterrupted sleep at night.

4. Adminstering diurectics before bedtime increases the likelihood of nocturia, which can interfere with the patient's normal sleep patterns.

5. Monitor serum electrolyte levels for imbalances.

5. Diuretics increase urination, placing the patient at greater risk for electrolyte imbalances.

Nursing diagnosis: *Impaired gas exchange related to pulmonary congestion*

GOAL: To improve gas exchange, as evidenced by improvements in the patient's activity level, vital signs, and diagnostic studies

Interventions

1. Elevate the head of the patient's bed to place him in semi-Fowler's position.

2. Administer oxygen as ordered.

3. Assess breath sounds and respiratory rate, rhythm, and depth.

Rationales

1. Lying flat shifts the abdominal organs toward the chest, making breathing more difficult.

2. Pulmonary congestion interferes with the exchange of oxygen and carbon dioxide across the alveolar-capillary membrane.

3. Pulmonary congestion usually is associated with adventitious breath sounds and abnormal respiratory patterns.

Nursing diagnosis: *Knowledge deficit related to management of chronic CHF*

GOAL: To increase the patient's and family's knowledge about chronic CHF, including factors that precipitate acute episodes, procedures for monitoring health status, and dietary, medication, and exercise regimens

Interventions

1. Assess the learning needs of the patient and family and the factors that influence learning.

2. Prepare a teaching plan that addresses precipitating factors, pathophysiology, diet, medications, and activities. Involve the patient and family when setting goals. Provide written guidelines.

3. Provide a general outline of permitted activities.

4. Evaluate the patient's social and financial needs, and make appropriate referrals.

5. Inform the patient and family about community resources that can provide assistance, such as a local chapter of the American Heart Association (AHA).

Rationales

1. Learning requires physical and emotional readiness. Assessing learning needs and influences increases the likelihood of a meaningful and successful teaching-learning process.

2. Patient and family participation in goal setting enhances their learning and retention. Written guidelines facilitate learning.

3. The patient may manifest anxiety and denial if he doesn't know activity limits or how to perform prescribed activities.

4. Social and financial problems can inhibit learning.

5. Such organizations can provide the patient and family with additional information and support.

Nursing diagnosis: *Activity intolerance related to decreased cardiac output and impaired gas exchange*

GOAL: To help the patient achieve an optimal level of mobility, free from dyspnea, pain, or dysrhythmias

Interventions

1. Involve the patient in setting activity goals, and plan gradual increases in activity. Monitor his heart rate, blood pressure, and respirations after periods of activity. Instruct him to discontinue activities that cause dyspnea, dysrhythmias, or vertigo.

2. Instruct the patient to rest before and after performing activities and for 1 hour after meals. Rest may include watching television, reading, napping, or listening to music.

3. Assess for and minimize adverse effects of medications. For example, instruct the patient with diuretic-induced hypokalemia to increase the amount of potassium in his diet.

4. Assess for changes in the patient's mental state during exercise.

Rationales

1. Increasing the patient's activity level helps improve his mobility. Monitoring his vital signs helps you measure his activity tolerance.

2. Rest prevents excessive energy expenditure and helps improve activity tolerance.

3. Some adverse effects can cause fatigue, thus limiting the patient's activity tolerance.

4. Although exercise can improve the patient's orientation, motivation toward self-care, and cognition, it also can cause cerebral hypoxia, resulting in restlessness, confusion, or irritability.

ASSOCIATED CARE PLANS
• Acute Myocardial Infarction
• Angina Pectoris
• Chronic Renal Failure
• Hypertension
• Ineffective Coping
• Sex and Sexuality
• Smoking Cessation

NETWORKING OF SERVICES
• Meals On Wheels
• durable medical equipment (DME) supplier
• Lifeline
• respiratory therapy (including oxygen therapy, as needed)
• cardiac rehabilitation program

CARE TEAM INVOLVED
• nurse
• doctor
• patient and family
• social worker
• dietitian
• exercise physiologist
• physical therapist
• occupational therapist
• religious advisor

IMPLICATIONS FOR HOME CARE
• patient's ability to function (mental status, mobility, self-care and other activities, support systems)
• family's ability to care for the patient at home
• home's appearance, physical facilities, safety

PATIENT EDUCATION TOOLS
• written instructions for taking pulse and monitoring daily weight
• written dietary restrictions and allowances
• written exercise and rest plan
• literature about each prescribed medication
• written description of adverse signs and symptoms that should be reported
• AHA literature
• written guidelines for oxygen use and safety measures, if applicable

DISCHARGE PLAN FROM HOME HEALTH CARE
Before discharge from home health care, the patient should:
• have written and verbal information about signs, symptoms, and precipitating causes of CHF
• have written instructions for monitoring daily weight
• know how to take his pulse (especially if he is taking cardiac glycosides) and know to consult the doctor before continuing medication if the pulse rhythm changes or the pulse is below 60 or above 110 beats/minute
• know the signs and symptoms of digoxin toxicity and hypokalemia
• have literature about each prescribed medication, including method of administration, dosage, action, and adverse effects
• know to check with the doctor, nurse, or pharmacist before taking other medications, including over-the-counter medications
• understand the rationale for fluid, caloric, or sodium restrictions; have information about food selection and

preparation; and know the sodium content of the water supply
• know to avoid smoking and smoky environments and persons with infections, especially respiratory infections
• have general guidelines for an activity and rest program
• have referrals for social and financial assistance, as needed
• have referrals to community counseling and information services, such as the AHA
• know to contact the doctor or nurse if he experiences:
—increased shortness of breath or dyspnea
—persistent palpitations or changes in pulse rhythm
—paroxysmal nocturnal dyspnea
—increased swelling of extremities, face, or abdomen
—persistent cough
—chest pain
—weight gain of more than 2 lb/day
• carry a card that lists his name and address, the names and addresses of his doctor and an emergency contact, the diagnosis, current medications and dosages, and allergies
• have an appointment for follow-up medical care.

SELECTED REFERENCES

Braunwald, E., et al. *Harrison's Principles of Internal Medicine*, 11th ed. New York: McGraw-Hill Book Co., 1987.

Braunwald, E., ed. *Heart Disease: A textbook of Cardiovascular Medicine*, 2nd ed. Philadelphia: W.B. Saunders Co., 1985.

Luckmann, J., and Sorenson, K. *Medical-Surgical Nursing: A Pathophysiologic Approach*, 3rd ed. Philadelphia: W.B. Saunders Co., 1987.

Shinn, J., and Douglas, M. *Advances in Cardiovascular Nursing*. Rockville, Md.: Aspen Systems Corp., 1985.

Weber, J. *Nurse's Handbook of Health Assessment*. Philadelphia: J.B. Lippincott Co., 1988.

CARDIOVASCULAR SYSTEM

Hypertension

DESCRIPTION AND TIME FOCUS

Hypertension, one of the most common chronic diseases in the United States, is defined for an adult as blood pressure consistently greater than 140/90 mm Hg. An average of two or more diastolic readings greater than 90 mm Hg or an average of two or more systolic readings greater than 140 mm Hg confirms hypertension. Based on the diastolic pressure, hypertension may be classified as mild, moderate, or severe.

Primary (essential) hypertension has no identifiable cause and accounts for about 90% of all hypertension cases. Secondary hypertension, caused by disease states or specific drugs, accounts for the remaining 10%.

The pathogenesis of essential hypertension is not clear but is believed to result from increased peripheral vascular resistance. Other theories include increased sympathetic drive or decreased parasympathetic drive, resulting in hemodynamic changes; alterations in sodium retention and transport, which affect extracellular fluid volume; and alterations in the metabolism of renin, angiotensin, or antidiuretic hormone. Age, race, family history, high sodium consumption, stress, and obesity have been identified as predisposing or contributing factors in essential hypertension development.

This clinical plan focuses on the patient recently diagnosed with essential hypertension or the hypertensive patient experiencing a recent exacerbation. The patient may have been hospitalized before referral to the home health agency. Home care involves monitoring progress toward blood pressure goals, assessing patient adherence to the prescribed regimen and evaluating its effectiveness, and teaching the patient behavior modifications to control blood pressure and eliminate risk factors.

■ Typical home health care length of service for a patient with hypertension without complications or changes in prescribed therapy: 4 weeks
■ Typical visit frequency: once weekly

HEALTH HISTORY FINDINGS

In a health history interview, the patient may report many of these findings:
• palpitations
• chest pain (possible with severe hypertension)
• occipital headache (typically worse on awakening and relieved on arising)
• light-headedness
• dizziness
• numbness and tingling in the extremities
• occasional nausea
• nocturia

• urinary frequency
• high dietary intake of sodium, fat, and calories
• low dietary potassium intake
• heavy alcohol use
• cigarette smoking
• high caffeine intake
• sedentary life-style
• emotional stress
• fatigue
• family history of hypertension, stroke, congestive heart failure, diabetes, or renal disease

PHYSICAL FINDINGS

In a physical examination, the nurse may detect many of these findings:

Cardiovascular
• blood pressure above 140/90 mm Hg

Neurologic
• retinal changes, such as sclerosis, constricted arterioles and retinal arteries, hemorrhaging, exudates, and papilledema

General
• obesity

DIAGNOSTIC STUDIES

The following studies may be performed to evaluate the patient's health status:
• urinalysis—before initiating therapy, then as indicated by symptoms; proteinuria indicates renal disease as a complication of long-standing hypertension or as a secondary cause of hypertension.
• hematocrit—before initiating therapy, then as indicated by symptoms; may be elevated in hypertension.
• fasting blood glucose—before initiating therapy, then routinely if patient is on diuretic; done to rule out diabetes. Diuretic therapy may elevate blood glucose levels.
• blood urea nitrogen (BUN) and serum creatinine—before initiating therapy, then routinely if patient is on diuretic; elevations indicate renal insufficiency, which can cause or result from hypertension. Slight rise in BUN level occurs with diuretic therapy.
• serum potassium—before initiating therapy, then routinely if patient is on diuretic; to rule out primary aldosteronism. Level will drop 0.5 to 1.5 mEq if patient is on diuretic. Hypokalemia is rarely a problem if the patient is taking less than 50 mg of hydrochlorothiazide daily.
• serum cholesterol and triglycerides—before initiating therapy, then routinely if patient is on diuretic or beta

blocker; to determine risk factors. Serum lipids may be slightly elevated after prolonged diuretic therapy and when using beta blockers.

• uric acid—before initiating therapy, then routinely if patient is on diuretic; level rises with diuretic therapy. Some patients may develop gout, necessitating hypouricemic therapy.

• serum calcium—before initiating therapy, then routinely if patient is on diuretic, to rule out hyperparathyroidism. Level may rise if patient is on diuretic.

• electrocardiography (ECG)—routinely in patients over age 40 and in younger patients with severe hypertension; left ventricular hypertrophy or myocardial ischemia indicates hypertensive cardiovascular disease.

Note: Additional diagnostic procedures may be ordered after initial screening if the patient is suspected of having secondary hypertension. These procedures would be specific to the underlying disease.

Nursing diagnosis: *Knowledge deficit related to essential hypertension and its treatment*

GOAL 1: To increase the patient's understanding of hypertension and its treatment

Interventions

1. Teach the patient about hypertension, including its possible causes, risk factors, treatments, and potential complications. Stress that hypertension is a chronic condition requiring ongoing monitoring and treatment.

2. Teach the patient how to take blood pressure readings, and encourage him to keep a record of daily readings. To obtain an accurate profile, instruct the patient to monitor blood pressure while in three positions: lying down, sitting, and standing.

3. Instruct the patient to report such symptoms as headache, fatigue, or lethargy.

4. Stress the importance of making appointments for follow-up monitoring and evaluation. Establish a reminder system.

Rationales

1. The patient's understanding of hypertension and its treatment improves his ability to cope with the disorder and promotes his compliance with the treatment regimen.

2. Blood pressure readings indicate the effectiveness of the prescribed therapeutic regimen. Maintaining normal blood pressure minimizes long-term complications. Involving the patient in health status monitoring promotes compliance and encourages responsibility.

3. Hypertensive patients have reported occipital headaches that are relieved on arising. The patient may also experience fatigue, which decreases as blood pressure stabilizes.

4. The patient must understand that hypertension is a chronic condition requiring regular monitoring and evaluation. Reminders let the patient know that someone is concerned.

GOAL 2: To help the patient minimize the life-style practices that aggravate his hypertension

Interventions

1. Provide a patient who smokes with information about health risks related to smoking. Encourage participation in a smoking cessation program.

2. If the patient drinks alcohol, explain the importance of limiting alcohol consumption.

3. If the patient is overweight, explain the correlation between obesity and high blood pressure. Provide the patient with a daily weight chart and instructions for measuring and recording his weight. Discuss safe and effective methods of weight loss.

4. Help the patient identify and become part of a positive social support network.

Rationales

1. Nicotine causes vasoconstriction, which temporarily raises arterial blood pressure and increases cardiovascular risk.

2. Heavy alcohol consumption elevates arterial blood pressure and increases cardiovascular risk.

3. An overweight patient must understand the correlation between obesity and high blood pressure so he can take steps to reduce his weight. Daily recording of weight is the best way to track weight loss or gain.

4. Life-style changes are usually difficult to achieve. Social support resources can help sustain desired life-style patterns.

Nursing diagnosis: *Noncompliance with the treatment plan related to the patient's reluctance to make life-style changes*

GOAL 1: To help the patient comply with the medication regimen and minimize adverse reactions

Interventions

1. Monitor all drugs taken by the patient.

2. Instruct the patient on the medication regimen, including method of administration, dosage, desired effect, and adverse reactions.

3. Establish a medication schedule linked to significant daily events. Provide the patient with a written schedule of drug names and the times they are to be taken.

4. Stress the importance of taking prescribed medications at the proper time. Tell the patient to consult the nurse or doctor before discontinuing any medication.

5. Tell the patient to notify the doctor of any adverse reactions to the medications.

6. Assess for signs of fluid retention, such as weight gain and edema.

Rationales

1. Adherence to the medication regimen is essential in controlling high blood pressure. Some drugs, such as cold medications, steroids, and oral contraceptives, elevate blood pressure.

2. Understanding the medication regimen fosters compliance.

3. The patient is less likely to omit a drug dose if he associates it with a daily activity, such as a meal or bedtime. A written schedule serves as a reminder and promotes compliance with the regimen.

4. Medications help maintain blood pressure within the normal (or specified) range, minimizing complications.

5. Antihypertensive drugs can produce potentially serious adverse reactions that may necessitate changes in dosage or medication. The patient is less likely to comply with a medication regimen that produces intolerable adverse reactions.

6. Fluid retention increases cardiac work load and output, thereby increasing blood pressure, and may indicate noncompliance with sodium restrictions or ineffective medication therapy.

GOAL 2: To help the patient comply with a low-sodium, low-fat, weight-control diet

Interventions

1. Assess patient and family attitudes about food, cooking methods, cultural practices, and personal preferences.

2. Provide the patient or food preparer with instructions on reducing sodium in the diet. Discuss foods to avoid, proper cooking methods, importance of reading labels, and use of sodium substitutes.

3. Encourage the patient to eat foods that contain potassium. Provide a list of high-potassium foods, and discuss the role potassium plays in hypertension.

4. Provide the patient or food preparer with instructions on reducing saturated fat in the diet. Discuss foods to avoid, proper cooking methods, importance of reading labels, and use of fat substitutes.

5. Instruct the patient to avoid beverages containing caffeine.

6. Determine the patient's need for a calorie-restricted diet and instruct him accordingly.

Rationales

1. Understanding the patient's motivations and personal dietary habits facilitates planning patient teaching.

2. Reducing sodium intake can decrease blood pressure. Some antihypertensive drugs cause fluid retention and require sodium restrictions to maintain their therapeutic effect.

3. Diuretic therapy can cause potassium depletion. The patient may require a dietary supplement if he develops hypokalemia.

4. Reducing saturated fat intake can help retard the atherosclerotic process and reduce the diet's caloric content.

5. Caffeine causes vasoconstriction, which increases peripheral vascular resistance.

6. A strong correlation often exists between body weight and blood pressure. Weight loss can result in lower blood pressure even when the body weight remains above the ideal.

Nursing diagnosis: *Anxiety related to hypertension and its effects*

GOAL: To reduce the patient's anxiety level

Interventions

1. Help the patient identify common stressors in his life and his typical responses to those stressors.

2. Explore with the patient techniques (such as progressive relaxation, self-coaching, and thought stopping) that can modify responses to stressful situations. Refer the patient for biofeedback therapy if appropriate.

3. Encourage the patient to adopt a program of regular physical exercise.

Rationales

1. Planning stress management requires an understanding of the patient's stressors and responses.

2. The body's psychophysiologic response to stress can result in a rise in blood pressure.

3. Regular exercise helps reduce stress, improve muscle tone, and promote weight control—all of which can help decrease blood pressure.

Nursing diagnosis: *Potential fluid volume deficit related to diuretic therapy*

GOAL: To maintain adequate fluid volume

Interventions

1. Assess body fluid status, including intake and output, weight, skin turgor, and edema.

2. Observe the patient for signs and symptoms of hypokalemia or hyponatremia.

3. Instruct the patient taking a non-potassium-sparing diuretic to maintain a high intake of potassium. Provide a list of potassium-rich foods, and suggest he use a salt substitute that contains potassium.

4. Advise the patient to maintain an adequate fluid intake during hot weather or strenuous activity.

Rationales

1. Diuretic therapy can cause excessive loss of body fluids, possibly resulting in hypotension.

2. Diuretic therapy reduces sodium and can cause potassium loss. Potassium-sparing diuretics reduce sodium.

3. A high-potassium diet will help offset potassium loss from use of non-potassium-sparing diuretics.

4. Diuretic therapy exacerbates normal fluid loss from diaphoresis. Dehydration enhances the potency of antihypertensive medications.

Nursing diagnosis: *Sexual dysfunction related to adverse effects of antihypertensive drugs*

GOAL: To minimize the patient's sexual dysfunction and promote return to normal sexual satisfaction

Interventions

1. Provide opportunities for the patient to express concerns regarding sexual function.

2. Assess the patient's past and current sexual function.

3. Discuss side effects of the antihypertensive therapy. Explain that these changes are not harmful and may lessen over time.

Rationales

1. Sexual concerns are not easily discussed. Trust promotes open communication.

2. This information helps determine the extent of the problem and provides a baseline for developing the nursing care plan.

3. Antihypertensive therapy may delay ejaculation or cause retrograde ejaculation. Lowering blood pressure may diminish erections. A female patient may have reduced vaginal lubrication. Anticipating these changes can reduce the patient's anxiety and help him prepare for altered sexual relations.

4. Help the patient and partner explore specific strategies to overcome sexual problems. Identify other life situations that affect sexual function.

5. Instruct the patient to contact the nurse or doctor if sexual problems persist.

4. Open communication between the patient and partner fosters support, understanding, and the development of alternative, satisfying sexual practices.

5. Changes in medications may be indicated.

ASSOCIATED CARE PLANS
- Cerebrovascular Accident
- Chronic Congestive Heart Failure
- Chronic Renal Failure
- Diabetes Mellitus
- Ineffective Coping
- Sex and Sexuality
- Smoking Cessation
- Substance Abuse

NETWORKING OF SERVICES
- Meals On Wheels
- smoking cessation program
- weight loss program
- American Heart Association (AHA)

CARE TEAM INVOLVED
- nurse
- doctor
- patient and family
- dietitian
- medical social worker

IMPLICATIONS FOR HOME CARE
- equipment and facilities for food preparation
- access to drinking water

PATIENT EDUCATION TOOLS
- list of high-sodium foods to avoid
- list of high-potassium foods to eat
- written medication schedule
- literature for each medication prescribed
- AHA literature
- relaxation tapes

DISCHARGE PLAN FROM HOME HEALTH CARE
Before discharge from home health care, the patient should:
- understand that hypertension is a chronic disease requiring life long treatment
- exhibit blood pressure readings consistently within normal or specified range
- be complying with prescribed medication regimen
- demonstrate adherence to a low-salt, high-potassium (unless contraindicated), low-fat diet
- know common side effects of therapy and appropriate management techniques
- know the dates and times of follow-up doctor appointments.

SELECTED REFERENCES
Carpenito, L. *Nursing Diagnosis: Application to Clinical Practice*, 2nd ed. Philadelphia: J.B. Lippincott Co., 1987.

Kochar, M., and Woods, K. *Hypertension Control for Nurses and Other Health Professionals*, 2nd ed. New York: Springer Publishing Co., 1985.

Lowenthal, D., and Swartz, C. "Hypertension Update for the 1980s," *Primary Care* 12(1):101-15, January 1985.

McDonald, M., and Gremm, R. "Compliance with Hypertension Treatment: Strategies for Improving Patient Cooperation," *Postgraduate Medicine* 77(8):233-42, June 1985.

McEntee, M., and Peddicord, K. "Coping with Hypertension," *Nursing Clinics of North America* 22(3):583-92, September 1987.

Moore, M. "Current Management of Hypertension," *American Family Physician* 32(12):129-36, December 1985.

CARDIOVASCULAR SYSTEM

Angina Pectoris

DESCRIPTION AND TIME FOCUS

Angina pectoris is the chest pain that occurs when coronary artery blood supply fails to meet myocardial oxygen demands. Coronary artery atherosclerosis is frequently the cause. However, physical exertion, exposure to cold, strong emotions, eating a large meal, tobacco use, sexual activity, and straining while urinating or defecating can also precipitate episodes.

Stable angina, the most common type, produces intermittent pain, is usually precipitated by physical exertion or emotional stress, and is relieved by rest or nitroglycerin therapy. The pain typically lasts 3 to 5 minutes and rarely lasts longer than 20 minutes.

Unstable or preinfarction angina lasts more than 20 minutes and increases in frequency, intensity, and duration over time. Episodes can be brought on by light exercise and may even occur during periods of rest or sleep. Angina lasting longer than 20 minutes that is not relieved by rest or nitroglycerin may indicate an impending myocardial infarction.

Prinzmetal's angina, usually caused by coronary artery spasm, occurs during rest and is associated with an elevated ST segment. Nocturnal angina is frequently caused by left ventricular failure. Angina decubitus occurs while the patient is lying down and is relieved by sitting or standing. Intractable or refractory angina is a severe, incapacitating form of angina not relieved by therapy.

With all types of angina pectoris, pain typically occurs in retrosternal or substernal regions and may radiate to other parts of the body. Angina patients may describe the pain as crushing, vise-like, heavy, choking, burning, squeezing, or sharp.

The geriatric patient may experience angina more readily in cold temperatures (because of reduction in subcutaneous fat) and may present different symptoms (because of changes in the neuroreceptors). Typical symptoms include weakness and fainting.

This clinical plan focuses on home care of the patient with angina pectoris.

■ Typical home health care length of service for a patient with newly diagnosed angina pectoris: 4 weeks

■ Typical visit frequency: once weekly

HEALTH HISTORY FINDINGS

In a health history interview, the patient may report many of these findings:
• substernal or retrosternal chest pain
• pain radiating to back, shoulders, neck, jaw, or inner aspects of arms, usually the left arm
• fatigue
• choking sensation
• weakness or numbness in arms and hands
• apprehension; sense of impending doom
• nausea
• heartburn or indigestion
• fainting
• hyperlipidemia
• history of hypertension
• tobacco use
• family history of cardiac disease
• history of cardiac disease
• obesity
• emotional stress or type A personality
• history of diabetes mellitus
• oral contraceptive use
• sedentary life-style
• urban life-style

PHYSICAL FINDINGS

In a physical examination, the nurse may detect many of these findings:

Cardiovascular
• tachycardia
• hypertension or hypotension

Respiratory
• dyspnea

Integumentary
• xanthelasma (caused by hyperlipidemia)
• pallor
• diaphoresis
• cool, clammy skin

General
• obesity

DIAGNOSTIC STUDIES

The following study may be performed to evaluate the patient's health status:
• electrocardiography (ECG)—periodically; may show ST segment changes during angina episodes

Nursing diagnosis: *Altered comfort: chest pain, related to myocardial oxygen imbalance*

GOAL: To help the patient achieve pain relief and reduce angina episodes

Interventions

1. Instruct the patient to decrease his activity by sitting or lying down when pain occurs.

2. Help the patient identify precipitating factors for angina attacks, such as emotional stress, physical exertion, exposure to cold temperatures, and overeating at a meal. Discuss strategies to modify these factors.

3. Encourage the patient and family to maintain as calm and quiet an environment as possible.

4. Assess the effectiveness of medications, such as nitroglycerin, that the patient may be taking.

5. Instruct the patient to notify the doctor if chest pain increases in frequency, intensity, or duration or if the medication does not relieve the pain.

Rationales

1. Decreasing activity during angina episodes reduces myocardial oxygen demand and alleviates pain.

2. Such discussion helps the patient determine the lifestyle changes he must make to decrease angina episodes and plan ways to make such changes.

3. A calm, quiet environment reduces stress. Stress stimulates the sympathetic nervous system, causing vasoconstriction that increases the heart's work load and can lead to angina.

4. Nitroglycerin and other nitrates are vasodilators that relieve anginal pain by reducing the heart's work load and oxygen demand. If nitroglycerin therapy is ineffective and pain continues, the doctor should be notified.

5. Increased or unrelieved chest pain may warrant a medication change and could indicate more serious cardiac problems.

Nursing diagnosis: *Activity intolerance related to development of chest pain on exertion*

GOAL: To help the patient achieve the highest level of activity tolerance possible within the constraints of the disease

Interventions

1. Assess the patient's level of activity intolerance by monitoring pulse rate and pain level before, during, and after an activity such as walking.

2. Teach the patient how to monitor his pulse rate and respiratory pattern.

3. Encourage the patient to alternate periods of rest and activity.

4. Instruct the patient to avoid overeating, excessive intake of caffeine or other stimulants, smoking, isometric exercises and Valsalva's maneuver, emotional stress, and exposure to extreme temperatures. Advise him to wait 2 hours after meals before exercising and to sit rather than stand when possible.

Rationales

1. This assessment provides baseline data for use in developing the nursing care plan.

2. The patient must know how to monitor vital signs to determine tolerable levels of activity. An abnormal pulse rate and respiratory pattern can indicate cardiac dysfunction.

3. Regular rest periods help the patient conserve energy and reduce fatigue and cardiac stress.

4. Avoiding these actions helps improve activity tolerance. Overeating increases cardiac work load during digestion. Caffeine and other stimulants increase heart rate and work load. Smoking causes vasoconstriction and raises carboxyhemoglobin levels, decreasing the amount of oxygen available to the myocardium. Isometric exercises and Valsalva's maneuver reduce coronary reserve and venous return. Stress increases epinephrine production, which increases the heart rate and causes vasoconstriction. Cold causes vasoconstriction, which increases the heart's work load, and heat causes vasodilation, which results in blood pooling. Exercise, which increases the need for blood flow to the myocardium, should be avoided during digestion, when blood is diverted to the GI tract. Sitting conserves energy and reduces blood pooling.

5. Instruct the patient to use nitroglycerin (if prescribed) before performing activities that commonly precipitate chest pain.

5. Nitroglycerin produces vasodilation and reduces the heart's work load, thus improving the patient's activity tolerance.

6. Help the patient develop a plan to progressively increase his activity.

6. Progressive increase in activity slowly increases the demand on the cardiovascular system, leading to increased strength and conditioning.

7. Instruct the patient to discontinue any activity if he experiences fatigue, chest pain, or shortness of breath.

7. These are symptoms of myocardial ischemia.

8. Evaluate the patient's activity tolerance before discharge from home health care.

8. Such evaluation measures the patient's progress and helps determine the need for altering the plan of care.

Nursing diagnosis: *Anxiety related to anticipation of chest pain*

GOAL: To help the patient reduce his anxiety level

Interventions

1. Encourage the patient to discuss his feelings. Use active listening skills during the discussion, and maintain a calm approach.

2. Help the patient identify sources of anxiety, such as fear of chest pain, fear of death from cardiac complications, or uncertainty about changes in life-style.

3. Identify the patient's present coping strategies, assess their effectiveness, and suggest alternate strategies if necessary.

4. Teach the patient relaxation techniques, such as guided imagery, pet therapy, music therapy, focused breathing, and progressive relaxation.

5. Instruct the patient to avoid products containing caffeine or other stimulants.

6. Provide positive reinforcement as the patient makes progress in reducing anxiety.

7. Evaluate the patient's progress in reducing anxiety before discharge from home health care.

Rationales

1. Such discussion helps decrease stress and stress-induced vasoconstriction. Active listening indicates an interest in the patient and encourages open, honest communication. A calm approach may reduce the patient's anxiety level.

2. Identifying sources of the patient's anxiety helps the nurse plan interventions to relieve anxiety.

3. These measures aid future planning and increase the patient's knowledge of coping strategies.

4. Relaxation techniques help the patient release energy and reduce anxiety.

5. Stimulants may increase symptoms of anxiety and cause arterial spasm and narrowing of coronary vessels.

6. Positive reinforcement encourages the patient to continue complying with the treatment plan.

7. Evaluation measures the patient's success in modifying his behavior and helps determine whether further interventions are needed.

Nursing diagnosis: *Knowledge deficit related to the disease process and disease management*

GOAL: To increase the patient's knowledge of angina and interventions to control it

Interventions

1. As necessary, teach the patient and family about the pathophysiology, causes, precipitating factors, and risk factors associated with angina. Be sure the patient fully understands the signs and symptoms he must report to the doctor.

Rationales

1. Knowledge in these areas promotes compliance with the treatment regimen, helps maximize the patient's level of functioning, and helps ensure prompt treatment of complications.

2. Instruct the patient to implement a diet low in fat, cholesterol, calories, and sodium and to eat high-fiber foods.

2. Such a diet can minimize certain risk factors associated with angina.

3. Explain the importance of regular aerobic exercise.

3. Regular aerobic exercise (at least three times a week) increases cardiovascular conditioning, which can help minimize certain risk factors associated with angina.

4. As necessary, teach the patient and family about the prescribed medication regimen, including method of administration, dosage, desired effect, and adverse reactions.

4. The patient's understanding of the medication regimen promotes his compliance.

5. Teach the patient how to monitor his pulse rate and rhythm.

5. The pulse rate and rhythm aid in assessing for adverse reactions to medications, measuring activity tolerance, and detecting complications.

6. Teach the patient about stress-reducing methods, such as regular exercise and biofeedback and massage therapy.

6. Stress-reducing methods help the patient minimize the effects of stress and anxiety and develop effective coping mechanisms.

7. Inform the patient who smokes of ways to quit smoking.

7. Smoking causes vasoconstriction and raises carboxyhemoglobin levels, reducing the amount of oxygen available to the myocardium.

8. Instruct the patient to keep scheduled follow-up appointments with the doctor.

8. The patient must understand the importance of ongoing care to good health.

9. Advise family members to learn how to perform cardiopulmonary resuscitation (CPR).

9. Performing CPR during the first 4 to 6 minutes of cardiac arrest can be crucial in saving the patient's life.

10. Inform the patient of available community resources, such as support groups, exercise clubs, and a local chapter of the American Heart Association (AHA).

10. Community resources can provide support and information that can help the patient cope with angina and encourage him to comply with the treatment plan.

Nursing diagnosis: *Sleep pattern disturbance related to anxiety and chest pain at night*

GOAL: To help the patient achieve a normal sleep pattern by reducing anxiety and chest pain

Interventions

1. Determine the patient's normal sleep pattern and bedtime rituals.

2. Help the patient identify possible causes of sleep disturbance, such as anxiety or the need to void during the night.

3. Discourage the patient from taking lengthy afternoon naps.

4. Advise the patient to eat a small evening meal and to avoid caffeine and other stimulants before bedtime.

5. Advise the patient to avoid strenuous physical or emotional activity before bedtime.

6. Teach the patient to use relaxation techniques before bedtime.

Rationales

1. This assessment provides baseline data for use in developing the nursing care plan.

2. The cause must be determined to plan care. Involving the patient fosters a sense of control and can reduce his anxiety.

3. Long naps may interfere with nocturnal sleep.

4. Large meals divert blood to the GI tract and may precipitate angina. Stimulants can interfere with sleep.

5. Strenuous activity can cause excess fatigue, which makes falling asleep more difficult.

6. Relaxation techniques can enhance the onset of sleep and improve the quality of sleep by reducing stress and anxiety.

Nursing diagnosis: *Sexual dysfunction related to chest pain, fear of chest pain, or the medication regimen*

GOAL: To help the patient maintain satisfying sexual relations within the limitations of the disease

Interventions

1. Obtain the patient's sexual history, and assess for indications of sexual dysfunction, such as diminished libido or impotence.

2. Encourage the patient to express his feelings, concerns, and knowledge about sexual function and angina and to include his partner in the discussions. Provide accurate information about the effects of sexual activity on the heart and correct any misconceptions they may have.

3. Teach the patient how anxiety, fatigue, and medications can affect sexual functioning.

4. Discuss the rationale for limiting sexual activity, and inform the patient and partner of techniques that reduce the heart's work load during sex. As appropriate, suggest using comfortable, relaxing sexual positions that permit unrestricted breathing; using sexual aids such as vibrators; and using alternatives to intercourse such as mutual masturbation.

5. Instruct the patient to discontinue sexual activity immediately if he develops chest pain or shortness of breath.

6. Instruct the patient on the use of nitroglycerin before sexual activity.

7. Tell the patient to notify the doctor if impotence persists.

8. Refer the patient to a sex therapist, if appropriate.

Rationales

1. This assessment provides baseline data for use in developing the nursing care plan.

2. An open discussion in which both partners participate enables you to correct misconceptions that have caused anxiety and inhibited sexual function.

3. Anxiety and fatigue can reduce stamina or cause angina. Medications can depress the central nervous system, decrease libido, and cause impotence.

4. These measures can reduce the patient's anxiety and help prevent angina during sexual activity—both of which can enhance sexual function and satisfaction.

5. The patient must recognize and react to signs and symptoms of complications.

6. Nitroglycerin can reduce the incidence of chest pain, thereby reducing anxiety and enhancing sexual activity.

7. Although impotence usually is temporary, the doctor may resolve the problem more quickly by adjusting the dosage or changing the medication.

8. A sex therapist can provide further information and guidance for a patient with serious sexual dysfunction.

Nursing diagnosis: *Altered health maintenance related to risk factors associated with cardiovascular disease*

GOAL: To help the patient eliminate or reduce personal risk factors

Interventions

1. Assess the patient's health history and current lifestyle for risk factors associated with cardiovascular disease, and evaluate the patient's knowledge of these risk factors.

2. Explain modifiable and nonmodifiable risk factors.

3. Help the patient identify personal risk factors, such as poor diet, sedentary life-style, high stress level, smoking, and excessive alcohol use.

Rationales

1. This assessment provides baseline data for use in developing the nursing care plan, including the patient teaching plan.

2. Increased knowledge of modifiable risk factors promotes compliance with the treatment plan.

3. Identification of personal risk factors helps the patient understand his susceptibility to coronary artery disease.

4. Explain the complications associated with cardiovascular disease, such as myocardial infarction, cerebrovascular accident, and renal failure.

4. This information can vividly demonstrate to the patient the possible consequences of maintaining his current life-style, which may provide incentive for change.

5. Help the patient perform a values clarification exercise if he resists changes in life-style.

5. Values clarification helps the patient identify important aspects of life and may provide support as he makes necessary life-style changes.

6. Help the patient establish realistic goals to decrease modifiable risks.

6. Setting realistic goals reduces the likelihood of patient frustration. Involving the patient in goal setting promotes compliance with the treatment plan.

Nursing diagnosis: *Noncompliance with the therapeutic regimen related to denial of diagnosis and necessary life-style changes*

GOAL: To improve the patient's compliance with the therapeutic regimen

Interventions

1. Encourage the patient to discuss his feelings, beliefs, and concerns about health and illness, angina, and life-style modifications.

2. Help the patient to identify possible causes of noncompliance, such as misinformation or lack of motivation, and to determine what constitutes compliance.

3. Explain the purpose of the therapeutic regimen and the benefits of complying with it.

4. Correct any misconceptions the patient may have about the disease, life-style changes, or the therapeutic regimen.

5. Include the patient's family in all aspects of the treatment plan, and provide positive feedback for compliant behavior.

6. As necessary, refer the patient to appropriate community resources, such as a local chapter of the AHA.

Rationales

1. This discussion can decrease the patient's anxiety and help you understand his perceptions of illness and the significance he places on life-style changes.

2. Such discussion involves the patient in the decision-making process and improves his understanding of what he's expected to do. Causes of noncompliance must be identified to plan future care.

3. This information promotes compliance.

4. Misconceptions may lead to noncompliance.

5. Family support and your encouragement enhance the patient's self-esteem and provide motivation to continue the treatment plan.

6. Community resources can improve the patient's compliance by helping him cope with the disease and life-style modifications.

Nursing diagnosis: *Altered nutrition: more than body requirements, related to sedentary life-style and lack of knowledge*

GOAL: To help the patient achieve and maintain a normal body weight

Interventions

1. Perform a comprehensive nutritional assessment.

2. Discuss factors causing the patient's obesity, and explain the relationship between obesity and coronary artery disease.

3. Collaborate with a dietitian to implement a diet that reduces risk factors and promotes weight loss. Consider the patient's food budget, religious and ethnic food preferences, and food preparation methods.

Rationales

1. A comprehensive assessment provides baseline data for use in developing the nursing care plan.

2. Such discussion increases the patient's knowledge of his condition and promotes compliance with the treatment regimen.

3. A dietitian can help with the therapeutic aspects of the diet. Input from the patient enhances weight control and promotes compliance with the dietary regimen.

4. Explain the importance of an exercise program to weight loss, and collaborate with the doctor to implement a regular exercise program.

4. Exercise promotes weight loss by enhancing the body's use of calories.

5. Help the patient set realistic weight loss goals (for example, 1 to 2 lb/week), and discuss normal weight fluctuations.

5. Involving the patient in setting realistic goals promotes long-term compliance and increases the likelihood of success. If the patient anticipates occasional fluctuations in weight, he's less likely to be frustrated by them.

6. Tell the patient to weigh himself at the same time each day, using the same scale and wearing similar clothing.

6. Weight monitoring helps to assess the effectiveness of the weight loss plan.

7. Encourage the patient to establish a reward system that excludes food, and provide positive reinforcement for weight loss and improved eating habits.

7. Rewards other than food divert the patient's attention from food and provide incentives to continue the weight loss program. Positive reinforcement increases the likelihood that the patient will repeat the desired behavior.

8. Refer the patient to community weight control programs.

8. These programs can offer encouragement and support in long-term weight control.

ASSOCIATED CARE PLANS
• Acute Myocardial Infarction
• Coronary Artery Bypass Grafting
• Ineffective Coping
• Pain
• Smoking Cessation

NETWORKING OF SERVICES
• cardiac rehabilitation program
• AHA
• Lifeline
• weight reduction support group
• smoking cessation support group
• vocational rehabilitation

CARE TEAM INVOLVED
• nurse
• doctor
• patient and family
• social worker
• nutritionist
• exercise physiologist

IMPLICATIONS FOR HOME CARE
• functional features of the home (stairs, location of bathroom)
• telephone (communication)

PATIENT EDUCATION TOOLS
• literature about diets low in sodium, cholesterol, fat, and calories
• smoking cessation literature
• literature for each medication ordered
• AHA literature
• literature on activity and exercise programs

DISCHARGE PLAN FROM HOME HEALTH CARE
Before discharge from home health care, the patient should:
• understand the cause of angina pectoris and possible precipitating factors for an attack
• identify personal stressors that may contribute to the problem and begin eliminating or minimizing them
• understand the medication regimen (including method of administration, dosage, desired effect, and adverse reactions) and special considerations of nitroglycerin use
• know ways to reduce the frequency of angina episodes
• understand the use of nitroglycerin before events that produce angina
• know the signs and symptoms of increasing coronary problems
• implement dietary modifications, such as reduced intake of fat, sodium, calories, and caffeine
• be participating in a smoking cessation program (if patient smokes)
• be enrolled in a weight reduction program (if patient is overweight)
• establish an exercise program
• keep telephone numbers for the doctor, home health agency, and ambulance service near the phone
• know the value of CPR training for all family members
• schedule a follow-up appointment with the doctor
• have a family member take a stress test to increase understanding of personal stressors and methods to reduce risk factors.

SELECTED REFERENCES

Campbell, C. *Nursing Diagnosis and Intervention in Nursing Practice,* 2nd ed. New York: John Wiley & Sons, 1984.

Carpenito, L. *Handbook of Nursing Diagnosis,* 2nd ed. Philadelphia: J.B. Lippincott Co., 1987.

Carpenito, L. *Nursing Diagnosis: Application to Clinical Practice,* 2nd ed. Philadelphia: J.B. Lippincott Co., 1987.

Doenges, M., et al. *Nursing Care Plans: Nursing Diagnoses in Planning Patient Care.* Philadelphia: F.A. Davis Co., 1984.

Gettrust, K., et al. *Applied Nursing Diagnosis: Guides for Comprehensive Care Planning.* New York: John Wiley & Sons, 1985.

Kim, M., et al. *Pocket Guide to Nursing Diagnoses,* 2nd ed. St. Louis: C.V. Mosby Co., 1987.

Lederer, J., et al. *Care Planning Pocket Guide: A Nursing Diagnosis Approach.* Menlo Park, Calif.: Addison-Wesley Publishing Co., 1988.

Taylor, C., and Cress, S. *Nursing Diagnosis Cards.* Springhouse, Pa.: Springhouse Corp., 1988.

Ulrich, S., et al. *Nursing Care Planning Guides: A Nursing Diagnosis Approach.* Philadelphia: W.B. Saunders Co., 1986.

CARDIOVASCULAR SYSTEM

Thrombophlebitis

DESCRIPTION AND TIME FOCUS
Thrombophlebitis is an acute venous disorder character-ized by venous inflammation and clot formation. It may occur in superficial veins (cephalic, basilic, saphenous) and in deep veins (tibial, popliteal, subclavian, vena cava, iliac, femoral). Thrombophlebitis usually is caused by venous stasis, vein wall trauma or changes, hyper-coagulability, or a combination of these factors.

This clinical plan focuses on the patient discharged home from an acute-care hospital after diagnosis and initial treatment of deep vein thrombophlebitis. The home setting provides a holistic environment for heal-ing in which the home health nurse can assess the pa-tient's response to therapeutic interventions, monitor for complications, and provide health education.

■ Typical home health care length of service for a patient with uncomplicated thrombophlebitis: 4 to 6 weeks

■ Typical visit frequency: once weekly

HEALTH HISTORY FINDINGS
In a health history interview, the patient may report many of these findings:
• pain (heavy sensation to severe cramping in affected part)
• prolonged bed rest or immobility
• occupation that requires long periods of sitting or standing
• history of cardiovascular disorders (congestive heart failure, myocardial infarction, varicose veins, venous in-sufficiency, previous thrombophlebitis)
• recent major surgery, accident, or major fracture
• pregnancy or recent delivery
• recent infection
• oral contraceptive use
• recently terminated anticoagulant therapy
• history of blood disorder (polycythemia vera or sickle cell disorder)
• history of cancer, especially of pancreas
• family history of vascular or coagulation disorders

PHYSICAL FINDINGS
In a physical examination, the nurse may detect many of these findings:

Cardiovascular
• edema in affected part
• redness, warmth, and tenderness of affected part
• prominent superficial veins in affected part
• fever and chills (less common)
• positive Homans' sign (sign is unreliable)
• palpable, firm, cordlike subcutaneous vein

General
• obesity

DIAGNOSTIC STUDIES
The following studies may be performed to evaluate the patient's health status:
• hematocrit and hemoglobin—usually weekly for 2 weeks, then monthly until discharge
• partial thromboplastin time (PTT), if patient is receiv-ing heparin—daily if heparin dose is being adjusted; otherwise, three times a week for 2 weeks, then weekly until discharge
• prothrombin time (PT), if patient is receiving an oral anticoagulant—usually twice weekly for 2 weeks, then weekly until discharge

---

Nursing diagnosis: *Altered tissue perfusion related to venous stasis*

GOAL 1: To increase venous flow by reducing blood pooling and edema in the affected leg

Interventions

1. Every visit, measure and record the circumference of the affected leg at a consistent place.

2. Instruct the patient to elevate the affected leg when sitting or lying down.

3. Tell the patient to avoid using a knee gatch or pillows under the knees, dangling the affected leg, crossing his legs, and wearing tight clothing.

4. Plan regular exercise periods for the patient, and have him wear antiembolism stockings while exercising. Tell him to avoid long periods of sitting or standing.

Rationales

1. Leg circumference provides an objective measure-ment of edema.

2. Elevation promotes venous return and reduces ve-nous pressure and edema, thereby reducing pain.

3. These actions compress the vein and hinder venous flow.

4. Exercise improves muscle tone and increases blood flow into veins. Antiembolism stockings compress capil-laries and small veins, forcing blood into large veins and reducing blood pooling.

5. Ensure that antiembolism stockings fit properly.

6. Assess the patient's diet and eating behaviors in relation to body weight.

7. Evaluate the patient's bowel habits, and help him avoid straining and constipation.

5. Improperly fitted stockings can constrict circulation.

6. Excess weight hinders venous flow by pressuring and constricting veins. The patient may benefit from modifications to his diet and eating patterns.

7. Straining and constipation can increase cardiac stress and reduce circulation. Increased intrathoracic pressure interferes with venous return to the heart.

GOAL 2: To prevent extension of the thrombus by decreasing blood viscosity

Interventions

1. Administer anticoagulant therapy, as ordered.

2. Monitor PTT or PT for abnormalities. (The therapeutic range is 1.5 to 2 times the normal.)

3. Monitor the patient's fluid intake and hydration status, and take measures to ensure adequate hydration.

4. Monitor the patient's response to a gradual reduction of the anticoagulant dosage.

Rationales

1. Anticoagulants interfere with various clotting factors and mechanisms.

2. Maintenance of therapeutic PT and PTT values will ensure proper blood viscosity and impede further clot formation.

3. Dehydration may cause hypovolemia and result in increased blood viscosity and hypercoagulability.

4. Anticoagulants must be withdrawn gradually to prevent rebound hypercoagulability.

Nursing diagnosis: *Altered comfort: pain, related to inflamed, distended vein and edema in the affected leg*

GOAL: To minimize the patient's discomfort and enhance his level of control

Interventions

1. Assess the effectiveness of analgesics if ordered.

2. Monitor the level of patient discomfort in relation to interventions to increase venous flow.

3. Demonstrate relaxation techniques—such as diversion, meditation, guided imagery, and music therapy—that the patient can use before or during medication therapy.

Rationales

1. Effective medication therapy reduces the patient's anxiety and increases confidence that discomfort can be controlled.

2. Discomfort should decrease as venous stasis and edema decrease.

3. Using relaxation techniques increases the patient's sense of control and enhances the therapy's effectiveness.

Nursing diagnosis: *Impaired skin integrity related to altered peripheral tissue perfusion*

GOAL 1: To prevent skin breakdown

Interventions

1. Inspect the skin of the affected leg and pressure points for signs of irritation or pressure.

2. Intervene to reduce venous stasis and edema (see "Altered tissue perfusion," Goal 1, above).

3. Provide meticulous skin care and hygiene. Turn the patient at least every 2 hours. Massage the trunk with lotion as indicated.

Rationales

1. Stasis and decubitus ulcers do not heal easily. Prevention is the most effective intervention.

2. Appropriate interventions improve circulation and preserve skin integrity.

3. Skin care removes bacteria and irritants and helps keep skin supple.

GOAL 2: To detect skin breakdown in early stages and promote healing

Interventions	Rationales
1. Assess for skin breakdown, noting location and stage of breakdown, tissue condition, contributing factors, size, shape, and drainage.	1. Early detection and assessment of skin breakdown guide the selection of appropriate treatments.
2. Gently cleanse the wound with mild soap and water. Avoid using hydrogen peroxide or povidone-iodine.	2. Cleansing removes dead tissue and bacteria without damaging new tissue. Hydrogen peroxide and povidone-iodine kill fibroblasts and retard healing.
3. Use selective debridement methods that remove only necrotic tissue and leave healthy tissue intact, such as surgical debridement, dry gauze impregnated with sodium chloride, and an occlusive or semiocclusive dressing.	3. Wound irrigations, wet-to-dry dressings, and chemicals (enzymes) can injure healthy or fragile new tissue.
4. Use an absorption product such as dextranomer absorption beads or granules, dry gauze impregnated with sodium chloride, gelatin-pectin wafer, hydrocolloid dressing, or hydrogel dressing.	4. Absorption products draw the exudate and drainage away from the wound, protect the surrounding skin, and provide a healthier environment for healing.
5. Monitor the size and depth of the ulcer, color and character of the tissue, and color, odor, and character of drainage.	5. Precise documentation provides accurate data for assessing the patient's response to treatment.
6. Assess for fever, purulent drainage, copious exudate without necrotic tissue, and surrounding cellulitis.	6. Clinical signs and symptoms identify wound infection. A wound culture usually is not helpful because skin ulcers are not always infected.

Nursing diagnosis: *Anxiety related to required life-style changes*

GOAL: To reduce the patient's anxiety to a comfortable coping level

Interventions	Rationales
1. Provide opportunities for the patient to discuss fears and concerns.	1. Discussion provides support and reduces stress.
2. Answer questions and provide needed information.	2. Accurate information improves the patient's level of understanding and sense of control.
3. Involve the patient in the care planning process by helping him set meaningful goals.	3. By participating in care planning, the patient begins to accept health care responsibilities.
4. Incorporate disease management into routine activities of daily living (ADLs).	4. Successfully integrating care into daily routines reinforces the patient's self-confidence and coping skills.
5. Provide frequent, positive reinforcement during the recovery process.	5. During recovery, progress often seems slow, and the patient may feel discouraged or depressed. Encouragement and positive reinforcement help the patient cope with anxiety inherent to a slow recovery.

Nursing diagnosis: *Knowledge deficit related to the disease process of deep vein thrombophlebitis*

GOAL 1: To help the patient and family understand and adapt to the treatment regimen and recommended life-style changes

Interventions

1. Assess the patient's and family's understanding of the disease, symptoms, causes, and complications.

2. Provide illustrations of the cardiovascular system and location of the patient's thrombophlebitis.

3. Explain the etiology of the disease and factors that caused the patient's thrombophlebitis.

4. Discuss potential complications, such as extension of the thrombus, pulmonary embolism, venous insufficiency, thrombophlebitis recurrence, and venous stasis ulcer.

Rationales

1. Identifying current levels of knowledge helps determine teaching priorities.

2. Knowledge of anatomy and physiology improves the patient's understanding of the disease and its potentially serious complications.

3. Accurate information helps prepare the patient to understand the treatment regimen and the need for life-style changes.

4. Knowledge about complications may improve compliance with the treatment regimen. A calm, accurate presentation of information reduces the patient's anxiety and corrects misconceptions the patient may have about his health.

GOAL 2: To explain the treatment regimen and achieve patient compliance

Interventions

1. Establish a schedule for elevating the affected body part.

2. Demonstrate the proper way to apply antiembolism stockings, and explain that the top should never be rolled down. Have the patient and caregiver demonstrate their understanding.

3. Establish an exercise regimen within allowed limits.

4. Plan activities to eliminate long periods of sitting or standing in home, work, and social situations.

5. Instruct the patient on the medication regimen, including method of administration, dosage, desired effect, and adverse reactions. Help the patient and caregiver make a medication schedule sheet that is easy to read and includes space to record medications taken.

6. Instruct the patient to maintain a daily fluid intake of 8 to 13 8-oz glasses (2 to 3 liters), unless restricted.

7. Outline a balanced diet that helps the patient maintain a normal weight. Help him keep a food intake record.

8. Discuss weight reduction programs, such as Weight Watchers, Diet Workshop, TOPS, and Overeaters Anonymous. Encourage the patient to select a program that meets personal needs.

9. Teach the patient skin hygiene, protection, and daily inspection.

Rationales

1. Elevation promotes circulation and decreases venous stasis.

2. Antiembolism stockings promote circulation and reduce edema. Improper application can constrict venous flow.

3. Moderate, regular exercise improves muscle tone and increases blood flow into the veins.

4. Prolonged immobility causes venous stasis.

5. Knowing the medication regimen and maintaining a record increase the patient's understanding, responsibility, and compliance.

6. Inadequate hydration can cause hypovolemia, increased blood viscosity, and impaired circulation.

7. A balanced diet promotes healing. Increased responsibility by the patient may promote compliance.

8. If the patient is obese, weight reduction will decrease circulatory stress and eliminate a risk factor associated with complications.

9. Skin is susceptible to injury and breakdown because of impaired circulation.

DRUG INTERACTIONS WITH SELECTED ANTICOAGULANTS

Drug (*Brand names*)	Effect on anticoagulant		
	dicumarol	heparin	warfarin
acetaminophen *(Tylenol)*	+		+
alkylating agents *(BiCNU, CeeNU, DTIC, Leukeran, Mustargen)*	+	+	+
allopurinol *(Zyloprim)*	+		
amiodarone *(Cordarone)*	+		+
anabolic steroids *(Halotestin, Virilon, Durabolin, Anavar, Depo-Testosterone)*	+		+
antilipemics *(Atromid-S, Choloxin)*	+		+
barbiturates	–		–
carbamazepine *(Tegretol)*	–		–
chloral hydrate	+/–		+/–
chloramphenicol *(Chloromycetin)*	+		+
cholestyramine *(Questran)*	*		*
cimetidine *(Tagamet)*	+		+
corticosteroids *(Decadron, SoluCortef)*			+
dicumarol		+	
diflunisal *(Dolobid)*	+		+
disulfiram *(Antabuse)*	+		+
ethacrynic acid *(Edecrin)*	+		+
ethchlorvynol *(Placidyl)*	–		–
glucagon	+		+
glutethimide *(Doriden)*	+/–		+/–
griseofulvin *(Fulvicin)*	–		–
haloperidol *(Haldol)*	–		–
heparin sodium	+		+
influenza vaccine	+		+
metronidazole *(Flagyl)*	+		+
nonsteroidal anti-inflammatory agents *(Clinoril, Feldene, Indocin, Ponstel, Butazolidin)*			
paraldehyde			–
phenytoin *(Dilantin)*	+		+
protamine sulfate		–	
quinidine	+		+
rifampin *(Rimactane)*	–		–
salicylates	+	+	+
sulfinpyrazone *(Anturane)*	+/–		+
sulfonamides	+		+
thyroid preparations	+		+
triclofos sodium	+/–		+/–
tricyclic antidepressants	+		
vitamin K	–		–
warfarin sodium *(Coumadine)*		+	

Table codes
(+) increases effect of anticoagulant
(–) decreases effect of anticoagulant
(+/–) increases or decreases effect of anticoagulant
(*) decreases effect of anticoagulant if given too close
together; give at least 6 hours apart

Nursing diagnosis: *Knowledge deficit related to anticoagulant therapy*

GOAL: To maintain a therapeutic level of anticoagulant and prevent complications

Interventions

1. Instruct the patient on the anticoagulant regimen, including method of administration, dosage, desired effect, and adverse reactions. Establish a record where the patient can document the doses taken.

2. Demonstrate techniques for heparin administration, as needed. Have the patient and caregiver demonstrate their understanding.

3. Monitor PT and PTT, and teach the patient their significance.

4. Monitor hemoglobin and hematocrit levels.

5. Review all prescribed and over-the-counter (OTC) medications being taken. Instruct the patient to consult with the doctor before adding or discontinuing any drug.

6. Monitor PT, PTT, and clinical findings closely when a medication is initiated or withdrawn.

7. Instruct the patient and caregiver to report signs or symptoms of bleeding, such as bleeding gums, nosebleed, petechiae, a bruise that continues to enlarge, hemoptysis, hematemesis, hematuria, bloody or tarry stools, excessive menstrual flow, or a cut that continues to bleed.

8. Teach methods of preventing injury and bleeding, such as using an electric shaver or depilatory instead of a blade razor, wearing protective footwear and not walking barefoot, using a soft-bristle toothbrush, using a thimble for needlework, and wearing gloves and using extreme caution when handling any sharp implement.

9. Identify an effective alternative birth control method for the patient using oral contraceptives or an intrauterine device (IUD). Possible alternatives include condoms and a diaphragm.

10. Instruct the patient and caregiver that anticoagulant therapy should be reduced gradually, never suddenly.

11. Instruct the patient and caregiver to notify the doctor if the patient experiences increased pain, tenderness, edema, or distention of superficial veins in the affected part. Monitor for fever, chills, or malaise.

Rationales

1. An anticoagulant must be taken regularly, at the same time each day, to be most effective.

2. Proper heparin administration improves absorption and minimizes complications.

3. PT and PTT should be maintained within the therapeutic range, generally 1½ to 2 times the normal range.

4. Decreased levels can signify undetected bleeding.

5. Many medications affect anticoagulant therapy, especially salicylates in OTC preparations (see *Drug interactions with selected anticoagulants*).

6. The anticoagulant dosage may require modification if an interaction occurs.

7. Signs and symptoms of bleeding may indicate excessive anticoagulation and the need to decrease the dose.

8. Minor cuts, bruises, or abrasions may result in severe bleeding and an increased risk of infection.

9. Oral contraceptive use can be a causative factor in thrombophlebitis. An IUD can cause irritation and bleeding.

10. Sudden withdrawal may cause rebound hypercoagulability.

11. Clinical data may indicate that anticoagulant therapy does not benefit the patient. The thrombus may be extending.

Nursing diagnosis: *Knowledge deficit related to potential pulmonary embolism*

GOAL: To identify early signs of pulmonary embolism and obtain prompt emergency care

Interventions

1. Discuss patient and family concerns about potentially life-threatening complications.

2. Instruct the patient and caregiver not to massage the affected body part or extremity.

3. Monitor for sternal chest pain, dyspnea, tachypnea, tachycardia, pleural friction rub, productive cough, blood-tinged sputum, distended neck veins, pallor, cyanosis, low-grade fever, restlessness, anxiety, and apprehension. Instruct the patient to notify the doctor immediately if he develops any of these signs or symptoms.

4. Establish a plan for obtaining prompt emergency care, and review the plan with all family members. Post a list of phone numbers for the doctor, ambulance service, and emergency department near the phone.

Rationales

1. Discussion reduces anxiety and promotes understanding of and compliance with the treatment regimen.

2. Massage may dislodge the thrombus.

3. Early detection of signs and symptoms permits prompt emergency intervention.

4. Establishing a plan decreases the likelihood of confusion and anxiety during a critical episode. Prompt care improves the patient's chances of recovery.

Nursing diagnosis: *Impaired home maintenance management related to recovery from deep vein thrombophlebitis*

GOAL: To provide necessary information and resources for a safe, health-promoting environment

Interventions

1. Assess the patient's home for safety hazards. Are pathways clear? Is furniture arranged so that sharp corners are not protruding? Does the bathtub have a rubber bath mat with firm suction? Do the bathtub, shower, and toilet have grab bars? Are telephones easily accessible?

2. Determine the patient's equipment needs, such as a hospital bed, bedside commode, walker, or shower bench.

3. Assess the patient's financial status, and refer him to medical social services as needed.

4. Evaluate the patient's need for support services, such as Lifeline, transportation, and Meals On Wheels.

5. Provide the patient with a list of community resources that can provide support services after discharge from home health care.

6. Establish a plan to ensure ongoing in-home or outpatient laboratory appointments after discharge from home health care.

Rationales

1. Preventing accidents and injuries, such as falls and bruises, is essential, especially if the patient is receiving anticoagulant therapy.

2. Appropriate durable medical equipment (DME) promotes safety during the patient's recovery at home.

3. The cost of health care supplies, equipment, and medications may create a strain on available financial resources. Anxiety about finances can impede the patient's recovery.

4. Appropriate support services enable the patient to maintain a safe level of independence.

5. Community resources can help the patient assume control of and responsibility for personal health care without feeling dependent on the home health agency.

6. The patient's PT or PTT must be monitored regularly if anticoagulant therapy is continued.

THROMBOPHLEBITIS PATIENT INFORMATION SHEET

■ Basic information

Thrombophlebitis is the inflammation of a vein, with a clot (thrombus) forming in the vein. It can occur in a vein near the skin's surface or deep in the body, although veins in the leg are most often affected. Thrombophlebitis poses two serious dangers. The clot can enlarge and completely block the vein, or part of the clot can break off and travel through the bloodstream to the lungs.

Thrombophlebitis is most often caused by blood pooling in a vein, a severe injury to the affected body part, or increased clotting of the blood. Major surgery, a severe accident, pregnancy or childbirth, bed rest or inactivity from a long illness, a job that requires long hours of sitting or standing, obesity, and oral contraceptive use increase the risk of thrombophlebitis.

■ Taking care of yourself

How well you take care of yourself will influence how fast your body heals. You must follow the advice of your doctor and nurse to heal the vein and prevent the clot from breaking loose.

You can help reduce blood pooling (stagnation) by:
• wearing elastic stockings when you are out of bed
• walking for a few minutes every couple of hours
• not crossing your legs
• elevating the affected body part when sitting or lying down.

Your medications have been selected to meet your special needs. Make sure to take them as ordered. The doctor may prescribe an anticoagulant, which keeps the blood thin enough to pass by the clot and keeps the clot from growing larger. Never start or stop any prescribed or over-the-counter medication without consulting your doctor. Many drugs can increase or decrease the power of your anticoagulant.

Call your doctor if you have:
• a nosebleed or bleeding gums
• a bruise that keeps getting bigger
• dark or hazy urine
• bloody or tarry stools
• constipation
• increasing pain, swelling, or tenderness in the affected part
• skin redness or pressure sore
• vomiting or coughing up blood
• a severe headache that won't stop
• abdominal pain
• chest pain
• rapid pulse
• difficult or rapid breathing
• general feeling of anxiety or apprehension
• questions about your medication or care.

Fill in these important names and phone numbers, and post this list by your telephone:

Home care agency: _____

Nurse: _____

Doctor: _____

Ambulance service: _____

Emergency department: _____

Drugstore: _____

ASSOCIATED CARE PLANS
• Cellulitis
• Chronic Congestive Heart Failure
• Fractured Hip
• I.V. Therapy
• Pain
• Teenage Pregnancy
• Total Hip Replacement
• Total Knee Replacement
• Total Parenteral Nutrition

NETWORKING OF SERVICES
• DME supplier
• Lifeline
• Meals On Wheels
• weight reduction program
• ambulance service or rescue squad
• transportation service
• laboratory service

CARE TEAM INVOLVED
• nurse
• doctor
• patient and family
• home health aide
• medical social worker
• volunteer

IMPLICATIONS FOR HOME CARE
• telephone, Lifeline (communication)
• fall prevention (ambulation aids, grab bars, rubber bath mat, sturdy footwear, shower bench)
• caution around sharp objects
• accident-proof environment (clearing pathways, moving furniture, padding sharp corners)
• assistance with ADLs

PATIENT EDUCATION TOOLS
• thrombophlebitis information sheet (See *Thrombophlebitis patient information sheet,* page 39.)
• literature for each prescribed and OTC medication
• instructions for using antiembolism stockings
• instructions and diagrams for administering subcutaneous injection (for patients receiving heparin)
• skin care instructions
• American Heart Association literature
• list of normal pulse and respiratory rates

DISCHARGE PLAN FROM HOME HEALTH CARE
Before discharge from home health care, the patient should:
• know how to apply antiembolism stockings correctly
• be participating in a weight reduction program, if appropriate
• have an established daily schedule of activity and exercise
• plan job, home, and social activities to eliminate long periods of sitting, standing, or immobility
• achieve stable, therapeutic PT or PTT
• schedule follow-up laboratory and doctor appointments
• have Lifeline in place, as needed
• post phone numbers for the doctor, ambulance service, and emergency department near the phone
• understand and state the medication regimen, including method of administration, dosage, desired effect, and adverse reactions
• know to consult the doctor before adding or discontinuing any medication, including OTC medications
• know how to prevent skin breakdown
• know the early signs and symptoms of skin breakdown
• be able to perform the treatment regimen to promote healing
• know how to reduce risk of accident or injury at home and at work
• have adaptive and safety equipment in place
• be able to cope effectively with anxiety
• know the causes of thrombophlebitis
• know the potential complications of thrombophlebitis and how to eliminate risk factors
• know the risks associated with oral contraceptive or IUD use and arrange alternative birth control methods, when appropriate
• know the signs and symptoms of anticoagulant side effects
• be able to safely administer heparin, if ordered
• know the signs and symptoms of pulmonary embolism.

SELECTED REFERENCES
Doenges, M.E., et al. *Nursing Care Plans: Nursing Diagnoses in Planning Patient Care.* Philadelphia: F.A. Davis Co., 1984.
Elkins, C.P. *Community Health Nursing: Skills and Strategies.* Bowie, Md.: Robert J. Brady Co., 1984.
Giving Cardiovascular Drugs Safely. Nursing Skillbook series. Springhouse, Pa.: Springhouse Corp., 1984.
Guzzetta, C.E., and Dossey, B.M. *Cardiovascular Nursing: Bodymind Tapestry.* St. Louis: C.V. Mosby Co., 1984.
Nursing89 Drug Handbook. Springhouse, Pa.: Springhouse Corp., 1989.

CARDIOVASCULAR SYSTEM
Coronary Artery Bypass Grafting

DESCRIPTION AND TIME FOCUS
Coronary artery bypass grafting (CABG) involves the grafting of a donor vessel (usually taken from the patient's saphenous vein) to relieve anginal pain caused by severe blockages in two or more coronary arteries. Typically, such blockages are caused by arteriosclerosis, in which fatty, fibrous plaques gradually narrow the lumen of coronary arteries, reducing blood flow to the myocardium and resulting in ischemia.

CABG usually is performed after other, more conventional treatments have failed. Therapy typically involves the use of nitrates (nitroglycerin, calcium channel blockers, and beta-adrenergic blockers) and angioplasty (if drug therapy produces limited success and angina recurs). Highly effective in relieving angina and improving functional exercise capacities, CABG is successful in 80% to 90% of all patients who have no other complications.

Patient care includes monitoring wound healing and assessing for signs and symptoms of cardiac decompensation. The postoperative phase at home also provides an ideal setting for patient teaching about life-style changes needed to maintain cardiac health.

This clinical plan focuses on the patient discharged home from an acute-care hospital after recovering from CABG for the treatment of a coronary blockage.
- Typical home health care length of service for a CABG patient without complications: 6 weeks
- Typical visit frequency: twice weekly for 2 weeks, then once weekly until discharge

HEALTH HISTORY FINDINGS
In a health history interview, the patient may report many of these findings:
- chest discomfort or pain
- angina with dyspnea and acute fatigue during exertion
- dyspnea on exertion
- paroxysmal nocturnal dyspnea
- orthopnea
- syncope
- vertigo
- epigastric discomfort and burning
- postprandial discomfort
- nausea and vomiting
- discomfort in back, shoulders, elbows, or hands lasting more than 5 minutes
- family history of arteriosclerosis
- history of hypertension
- tobacco use
- history of diabetes
- elevated triglyceride and cholesterol levels

PHYSICAL FINDINGS
In a physical examination, the nurse may detect many of these findings:

Cardiovascular
- hypertension or hypotension

Respiratory
- signs and symptoms of pulmonary edema: tachypnea, tachycardia, dependent crackles, cough

Integumentary
- cyanosis
- unexplained diaphoresis

General
- obesity

DIAGNOSTIC STUDIES
The following studies may be performed to evaluate the patient's health status:
- prothrombin time (PT) and partial thromboplastin time (PTT)—twice weekly for 3 weeks, then once weekly for a month, to detect coagulation problems
- plasma lipid studies—3 months after surgery, then monthly until normal

---

Nursing diagnosis: *Altered comfort related to sternal and incisional pain*

GOAL: To improve patient comfort

Interventions
1. Assess the quality and origin of the patient's pain.

2. Evaluate the effectiveness of the patient's prescribed pain medication.

Rationales
1. Accurate assessment of pain is the first step in planning interventions for its relief.

2. Such an evaluation indicates whether the patient is responding appropriately to the medication regimen.

3. Monitor the patient for increased temperature, incisional discomfort or redness, or sharp pain during respiration. Notify the doctor if these signs and symptoms occur.

4. Assess the patient's history of coping with pain, including his use of analgesics or other medications and their efficacy.

5. Suggest diversional activities to distract the patient from pain, using his past and present activity tolerances as guidelines.

6. Differentiate between coronary pain and pain secondary to sternal retraction, such as shoulder, neck, and scapular pain. Provide pain relief accordingly.

7. Promote nonpharmacologic interventions, such as guided imagery therapy, back and neck rubs, and pillows to improve comfort.

3. Infection, dehiscence, and sternal separation may occur as a result of CABG, causing additional pain. Notifying the doctor ensures prompt treatment.

4. Such assessment allows for reinforcement of positive coping behaviors to help alleviate discomfort. Knowing the patient's history of successful analgesic use provides important information about his tolerance for and dependence on analgesics.

5. Involving the patient in such activities diverts attention from discomfort and helps in developing a positive self-image by resuming activities associated with wellness.

6. Shoulder, neck, and scapular pain often accompany incisional discomfort secondary to postoperative sternal retraction. Although nitroglycerin fails to relieve this type of discomfort, analgesics and warm, moist packs may provide relief.

7. These interventions may reduce muscle tension that contributes to discomfort. They also promote rest, increasing the patient's ability to cope with discomfort.

Nursing diagnosis: *Altered cardiac output: decreased, related to cardiac dysrhythmias secondary to surgery*

GOAL: To optimize the patient's cardiac output

Interventions

1. Reinforce the importance of complying with the prescribed medication regimen, explaining to the patient the purpose and use of each medication ordered.

2. Monitor the patient for signs of dysrhythmias, and notify the doctor of any immediately.

3. Teach the patient to monitor his pulse rate, and tell him to keep a record for ongoing evaluation.

4. Teach the patient how to use nitroglycerin, if ordered. Stress the need to notify the doctor if the frequency of chest pain increases.

5. Instruct the patient to notify the doctor if shortness of breath, productive cough, edema (pedal or pretibial), or fatigue increases.

6. Instruct the patient to notify the doctor immediately if syncopal episodes increase.

Rationales

1. Strict adherence to the prescribed medication regimen helps optimize cardiac function. The patient's understanding of the purpose and use of each medication encourages compliance.

2. Dysrhythmias can damage the heart by reducing myocardial oxygenation; effects can be fatal. Dysrhythmias can also reduce oxygen flow to the brain, precipitating syncope.

3. Such monitoring is essential to detect any dysrhythmias that may occur between home care visits.

4. Chest pain, usually relieved by nitroglycerin, indicates continued coronary spasms, resulting in reduced myocardial oxygenation.

5. These are signs and symptoms of decompensating cardiac muscle, which may lead to pulmonary edema and reduced oxygenation of the blood.

6. Syncope may result from activities that increase myocardial oxygen demand. Frequent syncopal episodes may lead to dysrhythmias and decreased cardiac output.

Nursing diagnosis: *Potential for altered bowel elimination: constipation, related to analgesic use, decreased physical activity, and changes in diet*

GOAL: To promote elimination of soft stool at regular intervals

Interventions	Rationales
1. Assess the patient's bowel habits and use of medication or other methods to relieve constipation or diarrhea.	1. An evaluation of bowel habits reveals the patient's normal pattern of elimination. Whenever possible, remedies that the patient has used successfully in the past should be tried before introducing other treatments.
2. Examine the patient's abdomen for evidence of distention, pain on palpation, or hyperactive or hypoactive bowel sounds. If noted, immediately report these signs and symptoms to the doctor.	2. These signs and symptoms may signal bowel obstruction or paralytic ileus.
3. Remove impacted stools, if necessary.	3. Removal of impacted stools permits other stools to pass with little difficulty.
4. Stress the importance of adequate fluids and fiber in the daily diet.	4. Fluids keep stools soft and easy to eliminate. Fiber contributes bulk and increases the patient's need to defecate.
5. Evaluate for constipating effects all medications the patient is taking. Notify the doctor if effects persist.	5. Some medications can cause constipation secondary to smooth muscle relaxation or diuresis. When possible, other medications can be substituted to ease persistent constipation.
6. Instruct the patient to schedule regular, uninterrupted times for bowel movements.	6. Scheduling regular, quiet intervals for bowel movements helps to train the bowel to eliminate at specific times, thereby preventing constipation.

Nursing diagnosis: *Anxiety related to success of procedure, financial impact of disease, and proposed life-style changes*

GOAL: To minimize the patient's anxiety

Interventions	Rationales
1. Inform the patient about all aspects of his progress toward recovery.	1. Such knowledge as the progress of wound healing or blood pressure regulation helps alleviate the fear of cardiac decompensation.
2. As necessary, refer the patient to a medical social worker to help in obtaining financial assistance.	2. The high cost of hospitalization, coupled with the temporary loss of income, creates anxiety and stress for the patient. A medical social worker can help the patient manage hospitalization expenses and locate community financial resources to help during the recovery period.
3. Consult a nutritionist about necessary changes in the patient's diet. Be sure to include the patient's meal preparer in all discussions with the nutritionist.	3. Consulting a nutritionist ensures that the patient's meals are well balanced and contain necessary dietary changes required by his condition as well as his personal food preferences. Including the meal preparer in discussions helps increase the likelihood of compliance with the necessary changes.
4. Teach the patient the signs and symptoms of potential postoperative problems that require medical assistance.	4. Knowing the signs and symptoms of potential complications and when to seek help lessen the patient's fear of an emergency during the recovery period.
5. Instruct the patient to keep a daily food diary.	5. A daily food diary provides insight into the patient's compliance with dietary restrictions and need for further dietary adjustments.

6. Encourage the patient to express his fears concerning his condition and recovery.

6. Verbalizing fears helps reduce anxiety.

7. Encourage the patient to follow a progressive exercise program, as prescribed by the doctor. Review the program with the patient before he begins exercising.

7. Exercise increases cardiopulmonary capacity, may lower blood pressure and blood cholesterol levels, and may help reduce weight. Explaining and reinforcing these benefits may improve patient compliance.

8. Encourage the patient to begin resuming his normal activities, as tolerated.

8. Resuming preoperative activities improves the patient's self-esteem by diverting attention from his condition to more productive activities. The resulting positive feelings help promote relaxation and reduce anxiety.

9. If the patient smokes cigarettes, discuss methods of smoking cessation.

9. Cigarette smoking substantially increases the risk of myocardial infarction. Smoking cessation is of utmost importance in postoperative care of the CABG patient.

10. Assess the patient's stress level, and teach stress management techniques, including breathing exercises, self-hypnosis, and regular exercise.

10. Stress management effectively reduces blood pressure and heart rate, thereby reducing the work load of the heart.

Nursing diagnosis: *Potential sexual dysfunction related to fear of pain or death during intercourse or to the effects of drug therapy*

GOAL: To identify the cause of sexual dysfunction and help the patient overcome or cope with dysfunction

Interventions

1. Reassure the patient that sexual anxiety is common after CABG.

2. Conduct all sexually related discussions in a private, quiet setting. Maintain a concerned and nonjudgmental attitude when talking with the patient.

3. Obtain a sexual history.

4. Discuss the patient's feelings about the sexual dysfunction. Include the patient's partner in discussions whenever possible.

5. Compile a history of the patient's medication use, and explain the effects of specific medications on libido and sexual function.

6. Notify the doctor of the patient's dysfunction, and ask whether a change in medication is possible to alleviate the problem.

7. Discuss ways to reduce physical stress during sexual intercourse, such as altering regular positions.

Rationales

1. Understanding that fear and anxiety are common reactions after CABG may help reduce the patient's anxiety.

2. Privacy and concern can be reassuring to the patient when discussing such personal matters.

3. Knowing the patient's sexual history helps the nurse incorporate current limitations into usual sexual practices during cardiac healing. Compiling the history also creates a forum for discussing the patient's concerns about sexual practices.

4. Discussing the patient's feelings allows him to express fears, anxieties, and the impact of the dysfunction on his sexual relationship. Including the patient's partner in discussions allows the partner to ventilate feelings and share in deciding ways to alleviate the dysfunction.

5. Certain medications commonly prescribed postoperatively for CABG patients—such as diuretics, antihypertensives, and sedative-hypnotics—can have adverse physiologic or psychological affects on sexual function.

6. The doctor may choose to reevaluate the patient's medications or discontinue their use when sexual dysfunction occurs.

7. Minimizing the physical stress that sexual activity places on the heart helps reduce fears about resuming sexual relations.

8. Suggest alternative methods of sexual expression, such as mutual masturbation or massage, until the patient's dysfunction is resolved.

8. Alternatives allow the patient to choose physical expressions other than intercourse until the difficulty is resolved.

9. Refer the patient to a sex therapist, cardiac rehabilitation nurse, or other specialist if the dysfunction persists.

9. Persistent sexual dysfunction may require the help of a specially trained professional.

Nursing diagnosis: *Potential for diversional activity deficit related to fear of wound dehiscence and anticipated pain*

GOAL: To have the patient participate in diversional activities

Interventions

1. Assess the patient's usual diversional activities before CABG surgery, and discuss his current perception of personal strengths and weaknesses.

2. Review and discuss the benefits of diversional activities.

3. Suggest that the patient take prescribed pain-relief medication, such as nitroglycerin, before engaging in any activity that may cause chest pain.

4. Evaluate patient reports of activity-related pain or continued discomfort for potential problems.

Rationales

1. Such assessment and discussion allow the nurse to evaluate the patient's present ability to perform previously enjoyed activities and explain the need to modify certain activities. It also provides a forum for addressing the patient's questions and concerns.

2. Benefits include improved self-esteem and diversion from the patient's illness.

3. Pain-relief medications may comfort the patient during activities, permitting his total involvement without the reminder of chest pain.

4. Continuing, extreme discomfort or increasing pain during activities may indicate such problems as infection or wound dehiscence. Evidence of potential problems should be reported immediately to the doctor.

Nursing diagnosis: *Ineffective family coping related to disruption of the patient's household role during the acute recuperative phase*

GOAL: To promote the family's adjustment to the patient's temporary dependence role

Interventions

1. Explain to the patient and family that temporary role changes are normal and necessary after major surgery.

2. Assess the family's previous coping skills.

3. Encourage the patient and family to discuss their fears and anxieties about role changes.

4. Involve the family in planning role changes during the patient's recuperation.

5. Evaluate the potential effects of such medications as narcotics, sleeping medications, and antianxiety agents on the patient's mood or coping patterns.

Rationales

1. The patient and family may not realize that the patient's dependence is temporary and that he probably will resume his usual role after recovery.

2. Assessing coping patterns helps in evaluating the family's positive and negative behaviors. This allows for reinforcement of positive behaviors and an opportunity to suggest alternatives for negative behaviors.

3. Discussion may elicit ways that family members can alter their coping behaviors.

4. Involving the family in planning helps ensure their agreement with temporary role changes.

5. Some medications can alter consciousness, affecting the patient's ability to adapt successfully.

ASSOCIATED CARE PLANS
• Acute Myocardial Infarction
• Angina Pectoris
• Chronic Congestive Heart Failure
• Grief and Grieving
• Hypertension
• Ineffective Coping
• Pain
• Sex and Sexuality
• Smoking Cessation

NETWORKING OF SERVICES
• Meals On Wheels
• cardiac rehabilitation program
• community bookmobile

CARE TEAM INVOLVED
• nurse
• doctor
• patient and family
• medical social worker
• exercise physiologist
• massage therapist
• dietitian

IMPLICATIONS FOR HOME CARE
• telephone (communication)
• functional features of the home (stairs, location of bathroom)
• list of emergency numbers for ambulance service and hospital

PATIENT EDUCATION TOOLS
• documentation of patient's routine vital signs
• American Heart Association literature about life-style changes
• literature about dietary changes
• information about prescribed medications

DISCHARGE PLAN FROM HOME HEALTH CARE
Before discharge from home health care, the patient should:
• know signs and symptoms of potential cardiac problems and when to call for assistance
• know emergency phone numbers of ambulance service and hospital
• know the phone number of home health agency for questions, concerns, and follow-up care
• comply with prescribed dietary restrictions for fat, calories, sodium, and caffeine
• be participating in a smoking cessation program, if needed
• be participating in an exercise program
• exhibit positive coping behaviors to alleviate anxiety
• be participating in a stress reduction program, if needed
• involve family members in life-style changes
• know the date and time of follow-up appointments with the doctor
• know when he can resume sexual activity.

SELECTED REFERENCES
Burke, L.J., et al. "Nursing Diagnoses, Indicators, and Interventions in an Outpatient Cardiac Rehabilitation Program," *Heart & Lung* 15(1):70-81, January 1986.

Jader, G.C., and LeKander, B.J. "Open Heart Surgery: Caring for Bypass and Transplant Patients," *RN* 50(4):40-43, April 1987.

Jansen, K.J., and McFadden, P.M. "Postoperative Nursing Management in Patients Undergoing Myocardial Revascularization with the Internal Mammary Artery Bypass," *Heart & Lung* 15(1):48-54, January 1986.

Loan, T. "Nursing Interaction with Patients Undergoing Coronary Angioplasty," *Heart & Lung* 15(4):368-75, April 1986.

Nicklin, W.M. "Postdischarge Concerns of Cardiac Patients as Presented Via Telephone Callback System," *Heart & Lung* 15(3):268-72, March 1986.

RESPIRATORY SYSTEM
Pneumonia

DESCRIPTION AND TIME FOCUS
Pneumonia, an acute inflammation of the lung paren-
chyma involving the alveoli and bronchioles, is caused
by bacterial, viral, fungal, or protozoal infection. Classification depends on the location of the infection as well
as on the specific causative agent. Nursing measures
focus on improving the patient's oxygenation status,
thereby allowing for recuperation. The patient's home
provides an ideal environment for the home health
nurse to monitor for complications and conduct patient
teaching.

This clinical plan focuses on the patient discharged
home from an acute-care hospital after diagnosis, management, and treatment of pneumonia.

■ Typical home health care length of service for a
patient with pneumonia: 3 weeks

■ Typical visit frequency: twice weekly for 3 weeks,
then evaluate

HEALTH HISTORY FINDINGS
In a health history interview, the patient may report
many of these findings:
• chest discomfort or pain
• breathing difficulty
• headache
• nausea and vomiting
• abdominal pain
• muscle aches
• fatigue and weakness
• anorexia
• history of upper respiratory tract infection
• prolonged immobility
• chronic illness
• aspiration of gastric contents
• history of inhaling irritating gases
• tobacco use

PHYSICAL FINDINGS
In a physical examination, the nurse may detect many
of these findings:

Respiratory
• tachypnea
• cough
• sputum production
• dullness on chest percussion
• diminished breath sounds
• crackles
• pleural friction rub
• dyspnea
• nasal flaring
• intercostal and sternal retractions

Cardiovascular
• tachycardia
• hypertension

Integumentary
• diaphoresis
• cyanosis

General
• fever and chills
• restlessness

DIAGNOSTIC STUDIES
The following studies may be performed to evaluate
the patient's health status:
• chest X-ray—at any time, to identify pulmonary
infiltrates
• sputum for gram stain—at any time, to identify
causative organism
• sputum for culture and sensitivity—at any time,
to identify sensitivity of organism to specific drugs
• complete blood count (CBC)—when necessary, to
identify leukocytosis

Nursing diagnosis: *Impaired gas exchange related to exudate in alveoli and decreased functional lung surfaces*

GOAL: To improve gas exchange by ensuring adequate pulmonary ventilation

Interventions

1. Assess the patient for signs and symptoms of hypoxia, including irritability, tachycardia, increased blood
pressure, and tachypnea. Immediately report any such
findings to the doctor.

2. Auscultate the patient's lung fields for abnormal
sounds and report your findings.

Rationales

1. Signs and symptoms of hypoxia warrant prompt
medical attention to prevent complications such as respiratory failure.

2. Auscultation can reveal decreased ventilation and
perfusion of the lungs caused by secretions.

3. Instruct the patient on the purpose and use of bronchodilators, if ordered and indicated.

3. Bronchodilators help decrease spasms of the bronchial smooth muscles, thereby dilating the airways and improving gas exchange.

4. Teach the patient how to use supplemental oxygen, if ordered, and explain its purpose.

4. Supplemental oxygen may be necessary to ensure adequate oxygenation until airway and alveolar clearance are achieved.

5. Teach the patient the importance of adequate rest.

5. Rest decreases the body's oxygen demands and relieves a compromised respiratory system.

6. Instruct the patient to seek medical attention if he experiences increased dyspnea or fever.

6. Increased dyspnea or fever may indicate unresolved pneumonia or other complications, which may hamper gas exchange.

Nursing diagnosis: *Ineffective airway clearance related to tenacious sputum and poor cough effort*

GOAL: To promote airway clearance by thinning secretions and improving the patient's cough effort

Interventions

1. Instruct the patient to drink 8 or more 8-oz glasses (2 or more liters) of fluid (other than milk) each day to maintain adequate hydration.

2. Ensure that the patient is breathing humidified air.

3. Instruct the patient to cough and deep-breathe every hour; encourage him to splint the chest wall while doing so, to prevent pain, and to expectorate secretions into a tissue to enable evaluation of their amount and character.

4. Instruct the patient to rest between coughing sessions and to change position every 1 to 2 hours when awake.

5. Instruct the patient on the purpose and use of expectorants, if ordered.

6. Observe the characteristics of expectorated sputum, noting any significant changes in color, odor, consistency, or amount. Report any changes immediately.

Rationales

1. Adequate hydration helps thin secretions, enabling the patient to clear them more effectively. Milk products may thicken lung secretions.

2. A humid environment helps thin secretions, enabling the patient to clear them more effectively.

3. Proper coughing techniques facilitate movement of secretions upward into the major airways, where they can be expectorated or suctioned.

4. Resting and changing position help to decrease the fatigue associated with expectorating sputum, allowing more oxygen for cellular regeneration.

5. Expectorants help loosen secretions and aid their expectoration.

6. Sputum normally is thin and clear to white in color; blood-streaked, "rusty," or purulent sputum may indicate complications or another pulmonary disorder.

Nursing diagnosis: *Ineffective breathing pattern related to pleuritic pain and fatigue*

GOAL: To promote adequate oxygenation by minimizing the patient's discomfort and encouraging adequate rest

Interventions

1. Assess the patient for signs of respiratory distress, including increased respiratory rate, intracostal and sternal retractions, and nasal flaring. Report any such findings to the doctor.

2. Assess the patient's level of pain and anxiety.

Rationales

1. These signs and symptoms may signal a serious complication of pneumonia, such as hypoxemia, emphysema, sepsis, or pneumothorax.

2. Increased pain and anxiety can inhibit the patient from achieving full lung expansion on respiration, which in turn can contribute to atelectasis, inadequate airway clearance, and hypoxemia.

3. Teach the patient to splint the chest wall when coughing and deep breathing.

3. Splinting the chest with a pillow or the hands helps reduce pain during coughing and deep-breathing exercises, allowing the patient to achieve fuller lung expansion.

4. Instruct the patient to use pillows to elevate his head 45 degrees (Fowler's position).

4. Lying in Fowler's position improves ventilation and lung expansion by reducing the amount of pressure on the diaphragm.

5. Instruct the patient on the purpose and use of analgesics.

5. Analgesics help reduce pain and can help the patient achieve full lung expansion when breathing.

6. Instruct the patient on the purpose and use of cough suppressants.

6. Cough suppressants reduce the frequency of coughing, allowing the patient to rest more comfortably.

Nursing diagnosis: Altered body temperature: hyperthermia, related to fever from infection

GOAL: To prevent or control fever

Interventions

1. Teach the patient to use a thermometer correctly and to record accurate temperature readings.

2. Teach the patient about the need for increased fluid and caloric intake during periods of fever. Tell the patient and family to report any signs and symptoms of dehydration, such as mouth dryness, severe thirst, increased temperature, decreased urine output, and behavioral changes.

3. Instruct the patient on the purpose and use of antipyretics.

4. Instruct the patient on the purpose and use of prescribed antibiotics, stressing the importance of strict compliance with the antibiotic regimen.

5. Instruct the patient to seek medical attention if fever is unrelieved by antipyretics and antibiotics.

Rationales

1. Proper thermometer use and accurate temperature readings are essential to monitor the fever.

2. During periods of fever, increased fluid intake is necessary to replace body fluids lost through sweating and increased metabolism, and increased caloric intake is necessary to compensate for increased metabolism.

3. Antipyretics act on the hypothalamic heat-regulating center to reduce body temperature.

4. Antibiotics can prevent the reproduction of specific, sensitive microorganisms, thereby halting the spread of infection and reducing fever.

5. Additional medication may be necessary to destroy the causative organism.

Nursing diagnosis: Fluid volume deficit related to fever and decreased fluid intake secondary to fatigue

GOAL: To help the patient achieve and maintain normal fluid balance

Interventions

1. Assess the patient for signs and symptoms of dehydration, including poor skin turgor, dry mucous membranes, hypotension, decreased venous filling, and oliguria. Report such findings to the doctor.

2. Instruct the patient to drink 8 or more 8-oz glasses (2 or more liters) of fluid (other than milk) each day, unless contraindicated.

Rationales

1. These signs and symptoms indicate fluid volume deficit resulting from insufficient intake or from excessive loss related to fever or hyperventilation.

2. Adequate fluid intake is necessary to maintain hydration status while fighting infection. Milk products may thicken lung secretions, causing difficult expectoration and increased fatigue.

Nursing diagnosis: *Altered nutrition: less than body requirements, related to loss of appetite, fatigue, and dyspnea*

GOAL: To ensure the patient maintains adequate nutritional intake

Interventions

1. Monitor the patient's weight on each visit.

2. Assess the patient's diet by having the patient and family keep a food diary for 3 days and evaluating this diary.

3. Encourage the patient to eat small, frequent, high-protein and high-calorie meals

4. Instruct the patient to rest before meals.

Rationales

1. Progressive weight loss indicates insufficient caloric intake. If not reversed, this may lead to protein-calorie malnutrition, which can hinder vigorous respiratory effort and contribute to immune system impairment.

2. Because of fatigue or loss of appetite, the patient may not be ingesting sufficient calories and nutrients to meet his daily energy needs. Evaluating the patient's food diary helps the nurse identify whether this is the case.

3. Small, frequent meals are less overwhelming than a few large meals, which often cause stomach distention and increased pressure on the diaphragm, increasing the effort required to breathe. They also allow the patient to ingest more calories and nutrients over the course of the day.

4. Fatigue can discourage the patient from eating.

ASSOCIATED CARE PLANS
• Chronic Bronchitis
• Chronic Obstructive Pulmonary Disease
• Fractured Hip
• Kidney Transplant
• Pain
• Smoking Cessation
• Spinal Cord Injury

NETWORKING OF SERVICES
• Meals On Wheels
• durable medical equipment (DME) supplier

CARE TEAM INVOLVED
• nurse
• doctor
• patient and family
• homemaker
• medical social worker
• respiratory therapist

IMPLICATIONS FOR HOME CARE
• functional features of the home (stairs, location of bathroom, adequate cooking facilities)
• telephone (communication)
• support person

PATIENT EDUCATION TOOLS
• information on each prescribed medication
• literature from the American Lung Association

DISCHARGE PLAN FROM HOME HEALTH CARE
Before discharge from home health care, the patient should:
• know the medication regimen, including the method of administration, dosage, action, and adverse effects for each prescribed drug
• demonstrate the correct way to take his temperature
• know the signs and symptoms of recurring respiratory distress and infection
• demonstrate proper coughing and deep-breathing techniques
• understand the purpose of increased fluid intake and small, frequent meals until fatigue disappears
• have phone numbers of the home health agency and doctor.

SELECTED REFERENCES
Carpenito, L. *Nursing Diagnosis: Application to Clinical Practice.* Philadelphia: J.B. Lippincott Co., 1987.
Corbett, J. *Laboratory Tests and Diagnostic Procedures with Nursing Diagnoses,* 2nd ed. Norwalk, Conn.: Appleton & Lange, 1987.
Farzan, S., et al. *A Concise Handbook of Respiratory Diseases,* 2nd ed. East Norwalk, Conn.: Appleton & Lange, 1985.
Lederer, J., et al. *Care Planning Pocket Guide: A Nursing Diagnosis Approach,* 2nd ed. Reading, Mass.: Addison-Wesley Publishing Co., 1988.
Ulrich, S., et al. *Nursing Care Planning Guides: A Nursing Diagnosis Approach.* Philadelphia: W.B. Saunders Co., 1986.

Chronic Obstructive Pulmonary Disease

DESCRIPTION AND TIME FOCUS
Chronic obstructive pulmonary disease (COPD) results
from repeated acute bouts of emphysema, asthma, or
bronchitis. It is characterized by chronic inflammation
and destruction of the alveoli, resulting in an abnormal
exchange of oxygen and carbon dioxide. Primarily
caused by chronic tobbaco use, COPD also may be
caused by exposure to noxious stimuli, such as air and
chemical pollutants, over many years.

This clinical plan focuses on the patient discharged
home from an acute-care hospital after diagnosis, management, and treatment of COPD.

■ Typical home health care length of service for a
patient with COPD: 3 to 4 weeks

■ Typical visit frequency for a patient with acute exacerbation: three times weekly for 3 weeks, then twice
weekly until stable

■ Typical visit frequency for a terminal patient: daily
for 3 weeks

HEALTH HISTORY FINDINGS
In a health history interview, the patient may report
many of these findings:
• shortness of breath
• fatigue
• loss of appetite
• nausea
• insomnia
• headaches
• cigarette smoking
• history of working in coal mine or chemical plant
• history of recurrent respiratory infections

PHYSICAL FINDINGS
In a physical examination, the nurse may detect many
of these findings:

Respiratory
• barrel chest
• dyspnea
• wheezing
• cough producing thick sputum

Cardiovascular
• tachycardia
• atrial fibrillation
• jugular vein distention

Neurologic
• tremors (adverse effect of medication)

Integumentary
• cyanosis
• mottled skin

General
• anxiety
• depression
• confusion
• lethargy
• apprehension

DIAGNOSTIC STUDIES
The following studies may be performed to evaluate the
patient's health status:
• chest X-ray—with each exacerbation, to detect structural abnormalities, such as lung hyperinflation
• white blood cell (WBC) count—with each exacerbation, to detect abnormal elevations
• sputum specimens—with each exacerbation, to identify the causative organism
• capillary oximetry—monthly, to evaluate oxygen satu-
ration of arterial blood

Nursing diagnosis: *Impaired gas exchange related to inadequate airway clearance,
hypoxemia, fatigue, or difficulty breathing*

GOAL: To optimize gas exchange

Interventions

1. Each visit, assess the patient's respiratory rate and
rhythm, frequency and character of cough, amount and
character of sputum, temperature, skin color, and mental status.

2. Teach the patient proper breathing techniques, including relaxing shoulder and neck muscles, sitting in

Rationales

1. This assessment serves as a baseline for monitoring
acute exacerbations of COPD and for tracking disease
progression.

2. Relaxation and breathing exercises help conserve
the amount of available oxygen. Proper breathing max-

a comfortable chair, establishing a rhythmic breathing pattern, and using pursed-lip breathing (when indicated).

3. Teach the patient the proper breathing techniques to use when under stress, such as controlled coughing.

4. Instruct the patient to cough and deep-breathe every hour; encourage him to splint the chest wall while doing so, to prevent pain, and to expectorate secretions into a tissue to enable evaluation of their amount and character.

5. Help the patient establish a schedule for pacing activities of daily living (ADLs) based on the amount of time required for each activity and the amount of energy expended. Encourage energy conservation.

6. Administer oxygen, as needed, during periods of activity.

7. Teach the patient the purpose and correct use of respiratory devices, such as inhalers, humidifiers, and incentive spirometers.

8. Instruct the patient to perform postural drainage every 4 hours and immediately before meals.

9. Suction the patient, as needed.

imizes lung expansion while minimizing energy expenditure.

3. Such techniques help regulate the respiratory pattern and eradicate the shortness of breath commonly brought on by stress.

4. Proper coughing techniques facilitate movement of secretions upward into the major airways, where they can be expectorated or suctioned.

5. Pacing helps conserve oxygen while performing necessary ADLs.

6. A patient with COPD often needs supplemental oxygen to carry out routine activities.

7. Use of such devices, usually ordered every 2 to 6 hours as needed, helps facilitate gas exchange.

8. Postural drainage helps facilitate the drainage and elimination of secretions.

9. Occasional suctioning may be needed when other measures fail to alleviate thick secretions.

Nursing diagnosis: *Anxiety related to dyspnea or fear of complications*

GOAL: To relieve the patient's anxiety

Interventions

1. Assess the patient's current emotional status, especially his feelings about the disease and his breathing difficulties.

2. Encourage the patient to express his fears and anxieties. Try to help him find ways to deal with stress.

3. During dyspneic episodes, maintain a calm, reassuring attitude and encourage the patient to rely on learned coping skills.

Rationales

1. All emotions have an effect on breathing. Added stressors, such as worry about disease, may further impair breathing.

2. Expressing fears and anxieties and developing ways to deal with stress may help improve breathing.

3. Dyspnea can be stressful, especially to a COPD patient. A calm, reassuring attitude may reduce the patient's fear and encourage him to use the coping skills he has learned.

Nursing diagnosis: *Sleep-pattern disturbance: insomnia, related to nocturnal dyspnea, anxiety, and the stimulant effect of brochodilator medications*

GOAL: To help the patient minimize sleep disruption

Interventions

1. Identify the patient's usual sleep pattern before disease onset.

2. Encourage the patient to minimize the use of bronchodilators after 6 p.m.

Rationales

1. Identifying previous sleep patterns helps determine the patient's true sleep requirements.

2. Bronchodilators increase oxygen demand and have a stimulating effect that may keep the patient awake.

3. Reinforce the use of relaxation techniques before bedtime.

3. These techniques help promote more restful sleep by minimizing the body's demand for oxygen.

4. If appropriate, inform the patient that sexual relations before bedtime may help promote more restful sleep.

4. Orgasm helps promote sleep through the release of endorphins.

5. As ordered, instruct the patient and family to provide supplemental oxygen therapy throughout the night.

5. A patient with COPD may be unable to tolerate the decrease in oxygen supply normally brought on by sleep, and may require supplemental oxygen to prevent hypoxemia.

Nursing diagnosis: *Potential for injury related to failure to recognize signs and symptoms of acute illness*

GOAL: To teach the patient to recognize signs and symptoms of exacerbation and to seek prompt treatment

Interventions

1. Teach the patient and family the signs and symptoms of impending exacerbation, such as:
• changes in the amount, type, and color of sputum
• fever (based on the patient's baseline normal temperature)
• persistent disrupted sleep patterns, confusion, anxiety, or fatigue.

Rationales

1. Early detection of these signs and symptoms increases the chance of successful intervention to prevent exacerbation.

2. Instruct the patient and family to notify the doctor promptly if these signs and symptoms develop.

2. Prompt medical attention may be necessary to prevent exacerbation.

ASSOCIATED CARE PLANS
• Grief and Grieving
• Ineffective Coping
• Pneumonia
• Sleep Disorders

NETWORKING OF SERVICES
• Meals On Wheels
• durable medical equipment (DME) supplier
• respiratory therapy (if supplemental oxygen is ordered)
• pulmonary support group
• smoking cessation clinic

CARE TEAM INVOLVED
• nurse
• doctor
• patient and family
• home health aide
• physical therapist
• respiratory therapist
• occupational therapist

IMPLICATIONS FOR HOME CARE
• oxygen safety (if supplemental oxygen is ordered)
• maximum energy conservation
• small, frequent meals daily to promote adequate nutrition
• telephone, Lifeline (communication)

PATIENT EDUCATION TOOLS
• list of prescribed medications, dosage schedules, and adverse effects
• guidelines for safe use of oxygen (if supplemental oxygen is ordered)

DISCHARGE PLAN FROM HOME HEALTH CARE
Before discharge from home health care, the patient should:
• understand signs and symptoms of COPD, respiratory infection, and disease exacerbation
• understand the dangers of smoking, air and chemical pollutants, and respiratory infection
• understand and practice coughing and deep-breathing exercises
• know the principles of safe oxygen use (if supplemental oxygen is ordered)
• recognize possible adverse reactions to medications
• understand rest requirements
• know when to call the home health agency or the doctor
• understand the need to carry identification and a list of prescribed medications
• understand patterns of energy conservation and breathing techniques.

SELECTED REFERENCES

Burton, G., and Hodgkin, J., eds. *Respiratory Care: A Guide to Clinical Practice,* 2nd ed. Philadelphia: J.B. Lippincott Co., 1984.

Campbell, E. *Nursing Diagnosis and Intervention in Nursing Practice*, 2nd ed. New York: John Wiley & Sons, 1984.

Farzan, S., et al. *A Concise Handbook of Respiratory Diseases,* 2nd ed. East Norwalk, Conn.: Appleton & Lange, 1985.

Shapiro, B., et al. *Clinical Application of Respiratory Care*, 3rd ed. Chicago: Year Book Medical Publishers, 1985.

Ulrich, W., et al. *Nursing Care Planning Guides: A Nursing Process Approach*. Philadelphia: W.B. Saunders Co., 1986.

RESPIRATORY SYSTEM
Chronic Bronchitis

DESCRIPTION AND TIME FOCUS
Bronchitis, an inflammation of the mucosal lining of the tracheobronchial tree, may be acute or chronic. *Acute bronchitis*, characterized by partial obstruction of the bronchi by secretions or constriction, usually results from a viral infection of the upper respiratory tract. *Chronic bronchitis* involves chronic irritation of the tracheobronchial tree by inhaled irritants and recurrent respiratory tract infections. Chronic bronchitis is confirmed when cough and expectoration persist for at least 3 months each year for 2 consecutive years.

In chronic bronchitis, inflammation enlarges the mucous glands and increases the production of tenacious mucus. Cilia destruction compromises the integrity of the mucous blanket, the basic mechanism for transporting secretions to the upper airway. As a result, the patient must depend on the cough mechanism to clear secretions. Excessive coughing causes further bronchiole damage, however. Edema of the bronchial mucosa and increased mucus production narrow bronchioles and diminish airflow, especially during exhalation. This results in increased airway resistance, air trapping, and an increased effort required for breathing.

Because acute bronchitis rarely causes permanent lung damage, this clinical plan focuses on the patient with chronic bronchitis, who may or may not be experiencing an exacerbation of the disorder.

■ Typical home health care length of service for a patient with chronic bronchitis: 4 weeks

■ Typical visit frequency: twice weekly for 2 weeks, then once weekly for 2 weeks

HEALTH HISTORY FINDINGS
In a health history interview, the patient may report many of these findings:
• shortness of breath, particularly on exertion
• frequent productive cough that is worse in early morning and late evening
• copious, tenacious sputum, especially in morning
• anterior chest pain
• headache
• constipation
• fatigue
• activity intolerance, especially in cold weather
• insomnia
• history of smoking
• history of exposure to environmental toxins and irritants
• recurring respiratory tract infections
• history of asthma
• family history of bronchitis
• urban habitation

PHYSICAL FINDINGS
In a physical examination, the nurse may detect many of these findings:

Respiratory
• dyspnea
• tachypnea
• productive cough
• rhonchi that clear with cough
• wheezing on exhalation
• barrel chest
• use of accessory muscles
• restricted diaphragmatic excursion
• hyperinflation of lungs
• decreased expiratory flow rates
• dullness on percussion over areas of mucous plugs
• pulmonary hypertension
• hypoventilation

Cardiovascular
• tachycardia
• dysrhythmias
• palpitations secondary to cor pulmonale
• digital clubbing (late sign)

Neurologic
• mental status changes (late sign)
• tremors (late sign)

Gastrointestinal
• abdominal distention

Integumentary
• cyanosis
• peripheral edema

General
• obesity
• three-point posture

DIAGNOSTIC STUDIES
The following study may be performed to evaluate the patient's health status:
• sputum culture—on each exacerbation, to identify infectious organisms.

Nursing diagnosis: *Ineffective airway clearance related to edema of bronchial mucosa, excessive sputum production, and impaired ciliary movement resulting from chronic bronchial irritation or respiratory infection*

GOAL 1: To ensure early detection of exacerbation of bronchitis or respiratory infection

Interventions

1. Continually assess the character of the patient's cough and the quantity and character of respiratory secretions.

2. Monitor the patient's breath sounds and respiratory rate and rhythm.

3. Assess the patient for shortness of breath or dyspnea on exertion.

Rationales

1. Changes in the nature of cough and respiratory secretions may indicate exacerbation or respiratory infection.

2. An increase in rhonchi or wheezing may indicate an upper respiratory infection or an exacerbation of the patient's condition.

3. An increase in these conditions is often the first sign of exacerbation.

GOAL 2: To minimize bronchial mucosal edema and sputum production

Interventions

1. Instruct the patient and family to:

• avoid smoking and exposure to smoke

• avoid aerosols, ammonia cleansers, and chemical irritants

• reduce the amount of dust in the house by using electrostatic filters and damp dusting

• monitor outside air quality and avoid outdoor activity when air quality is poor

• use air-conditioning to reduce airborne irritants, especially during sleep

• stay indoors in very cold or windy weather

• wear a mask when exposure to respiratory irritants is unavoidable.

2. Teach the patient to correctly use inhalation bronchodilators.

Rationales

1. Teaching the patient and family to avoid respiratory irritants can help reduce bronchial mucosal edema and sputum production.
• Cigarette smoke is the most common respiratory irritant.

• Exposure to these products stimulates sputum production.

• Dust stimulates sputum production.

• Poor air quality can severely affect the patient's pulmonary status.

• Air-conditioning reduces the patient's contact with respiratory irritants.

• Cold air and wind can trigger bronchospasms.

• A mask will filter out some of the irritating substances.

2. Bronchodilators decrease bronchial mucosal edema and smooth muscle contraction.

GOAL 3: To help the patient effectively clear secretions from the airway

Interventions

1. Perform chest percussion and vibration at each visit, and teach the patient how to use postural drainage.

2. Instruct the patient to:
• use diaphragmatic breathing and controlled coughing

• maintain adequate hydration by consuming at least 8 8-oz glasses (2 liters) of fluids daily

Rationales

1. These measures enhance secretion drainage.

2. These measures enhance secretion clearance:
• Diaphragmatic breathing and controlled coughing help clear secretions.

• Adequate hydration helps liquify and remove secretions.

• drink warm liquids rather than cold liquids	• Warm liquids reduce the risk of bronchospasm and aid expectoration.
• use a humidifier to maintain moisture in the air, especially with forced-hot-air heating systems.	• Humid air reduces secretion viscosity and enhances removal of secretions.

Nursing diagnosis: *Ineffective breathing pattern related to decreased lung elasticity and compliance*

GOAL: To have the patient use breathing patterns that enhance gas exchange

Interventions

1. Monitor the patient's respiratory rate, depth, and rhythm on each visit. Encourage slow, deep breathing with prolonged exhalation.

2. Teach the patient measures to improve breathing patterns, such as:
• diaphragmatic breathing

• pursed-lip breathing

• use of the semi-Fowler's position

• use of the three-point posture—sitting and leaning forward with both elbows on a table.

3. Monitor for signs and symptoms of hypoxia (restlessness, tachycardia, impaired judgment) and hypercapnia (drowsiness, headache, confusion) resulting from poor gas exchange.

Rationales

1. A patient with chronic bronchitis tends to use rapid, shallow breathing as a result of dyspnea and anxiety. Slow, deep breathing maximizes lung expansion and enhances gas exchange.

2. The patient can use several methods to improve respiration:
• Diaphragmatic breathing strengthens the diaphragm and uses abdominal muscles to assist expiration.

• Pursed-lip breathing prolongs expiration and promotes emptying of lungs, which keeps airways open longer and allows more time for gas exchange.

• The semi-Fowler's position reduces the pressure exerted by abdominal organs on the lungs and eases the work of breathing.

• The three-point posture supports the body without strain and facilitates the use of accessory muscles of respiration, which eases the work of breathing.

3. Prompt recognition of hypoxia or hypercapnia is essential to prevent serious complications.

Nursing diagnosis: *Activity intolerance related to imbalance between oxygen supply and demand*

GOAL 1: To increase the patient's activity tolerance through energy conservation techniques

Interventions

1. On each visit, assess the patient's blood pressure, pulse rate, and respiratory rate during periods of rest and activity.

2. Question the patient about fatigue and weakness and any precipitating factors.

3. Assess the patient's cardiovascular, neurologic, and musculoskeletal systems for other possible causes of impaired activity tolerance.

Rationales

1. This assessment establishes baseline values to help determine the patient's tolerance for various activities.

2. To effectively plan interventions, the nurse must first determine factors impairing the patient's activity tolerance.

3. Many disorders can impair activity tolerance; all contributing factors must be considered during intervention planning.

4. Teach the patient energy conservation measures, such as:

• establishing priorities for scheduled activities
• scheduling rest periods after each activity
• stopping an activity at the first sign of fatigue
• sitting when possible and avoiding bending over
• pushing or sliding items rather than lifting them
• taking baths or using a shower chair
• dressing the lower part of the body while sitting on the bed to limit bending
• sitting and propping the elbows while shaving and combing hair.

4. Measures to conserve energy reduce the demands on a compromised respiratory system.

GOAL 2: To increase the patient's activity tolerance through physical conditioning

Interventions

1. Encourage the patient to participate in a regular exercise program, such as walking.

2. Instruct the patient to use diaphragmatic and pursed-lip breathing while exercising.

Rationales

1. Regular exercise improves physical conditioning, which enhances the delivery of oxygen to tissues and improves activity tolerance.

2. These breathing techniques help maintain adequate ventilation during exercise.

GOAL 3: To increase the patient's activity tolerance by promoting optimal function in other body systems

Interventions

1. Assess the patient's sleep patterns, and instruct him to establish a regular bedtime and to take measures to ensure a restful sleep.

2. Assess the patient's diet and nutritional status. If necessary, instruct the patient to eat small, frequent meals that are high in protein and calories and low in carbohydrates and other gas-producing foods.

3. Assess the patient's elimination patterns and intervene as necessary to prevent or treat constipation.

4. Monitor the patient's level of anxiety, and suggest stress-reducing measures as necessary.

Rationales

1. Adequate sleep is necessary for proper body function.

2. Lung hyperinflation from ineffective breathing limits stomach capacity. The increased work involved in ineffective breathing may increase caloric requirements. Carbohydrates form gas during digestion, which can interfere with abdominal breathing.

3. Constipation can cause abdominal distention, which may limit lung expansion.

4. Anxiety can cause ineffective breathing patterns.

Nursing diagnosis: *Potential for infection: respiratory, related to exposure to infection and improper infection-control measures*

GOAL: To promote patient compliance with measures to prevent respiratory infection and the spread of infection

Interventions

1. Instruct the patient to have influenza and pneumococcal vaccinations yearly and to avoid crowds and people with respiratory infections.

2. Teach the patient and family proper hand-washing techniques and proper disposal of tissues and other contaminated items.

Rationales

1. These actions reduce the patient's risk of respiratory infection.

2. These actions help prevent the spread of infection.

ASSOCIATED CARE PLANS
• Chronic Obstructive Pulmonary Disease
• Ineffective Coping
• Pain

NETWORKING OF SERVICES
• pulmonary rehabilitation program
• respiratory therapy (if supplemental oxygen is ordered)
• Meals On Wheels
• durable medical equipment (DME) supplier
• Christmas Seal League
• homemaker services

CARE TEAM INVOLVED
• nurse
• doctor
• patient and family
• medical social worker
• respiratory therapist
• physical therapist

IMPLICATIONS FOR HOME CARE
• control of environment
• oxygen safety (if supplemental oxygen is ordered)
• regulation of activity

PATIENT EDUCATION TOOLS
• literature from Christmas Seal League
• literature on each medication and inhalant ordered
• guidelines for safe use of oxygen (if supplemental oxygen is ordered)
• physical therapy guidelines

DISCHARGE PLAN FROM HOME HEALTH CARE
Before discharge from home health care, the patient should:
• be able to explain the disease and methods to slow its progression
• demonstrate proper techniques for controlled coughing and pursed-lip and diaphragmatic breathing
• be participating in a smoking cessation program, if needed
• be participating in a pulmonary rehabilitation program
• understand signs of exacerbation or respiratory infection and know when to seek medical assistance
• understand factors that precipitate exacerbations
• understand personal stressors and have a plan for coping with stress
• verbalize energy conservation measures
• verbalize dietary modifications
• know phone numbers of the home health agency and ambulance service
• know the date and time of the next doctor appointment.

SELECTED REFERENCES
Burton, G., and Hodgkin, J., eds. *Respiratory Care: A Guide to Clinical Practice,* 2nd ed. Philadelphia: J.B. Lippincott Co., 1984.
Campbell, E. *Nursing Diagnosis and Intervention in Nursing Practice,* 2nd ed. New York: John Wiley & Sons, 1984.
Farzan, S., et al. *A Concise Handbook of Respiratory Diseases,* 2nd ed. East Norwalk, Conn.: Appleton & Lange, 1985.
Shapiro, B., et al. *Clinical Application of Respiratory Care,* 3rd ed. Chicago: Year Book Medical Publishers, 1985.
Ulrich, W., et al. *Nursing Care Planning Guides: A Nursing Process Approach.* Philadelphia: W.B. Saunders Co., 1986.

Lung Cancer

DESCRIPTION AND TIME FOCUS
Classified according to cell type, lung cancers include epidermoid, small cell, and large cell cancers and adenocarcinomas. Treatment options vary according to the cell type and extent of the tumor and may include surgery, radiation therapy, chemotherapy, and immunotherapy individually or in combination. Even with treatment, however, lung cancer carries a high mortality rate.

This clinical plan focuses on the patient discharged home from an acute-care hospital after initial diagnosis and treatment of lung cancer. Care provided by the home health nurse includes monitoring for complications, providing patient teaching, and providing support for the patient and family as decisions are made concerning further treatment.

■ Typical home health care length of service for a patient with lung cancer: 6 weeks

■ Typical visit frequency: two visits weekly for 2 weeks, then one visit weekly for 4 weeks

HEALTH HISTORY FINDINGS
In a health history interview, the patient may report many of these findings:
• recent weight loss, increasing fatigue, or weakness
• chest tightness or pain
• dysphagia
• nausea
• anorexia
• history of chronic tobacco use
• prolonged occupational exposure to such materials as asbestos, petroleum distillates, tar coal distillates, or radiation
• history of exposure to significant air pollution
• family history of lung cancer
• history of respiratory infections
• history of pulmonary disease

PHYSICAL FINDINGS
In a physical examination, the nurse may detect many of these findings:

Respiratory
• frequent cough (productive or nonproductive)
• hemoptysis
• dyspnea on minimal exertion
• diminished breath sounds
• wheezing
• hoarseness

Cardiovascular
• tachycardia
• digital clubbing

Neurologic
• peripheral neuropathy
• polymyositis

Integumentary
• dermatomyositis
• enlarged cervical and axillary lymph nodes

Musculoskeletal
• hypertrophic pulmonary osteoarthropathy
• arthralgias

General
• weight loss

Note: Neurologic, integumentary, and musculoskeletal findings result from the release of hormones and other chemicals from tumor cells.

DIAGNOSTIC STUDIES
The following studies may be performed to evaluate the patient's health status:
• lung tomography—any time after initial diagnosis, to determine tumor size
• computed tomography (CT) scan—any time after initial diagnosis, to detect metastasis or lymph node involvement
• complete blood count (CBC) and lymphocyte count—any time after initial diagnosis, to determine extent of anemia and immunosuppression

---

Nursing diagnosis: *Impaired gas exchange related to loss of healthy pulmonary tissue*

GOAL : To promote optimal gas exchange

Interventions
1. On each visit, assess the patient's breathing patterns and strength of cough.

Rationales
1. Pain and fatigue may lead to shallow respirations and a poor cough effort, increasing the risk of atelectasis and further loss of healthy pulmonary tissue.

2. Observe the patient for reduced breath sounds, changes in skin color, darkening of mucous membranes, increased dyspnea, fever, increased heart rate, or sudden confusion.

2. These signs of impaired gas exchange may develop as tumor growth, atelectasis, pleural effusion, or respiratory infection further decrease capillary membrane efficiency and severely compromise systemic oxygenation.

3. Teach the patient deep-breathing and forced coughing techniques and, if appropriate, how to use an incentive spirometer.

3. Effective deep breathing and coughing and use of an incentive spirometer can increase lung expansion and promote optimal gas exchange.

4. Carefully assess the patient's breath sounds before and after deep breathing during each visit, and record your findings.

4. The effectiveness of breathing exercises can best be assessed by repeated evaluation of breath sounds.

5. Teach the patient techniques of positioning (side-lying, semi-Fowler's) and the need for frequent position changes to promote gas exchange.

5. Gravity and pooling of secretions can further limit the amount of usable lung tissue. Movement can counter these effects.

6. Evaluate the ventilation and humidity of the environment and increase as necessary.

6. Adequate ventilation and humidity in the environment help ease the work of breathing and facilitate gas exchange.

Nursing diagnosis: *Ineffective airway clearance related to fatigue and pain*

GOAL: To maximize the patient's airway clearance and prevent pooling of secretions

Interventions

1. Monitor the patient's hydration status. Explain the need for adequate fluid intake, and encourage a daily intake of 8 to 13 8-oz glasses (2 to 3 liters), unless contraindicated.

Rationales

1. Adequate hydration loosens and thins secretions, enabling the patient to clear airways with less effort.

2. Teach the patient techniques of productive coughing, such as splinting the abdomen with a pillow and taking deep breaths before each cough.

2. Productive coughing techniques effectively clear airways; splinting helps reduce pain from coughing.

Nursing diagnosis: *Activity intolerance related to general weakness and decreased pulmonary reserve*

GOAL: To maximize the patient's activity tolerance

Interventions

1. Assess the patient's blood pressure, pulse rate, and respiratory rate before and after activity during each visit.

Rationales

1. The nurse can use this assessment data to determine the patient's activity limitations. Markedly increased blood pressure, pulse rate, and respiratory rate after activity indicate an imbalance between oxygen supply and oxygen demand.

2. Teach the patient energy conservation measures, such as separating activities of daily living (ADLs) into single tasks, resting between each task, spacing tasks throughout the day, and resting 2 hours each day. Encourage the use of an aide to help with bathing and dressing.

2. Such energy conservation measures help the patient maintain a balance between oxygen supply and demand and increase activity tolerance.

Nursing diagnosis: *Altered nutrition: less than body requirements, related to hypermetabolic state and anorexia*

GOAL: To ensure adequate nutrition to meet the patient's increased metabolic requirements

Interventions	Rationales
1. Have the patient keep a food diary for several days.	1. The food diary helps the nurse assess the patient's nutritional patterns and then develop realistic plans and goals. Nutritional interventions are effective only when the patient's eating habits and preferences are taken into consideration.
2. Increase the patient's daily intake of protein and calories.	2. Because lung cancer often causes a hypermetabolic state, the patient must consume increased amounts of protein and calories to prevent malnutrition and maintain an adequate energy level.
3. Combat anorexia by providing small, frequent meals, nutritional supplements, and high-protein snack foods, such as cheese cubes and peanut butter and crackers.	3. Anorexia associated with cancer is caused in part by fatigue while eating. Small meals and snacks are easy to eat and require minimal energy expenditure.

Nursing diagnosis: *Altered health maintenance related to immunosuppression*

GOAL: To promote optimal health status

Interventions	Rationales
1. Assess the patient for signs of infection—fever, night sweats, sudden increases in lymph node size, and changes in sputum color or consistency—during each visit.	1. Most patients with lung cancer have some degree of immunosuppression, predisposing them to a host of common viral and bacterial infections. Any signs of infection require immediate attention.
2. Teach the patient the importance of avoiding crowds and any family member with an illness. Teach the patient's family about the need for thorough hand washing by all people before coming in contact with the patient.	2. Because immunosuppression leaves the patient with very little defense against infection, the patient's exposure to potential sources of infection must be minimized.

Nursing diagnosis: *Impaired home maintenance management related to long-term illness*

GOAL: To adapt the patient's home environment to ensure safe and convenient home maintenance

Interventions	Rationales
1. Evaluate the patient's home for overall safety, location of telephones, the need for stair climbing, and accessibility of the bathroom and kitchen.	1. A safe and convenient home environment will increase the patient's sense of independence and ability to perform ADLs.
2. Evaluate the patient's support systems and need for financial assistance, equipment, and community resources. Refer the patient to a medical social worker if indicated.	2. Support systems and community resources can help the patient remain at home. He may need assistance to obtain necessary services.

Nursing diagnosis: *Powerlessness related to loss of control over life-style*

GOAL: To minimize the patient's feelings of powerlessness and loss of control

Interventions	Rationales
1. Assess the patient's degree of anger, fear, and resentment and his ability to make choices.	1. The patient may be supervised by several health care professionals and have multiple appointments and treatments scheduled. The patient may transfer anger, fear, and resentment over the disease and treatment to the health care team.
2. When appropriate, let the patient make choices on treatment options; for example, type of analgesic or food choices. If the patient appears unable to do so, assist with decision making.	2. Some patients are paralyzed by anger and cannot make choices. Others need to be involved in decision making as much as possible. The nurse must accommodate changes in the patient's perspective as she works with the patient and family.

ASSOCIATED CARE PLANS
• Grief and Grieving
• Hospice
• Ineffective Coping
• Pain

NETWORKING OF SERVICES
• Lifeline
• Meals On Wheels
• durable medical equipment (DME) supplier
• respiratory therapy (if supplemental oxygen is ordered)
• community support groups
• American Cancer Society
• transportation services

CARE TEAM INVOLVED
• nurse
• doctors (pulmonary, oncology, and radiology specialists)
• patient and family
• medical social worker
• home health aide

IMPLICATIONS FOR HOME CARE
• functional features of the home (stairs, location of bathroom and kitchen)
• telephone, Lifeline (communication)
• oxygen safety (if supplemental oxygen is ordered)

PATIENT EDUCATION TOOLS
• dietary information
• American Cancer Society literature about treatment of lung cancer
• literature about each prescribed drug
• list of signs and symptoms of infection and respiratory failure
• guidelines for safe use of oxygen (if supplemental oxygen is ordered)

DISCHARGE PLAN FROM HOME HEALTH CARE
Before discharge from home health care, the patient or family should:
• have the phone numbers of the doctor, emergency medical service, oxygen supplier (if applicable), home health agency, and local American Cancer Society
• understand the prescribed medication regimen and have a written dosage schedule and list of adverse effects
• explain activity restrictions and energy conservation measures
• know signs and symptoms of respiratory failure
• know signs and symptoms of infection
• explain dietary needs and plans for meeting those needs
• list foods high in protein and calories
• be familiar with care and use of oxygen equipment, if prescribed
• write down the dates and times of follow-up appointments for evaluation and treatment
• have a plan for transportation to appointments.

SELECTED REFERENCES
Birmingham, J. *Home Care Planning Based on DRGs*. Philadelphia: J.B. Lippincott Co., 1986.
Donavan, M., and Pierce, S. *Cancer Care Nursing*. East Norwalk, Conn.: Appleton & Lange, 1984.
Eliopoulos, C. *A Guide to the Nursing of the Aged*. Baltimore: Williams & Wilkins Co., 1987.
Groenwald, S. *Cancer Nursing Principles and Practice*. Boston: Jones and Bartlett Publishers, 1987.
Iyer, P., et al. *Nursing Process and Nursing Diagnosis*. Philadelphia: W.B. Saunders Co., 1986.

Tuberculosis

DESCRIPTION AND TIME FOCUS
Tuberculosis is an infectious disease caused by *Mycobacterium tuberculosis* and characterized by pulmonary infiltrates, formation of granulomas with caseation, fibrosis, and cavitation. Infected persons transmit the disease through airborne droplet nuclei ejected during sneezing, coughing, speaking, or singing. Infectious droplet nuclei are inhaled and deposited in the alveoli. Susceptible persons may then develop the disease. Persons who produce sputum containing many tubercle bacilli are considered highly infectious.

Although morbidity and mortality from tuberculosis have steadily declined in the United States, tuberculosis remains an important public health problem in certain population groups. Incidence is increasing in the elderly population, with nearly a third of reported tuberculosis disease cases occurring in persons ages 65 and over. Other populations at risk include younger persons of economically disadvantaged backgrounds and foreign-born persons and homeless persons of all ages.

Tuberculosis can be prevented and cured. Many cases of tuberculosis could be prevented by identifying infected and potentially infected persons and administering preventive therapy. Cure relies on strict patient compliance with the prescribed treatment or prevention regimen. The regimen can be flexible to promote patient compliance.

This clinical plan focuses on the patient at home with infectious tuberculosis. Unless the patient is acutely ill from tuberculosis or a concurrent disease, hospitalization usually is not required. A patient who complies with the prescribed treatment usually will demonstrate improvement after a few weeks of treatment.

■ Typical home health care length of service for a patient with tuberculosis: varies according to the treatment; may be as short as 6 months or longer than 12 months if the patient is noncompliant or if the tuberculosis organism proves nonsusceptible to prescribed medication

■ Typical visit frequency: once weekly for 4 weeks while establishing compliance with treatment or preventive therapy; once every 2 weeks for 4 weeks to observe for adverse reactions, collect specimens, and confirm compliance; then monthly until the regimen is completed to observe for adverse reactions, collect specimens, and confirm compliance

HEALTH HISTORY FINDINGS
In a health history interview, the patient may report many of these findings:
• difficulty breathing
• chest pain
• night sweats
• anorexia
• weight loss
• malaise
• fatigue and weakness
• irregular menses
• history of prolonged immunosuppressive or corticosteroid therapy
• history of gastrectomy
• history of diabetes
• history of silicosis
• history of hematologic or reticuloendothelial disease, such as leukemia or Hodgkin's disease
• history of human immunodeficiency virus (HIV) infection that has not progressed to acquired immunodeficiency syndrome (AIDS); may cause tuberculosis infection to progress to distuberculosis
• economically disadvantaged
• urban habitation
• foreign born

PHYSICAL FINDINGS
In a physical examination, the nurse may detect many of these findings:

Respiratory
• dyspnea
• productive cough
• hemoptysis

Integumentary
• lymph node enlargement

Renal and urinary
• signs of urinary tract infection (with no evidence of common bacterial pathogens)

General
• cachexia
• fever and chills

DIAGNOSTIC STUDIES
The following studies may be performed to evaluate the patient's health status:
• tuberculin skin test (Mantoux)—significant when induration is 10 mm or more (5 mm if the patient is a close contact of an infected person)
• chest X-ray—standard anterior, posterior, and lateral views to detect changes compatible with tuberculosis (cavities and small, diffuse nodules)
• bronchography (pleural biopsy, lung biopsy, bronchospirometry, and fiberoptic bronchoscopy)—to confirm diagnosis of pulmonary tuberculosis
• gastric washings (gastric aspiration of swallowed respiratory secretions)—to obtain specimens for examination

• surgical biopsies—for tissue examination and cultures of other affected sites
• sputum smears (acid-fast stain)—to determine the presence of *M. tuberculosis* and to indicate the number of organisms being excreted; also to determine the in-

fectiousness and mark the effectiveness of treatment
• sputum cultures—to identify the tubercle bacilli, confirm the diagnosis of tuberculosis, and determine drug sensitivities

Nursing diagnosis: *Altered health maintenance related to disease management*

GOAL: To minimize the spread of tuberculosis in the patient's family and community

Interventions

1. Identify any persons who may have been infected by the patient.

2. Identify those persons who have come in contact with the patient but who are not infected.

3. Identify the source of the patient's infection (*index case*—a person with active untreated tuberculosis who is infecting others).

4. Report all persons with active disease or with infection to state and local health departments, following appropriate protocol.

Rationales

1. Persons exposed to the patient must undergo Mantoux skin testing to determine whether they have been infected and should begin preventive therapy.

2. These persons will need reassurance that they are not infected. In many cases, they also will need a permit from a doctor or state health department (regulations vary among states) enabling them to return to work or school.

3. The infection source is especially important to patient contacts who have children under age 5. Young children are especially prone to developing tuberculosis if infected.

4. This information aids evaluation of the current status of tuberculosis locally and statewide. Statistics are required by the Centers for Disease Control in Atlanta.

Nursing diagnosis: *Potential noncompliance related to lack of signs and symptoms and lack of patient understanding of disease and treatment regimen*

GOAL: To have the patient comply with treatment for several months after symptoms disappear, and to have infected persons undergo preventive therapy even though no signs or symptoms of illness exist

Interventions

1. Plan frequent visits to the patient's home.

2. Monitor the patient for adverse reactions to prescribed medications, such as GI upset, dyspnea, optic neuritis, skin rash, vertigo, and tinnitus. Report any reactions to the doctor, who may adjust the medication regimen.

3. Teach the patient and caregiver techniques of disease management and preventive therapy, including:
• covering the mouth and nose with a tissue when coughing, sneezing, or laughing
• using an exhaust fan to expel air from the patient's room
• avoiding drinking raw milk, which can carry infectious organisms.

4. With the patient's cooperation, collect sputum specimens at 2- to 4-week intervals.

Rationales

1. Frequent visits facilitate regular monitoring of the patient's understanding of and compliance with the treatment regimen.

2. Adverse reactions may reduce the patient's willingness to comply with the medication regimen.

3. The patient and caregiver need to understand management and preventive measures and their importance in order to comply with them.

4. Sputum specimens are required to determine the effectiveness of medications and the infectiousness of the patient.

5. If necessary, adjust the patient's daily medication regimen to meet the demands of his schedule.

5. The regimen can be modified from daily to twice-weekly administration if necessary, which may help improve compliance.

6. Involve the patient and caregiver in the care planning process.

6. Patient and caregiver participation in care planning increases the likelihood that the patient will comply with the treatment regimen.

7. Encourage the patient to dispose of used tissues following standard disposal methods for infectious waste.

7. Knowing and using the proper tissue disposal method helps improve the patient's sense of self-control and also prevents the spread of infection.

Nursing diagnosis: *Potential social isolation related to a communicable disease diagnosis*

GOAL: To increase the patient's interaction with family, friends, and community

Interventions

1. Approach the patient with an accepting, positive attitude, and offer support to eliminate anxiety caused by fear of rejection.

2. Assess and document the patient's expressed feelings about self-image.

3. Encourage the patient to share feelings and emotions.

4. Encourage the patient to maintain contact with friends and relatives through frequent telephone calls or visits.

Rationales

1. The patient needs to experience acceptance from others in order to maintain a positive self-image and interact effectively with others.

2. Documenting the patient's concept of self helps the nurse develop an appropriate plan of care.

3. This encourages open, honest communication, which will enhance the patient's interactions with others.

4. Contact with others diminishes the patient's feelings of isolation and improves his self-image.

Nursing diagnosis: *Potential for injury related to adverse effects of antituberculosis medication*

GOAL: To determine the patient's medication intolerances and, if necessary, help the patient and caregiver adjust the medication regimen

Interventions

1. Assess the patient for adverse reactions to antituberculosis medication, such as GI upset, dyspnea, optic neuritis, skin rash, vertigo, and tinnitus. Promptly report any reactions to the doctor.

2. Discuss with the doctor any adjustment to the patient's antituberculosis medication regimen.

3. Teach the patient and caregiver about possible adverse reactions to new medications, when to report reactions, and the importance of scheduled doctor appointments.

Rationales

1. Early detection of adverse reactions allows adjustment of the medication regimen to eliminate or minimize reactions before they cause serious problems.

2. The nurse must understand medication adjustments to effectively assess the patient for adverse reactions.

3. Continuing to update the patient's and caregiver's knowledge of the treatment helps ensure compliance and efficacy.

Nursing diagnosis: *Ineffective breathing pattern related to fatigue*

GOAL: To maximize the patient's oxygen use through energy conservation measures

Interventions	Rationales
1. Teach the patient how to conserve oxygen through proper positioning (for example, sitting with elbows on a table [three-point posture] and lying in semi-Fowler's position) and relaxation of neck and shoulder muscles.	1. Conservation of oxygen will reduce anxiety and encourage full lung expansion.
2. Teach the patient deep-breathing exercises to coordinate breathing with activity.	2. The patient should understand that inhalation requires muscle work and energy expenditure. Breathing exercises help reduce the work of breathing.
3. Plan the patient's activities to coincide with periods of maximum oxygenation.	3. Planning activities to coincide with periods of maximum oxygenation will increase the patient's activity tolerance, which will have the added benefit of enhancing his self-image and feelings of independence.

ASSOCIATED CARE PLANS
• Acquired Immunodeficiency Syndrome
• Chronic Bronchitis
• Chronic Obstructive Pulmonary Disease
• Grief and Grieving
• Ineffective Coping
• Malnutrition
• Pneumonia
• Smoking Cessation

NETWORKING OF SERVICES
• state and local health departments
• Centers for Disease Control
• American Lung Association
• American Thoracic Society
• Lifeline
• Meals On Wheels
• respiratory therapy
• durable medical equipment (DME) supplier

CARE TEAM INVOLVED
• nurse from local home health agency
• nurses from state and local health departments
• doctor (pulmonary specialist)
• patient and family
• public health advisor
• laboratory technician
• X-ray technician
• respiratory therapist
• physical therapist
• home health aide
• medical social worker

IMPLICATIONS FOR HOME CARE
• functional features of the home (single, well-ventilated room for the patient)
• masking when others are present until sputum is smear-negative
• telephone (communication)
• oxygen safety (if supplemental oxygen is ordered)
• proper containers for contaminated waste disposal

PATIENT EDUCATION TOOLS
• literature about tuberculosis and infection
• literature about treatment and preventive therapy
• list of prescribed medications, dosage schedules, and possible adverse reactions
• literature from the American Lung Association, American Thoracic Society, Centers for Disease Control, and state and local health departments
• guidelines for safe use oxygen (if supplemental oxygen is ordered)

DISCHARGE PLAN FROM HOME HEALTH CARE
Before discharge from home health care and the state and local Tuberculosis Control Program, the patient should:
• be smear- or culture-negative on sputum (or other) specimens submitted
• be complying with the treatment or preventive therapy
• have a chest X-ray indicating no active disease (or a normal X-ray for preventive therapy)
• know the signs and symptoms of tuberculosis in the event of relapse
• understand the need for follow-up doctor appointments

• know the date of the next follow-up doctor appointment
• be alert to the health status of close contacts
• be certain that close contacts are familiar with the signs and symptoms of tuberculosis and know the value of skin testing
• list prescribed antituberculosis medications and dosage schedules
• understand the need to report adverse reactions caused by antituberculosis medications
• have telephone numbers of doctor, home health agency, and state and local health departments
• post emergency telephone numbers by the phone
• obtain the doctor's approval to return to work.

SELECTED REFERENCES

American College of Chest Physicians Consensus Conference. *Chest (Supplement)* 87(2):115s-49s, February 1985.

American Lung Association. *Treatment of Tuberculosis and other Mycobacterial Diseases; Control of Tuberculosis*. New York: American Lung Association, 1983.

Farzan, S., et al. *A Concise Handbook of Respiratory Diseases,* 2nd ed. East Norwalk, Conn.: Appleton & Lange, 1985.

Snider, D. *Improving Patient Compliance in Tuberculosis Treatment Programs*. Atlanta: U.S. Department of Health and Human Services, Centers for Disease Control, February 1985.

U.S. Department of Health and Human Services, Public Health Service, Centers for Disease Control. *TB Notes*. Atlanta: Summer 1987.

NEUROLOGIC SYSTEM

Parkinson's Disease

DESCRIPTION AND TIME FOCUS

Parkinson's disease is a progressive neurologic syndrome affecting the brain centers that regulate movement and muscle tone. It is characterized by impaired movement, muscle rigidity, and tremors, which are most severe during rest and decrease with activity. In most cases, the etiology of Parkinson's disease is not known. However, a few cases have been related to carbon monoxide and manganese poisoning, and others may be induced by high-dose tricyclic antidepressant therapy.

A five-stage classification system is used to evaluate the extent of the disease. In Stage I, the patient has unilateral, mild involvement and is not disabled. In Stage II, the patient has bilateral involvement and minimal disability. In Stage III, the patient has impaired posture and gait and mild to moderate disability with a significant degree of slowness. In Stage IV, the patient has marked bradykinesia, rigidity, and festination. In Stage V, the patient cannot walk and is confined to a bed or a wheelchair.

This clinical plan focuses on the patient discharged home after inpatient treatment of Parkinson's disease. The patient's home is an ideal setting for teaching the patient and family about the nature of the disease and its treatment and monitoring for progressive disease symptoms. Treatment focuses on drug and physical therapy. Drug therapy usually involves levodopa, given in increasing doses to control symptoms. Other drugs used include amantadine, bromocriptine and other ergot alkaloids, and anticholinergics. Nursing care goals include maintaining or improving the patient's current level of functioning and helping the patient become as independent, knowledgeable, and symptom-free as possible.

■ Typical home health care length of service for a patient with Parkinson's disease: 8 weeks, or until stable

■ Typical visit frequency: twice weekly for 8 weeks, or until stable

HEALTH HISTORY FINDINGS

In a health history interview, the patient may report many of these findings:
• fatigue
• frequent falls
• muscle aches and pain
• stiffness and heaviness in legs
• confusion
• depression
• restlessness and insomnia
• dysphagia
• anorexia
• weight loss
• constipation
• urinary incontinence
• history of carbon monoxide or manganese poisoning
• prolonged use of tricylclic antidepressants

PHYSICAL FINDINGS

In a physical examination, the nurse may detect many of these findings:

Neurologic
• "pill-rolling" tremor
• akinesia or bradykinesia
• dysarthria, with soft, low- or high-pitched, monotone voice
• festinating gait (shuffling, propulsive)
• masklike facial expression with unblinking eyes
• increased salivation, possibly with drooling
• increased lacrimation
• loss of postural reflexes

Gastrointestinal
• decreased bowel sounds

Integumentary
• excessive sweating
• flushed, oily skin

Musculoskeletal
• muscle rigidity ("lead pipe" or "cogwheel" rigidity)
• stooped posture

Renal and urinary
• signs of urinary tract infection

DIAGNOSTIC STUDIES

No routine studies are performed.

Nursing diagnosis: *Self-care deficit: feeding, bathing/hygiene, dressing/grooming, toileting, related to neuromuscular impairment*

GOAL: To help the patient achieve and maintain the highest possible level of self-care functioning

Interventions

1. Assess the patient's ability to feed, bathe, dress, and groom himself and to perform toileting activities independently.

2. Based on the patient's abilities, encourage independence in performing ADLs.

3. Assist the patient with ADLs only as needed.

4. Arrange a consultation with an occupational therapist, as necessary.

Rationales

1. The neuromuscular impairment associated with Parkinson's disease often impairs the patient's ability to perform activities of daily living (ADLs). The nurse needs to determine the nature of this impairment to plan appropriate interventions.

2. Performing ADLs within his abilities promotes the patient's sense of confidence and self-esteem, which contributes to increased self-care functioning.

3. Assisting the patient only when he needs help encourages independence. The patient's knowledge that help is available when needed encourages him to try activities and reduces frustration when he encounters difficulties.

4. An occupational therapist may be able to suggest alternative methods of performing certain ADLs and can provide specially adapted equipment, such as hairbrushes, toothbrushes, kitchen utensils, dishes and cups, appliance knobs, elevated toilet seats, and grab bars, to enable the patient to perform ADLs more independently.

Nursing diagnosis: *Impaired physical mobility related to muscle rigidity, weakness, and tremors*

GOAL: To help the patient achieve and maintain the maximum level of mobility possible within disease limitations

Interventions

1. Each visit, perform range-of-motion exercises (active or passive, as appropriate) for the patient's arms and legs. Teach the patient and family these exercises, and encourage them to perform the exercises daily.

2. Teach the patient other simple methods of improving mobility, such as rocking from side to side to simulate leg movement.

3. As appropriate, develop and implement a simple exercise program, such as walking, that the patient can perform daily.

4. Consult with an occupational therapist and a physical therapist, as needed, for help in developing an exercise program for the patient.

Rationales

1. Regular range-of-motion exercises help prevent muscle contractures and other complications of prolonged immobility.

2. These techniques also can help prevent complications of prolonged immobility.

3. Regular exercise decreases bone demineralization and reduces muscle atrophy.

4. These therapists can evaluate the patient's muscle strength, joint flexibility, and overall physical capabilities to tailor an individualized exercise program that he can perform and that will help improve mobility.

Nursing diagnosis: *Altered nutrition: less than body requirements, related to dysphagia*

GOAL: To ensure that the patient maintains sufficient caloric intake

Interventions	Rationales
1. Monitor the patient's caloric intake and weight on each visit.	1. Adequate caloric intake is required to meet the body's energy demands and maintain adequate body weight. Weight loss usually indicates inadequate caloric intake.
2. Assess the patient's ability to chew and swallow.	2. Reduced laryngeal closure or difficulty with lip control, chewing, or swallowing can cause the patient to aspirate food and discourage him from eating.
3. Teach the patient the following measures for eating: • sit upright and relax • cut food into small portions and take small bites • eat slowly and chew food thoroughly • drink fluids during meals.	3. These measures will help reduce dysphagia and decrease the risk of aspiration, which will encourage the patient to eat more.
4. Consult a dietitian as needed.	4. A dietician can recommend an individualized diet regimen for the patient, help the family modify menus to accommodate the patient's needs, and suggest measures to reduce dysphagia and increase the patient's caloric intake.

Nursing diagnosis: *Altered bowel elimination: constipation, related to loss of muscle tone and immobility*

GOAL: To prevent or treat constipation

Interventions	Rationales
1. Assess the patient's bowel elimination patterns.	1. Neuromuscular impairment and inactivity may result in constipation.
2. Recommend that the patient increase his intake of dietary fiber and fluids. Encourage a fluid intake of at least 8 8-oz glasses (2 liters) per day.	2. Adequate fiber and fluid intake helps prevent constipation.
3. Encourage the patient to use stool softeners as necessary.	3. Stool softeners may help the patient maintain a normal elimination pattern.
4. Check the patient's bowel for impacted stool and remove when necessary.	4. Stool impaction can cause constipation.

Nursing diagnosis: *Knowledge deficit related to disease effects and progression and the prescribed medication regimen*

GOAL: To improve the patient's and family's understanding of the disease and medication regimen

Interventions	Rationales
1. Discuss the symptoms and progressive nature of Parkinson's disease with the patient and family. Provide them with written information as available.	1. An understanding of the disease effects and progression will help the patient and family cope with the disease.
2. Provide the patient and family with information about local Parkinson's disease support groups.	2. Support groups can provide additional information and assistance.

3. Reinforce the doctor's instructions about the prescribed medication regimen, including dosage schedule and adverse effects to report. If possible, provide written instructions.

3. The patient's understanding of the medication regimen helps promote compliance; knowledge of adverse effects helps ensure safe and effective drug therapy.

Nursing diagnosis: *Impaired verbal communication related to impaired facial muscle movement*

GOAL: To help the patient communicate effectively

Interventions

1. Assess the patient's speech for intelligibility.

2. Teach the patient methods to help improve intelligibility of speech, including:
• practicing speech exercises, such as speaking slowly and as distinctly as possible in front of a mirror or into a tape recorder
• breathing deeply before speaking
• using a telephone amplifier to enhance telephone conversation.

3. If the patient's speech is unintelligible, suggest alternatives to verbal communication, such as a spelling board or picture-and-symbol message board.

4. Refer the patient to a speech therapist if necessary.

Rationales

1. Parkinson's disease often causes dysarthria, characterized by slurred, slow (or occasionally rapid) speech and a soft, low- or high-pitched, monotone voice.

2. These methods can help the patient with slight to moderate dysarthria maintain verbal communication.

3. These devices can help a patient with severe dysarthria maintain communication with caregivers, family, and friends. Remember that the patient also may find written communication difficult or impossible because of tremor and bradykinesia.

4. A patient learning new methods of communication often requires special assistance.

Nursing diagnosis: *Impaired home maintenance management related to neuromuscular impairment and decreased mobility*

GOAL: To optimize the home's safety and functional features

Interventions

1. Assess the patient's home for potential safety hazards, such as slippery floors, sliding rugs, poor lighting, broken chairs, exposed electrical and telephone cords, and general clutter. Take steps to eliminate as many hazards as possible.

2. Determine the patient's needs for durable medical equipment and assistive devices, such as a cane, walker, shower chair, elevated toilet seat, and specially adapted kitchen utensils and tools. Help the patient secure needed equipment and devices.

3. Evaluate the patient's need for home support services, and arrange for appropriate services if necessary.

Rationales

1. Ensuring a safe home environment enhances the patient's ability to perform ADLs and function independently.

2. Such equipment and devices can improve the patient's ability to perform ADLs and alleviate anxiety.

3. The patient may require a home health aide to provide personal care during the transition period from hospital to home, and in later disease stages as impairment worsens. A patient with limited financial resources may benefit from consultation with a social service worker, who can secure available financial aid.

ASSOCIATED CARE PLANS
• Hospice
• Ineffective Coping
• Malnutrition

NETWORKING OF SERVICES
• Meals On Wheels
• Parkinson's disease support group
• durable medical equipment (DME) supplier

CARE TEAM INVOLVED
• nurse
• doctor
• patient and family
• home health aide
• physical therapist
• occupational therapist
• speech therapist
• medical social worker
• dietitian

IMPLICATIONS FOR HOME CARE
• functional features of the home (such as ramps, elevated toilet seat and shower chair in bathroom, and telephone amplifier)
• exercise and rehabilitation programs

PATIENT EDUCATION TOOLS
• information on prescribed medications, including dosage schedules and possible adverse effects
• individualized diet plan
• written instructions from therapists involved in care
• National Parkinson's Foundation literature

DISCHARGE PLAN FROM HOME HEALTH CARE
Before discharge from home health care, the patient should:
• have a list of medications, dosage schedules, and possible adverse effects
• understand dietary requirements and modifications
• know signs and symptoms of disease progression
• have the telephone number of the home health agency for follow-up
• know the dates and times of scheduled follow-up appointments with the doctor or therapists
• establish a daily exercise program
• have appropriate assistive devices or equipment to aid in ADLs.

SELECTED REFERENCES
Adams, R., and Victor, M. *Principles of Neurology*, 3rd ed. New York: McGraw-Hill Book Co., 1985.
Dzuna, J. "Alterations in Mentation: Nursing Assessment and Intervention," *Journal of Neurosurgical Nursing* 17(1):166-70, February 1985.
Lannon, M., et al. "Comprehensive Care of the Patient with Parkinson's Disease," *Journal of Neuroscience Nursing* 18(3):121-31, June 1986.
Norberg, A. and Winblad, B. "A Model for the Assessment of Eating Problems in Patients with Parkinson's Disease," *Journal of Advanced Nursing* 12(4):473-81, July 1987.
Schafer, S. "Modifying the Environment," *Geriatric Nursing* 6(3):157-59, May/June 1985.
Scott, C., Carol, F., and Williams, B. *Communication in Parkinson's Disease*. Rockville, Md.: Aspen Systems, 1985.
Yanko, J. "What Your Patient Should Know About Parkinson's Disease," *Nursing88* 18(1):32p-32s, February 1988.

NEUROLOGIC SYSTEM
Spinal Cord Injury

DESCRIPTION AND TIME FOCUS
Spinal cord injuries usually result from accidents, such as automobile accidents, falls, gunshot wounds, and diving or other sports-related mishaps. Physical disability from spinal cord injury varies depending on the type of injury sustained and the level at which the spinal cord is injured. In general, the higher the level of injury, the greater the resulting disability.

A spinal-cord-injured patient must make great physical and psychosocial adjustments to adapt to a newly restricted life-style. The patient often finds psychosocial adjustment particularly difficult and typically requires much emotional support. Home health care centers on maximizing the patient's functional independence. The home should be adapted to facilitate accessibility before the patient returns from the hospital. Ongoing assessment after the patient returns will ensure adequate adaptation, and ongoing collaboration between the nurse and patient will help the patient achieve the maximum level of functioning possible.

This clinical plan focuses on the patient discharged home from an acute-care hospital after treatment of and rehabilitation for a spinal cord injury.

■ Typical home health care length of service for a patient with spinal cord injury: 8 weeks

■ Typical visit frequency: three times weekly, gradually decreasing to once weekly and then once monthly until discharge criteria are met

HEALTH HISTORY FINDINGS
In a health history interview, the patient may report many of these findings:
• history of spinal trauma
• constipation
• diarrhea
• sexual dysfunction (*males*: inability to experience orgasm or ejaculate, erectile difficulty, reflexogenic erections; *females*: inability to experience orgasm, irregular menstruation, altered vaginal lubrication)
• history of urinary tract infection, renal calculi, hydronephrosis, epididymitis, urethral diverticuli, or renal failure
• grief reaction
• altered self-image
• increased emotional stress
• changes in life-style
• changes in occupation
• disruption of developmental tasks

PHYSICAL FINDINGS
In a physical examination, the nurse may detect many of these findings:

Neurologic
• loss of sensation (location and degree depend on type and severity of spinal cord lesion)
• pain at the level of the injury
• autonomic dysreflexia
• spinal automatisms

Cardiovascular
• impaired circulation in denervated tissue
• orthostatic hypotension
• bradycardia
• deep vein thrombosis

Respiratory
• impaired cough response
• poor clearance of respiratory secretions
• reduced vital capacity
• respiratory fatigue
• pulmonary congestion

Gastrointestinal
• stress ulcers
• fecal impaction
• paralytic ileus

Integumentary
• skin breakdown

Musculoskeletal
• muscle atrophy below level of injury
• muscle spasms
• muscle shortening
• tendon contractures
• ankylosis of joints
• footdrop, wristdrop

Renal and urinary
• neurogenic bladder

General
• overweight or underweight

DIAGNOSTIC STUDIES
The following studies may be performed to evaluate the patient's health status:
• urinalysis, culture and sensitivity—once a week or as ordered, to monitor for urinary tract infection

Nursing diagnosis: *Self-care deficit related to partial or total paralysis from spinal cord injury*

GOAL: To help the patient maximize independence in all activities of daily living (ADLs)

Interventions

1. Before the patient is discharged from the hospital, assess the home environment to determine if it is adequately adapted for maximum independence. Check such items as interior and exterior wheelchair accessibility, doorway widths, bathroom facilities, doorknob levels, phone accessibility, counter heights, and appliances.

2. Collaborate with the patient, caregiver, and appropriate community services to make necessary adaptations.

3. Assess the patient's need for assistive devices, such as a transfer board, adapted utensils, dressing aids, or Lifeline (if the patient will be alone). Collaborate with the patient and caregiver to obtain needed items.

4. Assess the patient's plan for transportation. If the patient or caregiver owns a vehicle and the patient can use hand controls, help them arrange appropriate vehicle adaptations. If a vehicle is not available, or the patient cannot use hand controls, help the patient contact appropriate community services to secure transportation when needed.

5. Assess the patient's use of assistive devices and community services. Encourage the use of all available resources.

Rationales

1. An adequately adapted home facilitates maximum independence within the limits of the patient's disability.

2. Involving the patient in decisions about necessary adaptations increases the patient's feeling of independence.

3. Assistive devices increase independence by letting the patient perform many activities that would otherwise be impossible.

4. Access to transportation maximizes the patient's independence. Lack of transportation can produce feelings of isolation.

5. The patient may need encouragement to use all available resources; doing so will maximize independence.

Nursing diagnosis: *Impaired physical mobility related to neuromuscular deficit resulting from spinal cord injury*

GOAL 1: To prevent musculoskeletal complications, such as contractures, footdrop, and wristdrop

Interventions

1. Perform active or passive range-of-motion (ROM) exercises at regular intervals.

2. Assess the patient's muscles and joints routinely to detect musculoskeletal complications. If complications are detected, increase the frequency of ROM to the affected area and refer the patient to the doctor and a physical therapist. Teach the patient the signs and symptoms of musculoskeletal deformity.

3. Assess the patient's use of assistive devices or braces designed to prevent footdrop or wristdrop.

4. Encourage the patient to perform as much activity as is tolerable, using all functional muscles.

Rationales

1. Routine movement of muscles and joints helps prevent musculoskeletal complications.

2. Early detection of musculoskeletal complications allows prompt attention to prevent permanent deformity.

3. The proper use of assistive devices or braces can help prevent footdrop and wristdrop.

4. Physical activity helps prevent musculoskeletal deformities. Maintaining the functional ability of nonaffected muscles improves overall ability.

5. Teach the patient the causes of muscle spasms and factors that stimulate spasticity. Explain possible treatments for spasms, including medications as appropriate.

5. Understanding the cause of spasticity helps the patient cope with this problem. Factors that stimulate spasms include skin breakdown, tight-fitting clothes, and infection. Avoiding these can reduce the incidence of spasm. Treatments for spasms include analgesic and antispasmodic medications, stretching exercises, massage, and warm baths.

6. Explain that spasms are involuntary and do not represent an improvement in neuromuscular function.

6. By simulating voluntary movement, muscle spasms may cause the patient to develop false hope for return of neuromuscular function.

GOAL 2: To prevent patient injury from falls related to incorrect transfer techniques

Interventions

1. Assess the patient's ability to perform safe transfers to and from a wheelchair, bed, or car. Teach the patient and caregiver correct transfer procedures and assist when necessary.

2. Teach the patient and caregiver the correct use of transfer assistive devices, such as a transfer board.

3. Assess the home for unsafe conditions; for example, a doorway with a high sill that can upset a wheelchair. Help the patient arrange for home modifications that improve safety.

4. Assess the patient's need for Lifeline and, if necessary, help the patient obtain this service.

Rationales

1. Using proper transfer techniques helps prevent accidents and injury.

2. The correct use of assistive devices helps prevent accidents and injury.

3. Modifying unsafe conditions in the home helps prevent accidents and injury.

4. A patient who lives alone or is left alone for considerable periods may require Lifeline, which enables the patient to notify rescue services immediately during an emergency. Falls and other accidents can result in serious injury or even death if the patient cannot get prompt help.

GOAL 3: To prevent cardiopulmonary complications, such as pneumonia, orthostatic hypotension, deep vein thrombosis, and autonomic hyperreflexia

Interventions

1. Teach the patient deep-breathing exercises and the use of an incentive spirometer. Provide chest physiotherapy at regular intervals, determined by the severity of respiratory compromise. Encourage the patient to change positions every 1 to 2 hours.

2. As appropriate, teach the patient and caregiver tracheostomy care or mechanical ventilator care. Assist in this care if needed.

3. Teach the patient to change position slowly.

4. Teach the patient the proper use of abdominal binders and elastic stockings, when applicable.

5. Teach the patient and caregiver the classic signs and symptoms, common causes, and treatment of autonomic hyperreflexia. Classic signs and symptoms of autonomic hyperreflexia include facial flushing, severe headache, diaphoresis above the injury level, bradycardia, and hypertension. Causes include any noxious stimuli, such as a distended bladder. Treatment includes finding and eliminating causes and having the patient sit upright as much as possible.

Rationales

1. Pooling of respiratory secretions can lead to respiratory infection and pneumonia. Frequent position changes and movement of air and secretions help prevent these problems.

2. Proper care of a tracheostomy or mechanical ventilator helps prevent respiratory infections and complications.

3. Moving slowly when changing position helps prevent orthostatic hypotension.

4. These devices prevent pooling of blood in the abdomen and legs, which can lead to orthostatic hypotension and deep vein thrombosis.

5. Prompt recognition and intervention is necessary to prevent further complications.

GOAL 4: To maintain maximum patient independence and function

Interventions

1. Encourage the patient to engage in recreational activities as his abilities allow; assist when necessary. Refer the patient to a recreational therapist, if needed.

2. Encourage the patient to engage in a desired, meaningful vocation. Refer the patient to a vocational counselor, if needed.

3. Encourage the patient's involvement in community activities and spinal-cord-injury support groups and services.

Rationales

1. Recreational activities foster independence and enjoyment.

2. A desired, meaningful vocation fosters independence, activity, and sense of purpose.

3. Involvement with other spinal-cord-injured patients can encourage independence.

Nursing diagnosis: *Potential impaired skin integrity related to immobility and reduced sensation resulting from spinal cord injury*

GOAL: To prevent skin breakdown

Interventions

1. Teach the patient to change position at least once every 1 to 2 hours. If some mobility is present, teach the patient to shift weight every 30 minutes while in a wheelchair and relieve weight by leaning forward.

2. Teach the patient to use assistive devices that relieve pressure, such as an air mattress, heel and elbow protectors, and a wheelchair cushion.

3. Teach the patient proper nutrition and hygiene measures.

4. Teach the patient and caregiver to assess the entire skin surface daily for signs of skin breakdown.

5. Teach the patient and caregiver to massage areas of potential breakdown and to reduce pressure on these areas.

6. Teach the patient to wear loose-fitting clothes and ensure that assistive devices are fitted properly.

7. Teach the patient to avoid touching very hot or cold surfaces with body areas having decreased sensation.

Rationales

1. Frequent movement increases blood circulation to pressured areas, which helps prevent skin breakdown.

2. These devices reduce pressure, which helps prevent skin breakdown.

3. Proper nutrition provides the body with the nutrients needed to maintain skin integrity. Proper hygiene prevents the accumulation of waste products on the skin that can lead to breakdown.

4. Early detection of signs of skin breakdown enables interventions to help prevent breakdown.

5. Massage and relief from pressure increase blood circulation to affected areas, which promotes skin integrity.

6. Constrictive clothing or improperly fitted assistive devices can predispose the patient to skin breakdown in pressured areas.

7. The patient will not feel an injury in areas of decreased sensation and skin breakdown may result.

Nursing diagnosis: *Altered urinary elimination patterns related to neurogenic bladder resulting from spinal cord injury*

GOAL: To facilitate adequate urinary elimination

Interventions

1. If possible, teach the patient and caregiver techniques to encourage urination without using a catheter, such as Credé's maneuver, Valsalva's maneuver, and rectal stretch.

Rationales

1. Avoiding catheter use decreases the risk of urinary tract infection.

2. If intermittent catheterization is ordered and the patient's condition permits, teach the patient and caregiver proper techniques for intermittent catheterization.

2. Proper catheterization techniques help prevent urinary tract infection.

3. Teach the patient and caregiver to monitor fluid intake and output, and explain the importance of maintaining the prescribed fluid intake.

3. Fluid restrictions during intermittent catheterization help prevent excessive bladder distention. Increased fluid intake promotes adequate urine output, which helps prevent renal calculi and infection. The patient must monitor intake and output to detect and prevent fluid imbalance.

4. Teach the patient and caregiver the signs and symptoms of bladder distention.

4. Avoiding bladder distention helps prevent urinary and renal complications, such as hydronephrosis, pyelonephrosis, and stretching of the bladder.

5. If an external urine collecting device is ordered, instruct the patient and caregiver in proper use and application. Assist as needed.

5. Urine leakage and skin breakdown can result from an improperly applied device or waste products on the skin.

6. If long-term use of an indwelling (Foley) catheter is ordered, change the catheter every 4 to 6 weeks or more often if needed.

6. Periodically changing the catheter helps prevent infection and an excessive build-up of sediment that can block urine flow.

7. Teach the patient and caregiver the proper use of equipment related to long-term indwelling catheter use.

7. Using equipment properly facilitates adequate urine flow and helps prevent infection. The patient should know to keep the collection bag below bladder level, how to irrigate the catheter, and how to anchor the catheter and change bags when irrigation is indicated.

Nursing diagnosis: *Altered bowel elimination: constipation, related to neurologic damage resulting from spinal cord injury*

GOAL: To facilitate regular bowel movements

Interventions

1. Collaborate with the patient to determine the best time of day for bowel evacuation. Teach the patient to attempt evacuation at the same time every 1, 2, or 3 days—depending on the patient's bowel habits before spinal cord injury.

2. Based on the level of spinal cord damage, determine an effective method of bowel evacuation for the patient. Methods include digital removal of stool and rectal suppositories. Explain the reason for choosing the selected method.

3. Teach the patient or caregiver the proper method for digitally removing stool or using rectal suppositories and enemas. (*Note:* Enemas are not indicated for long-term bowel management.)

4. Encourage the patient to maintain an adequate fluid and dietary fiber intake and to be as physically active as possible.

Rationales

1. Determining and following a consistent bowel evacuation routine facilitates regular evacuations and bowel continence, which helps promote the patient's sense of independence and self-confidence.

2. The optimum method of evacuation depends on the level and severity of the patient's spinal cord damage. Explaining the rationale for selecting a particular method encourages the patient to comply with the bowel management program.

3. Using these methods properly facilitates bowel evacuation.

4. These interventions facilitate bowel movements and help prevent constipation.

ASSOCIATED CARE PLANS
• Grief and Grieving
• Ineffective Coping
• Malnutrition
• Neurogenic Bladder
• Pain
• Sex and Sexuality
• Urinary Tract Infections

NETWORKING OF SERVICES
• Lifeline
• durable medical equipment (DME) supplier
• Meals On Wheels
• respiratory therapy (if the patient is dependent on a mechanical ventilator or oxygen)
• local support groups for spinal-cord-injured persons
• handicapped transportation services
• vocational rehabilitation services

CARE TEAM INVOLVED
• nurse
• doctor
• patient and family
• family therapist
• medical social worker
• home health aide
• professional homemaker
• occupational therapist
• recreational therapist
• physical therapist
• vocational counselor
• rehabilitation nurse

IMPLICATIONS FOR HOME CARE
• functional features of the home (wheelchair ramps, elevator chairs, location of bathroom and kitchen)
• accessible telephone
• respiratory safety (if using a mechanical ventilator or oxygen)
• appropriate assistive devices

PATIENT EDUCATION TOOLS
• list of signs and symptoms of urinary tract infection, skin breakdown, respiratory infection, deep vein thrombosis, contractures, footdrop, wristdrop, and autonomic dysreflexia
• literature from:
National Spinal Cord Injury Association
Paralyzed Veterans of America (if applicable)
National Wheelchair Association
Regional Model Spinal Cord Injury System Rehabilitation Services Administration
National Institute of Handicapped Research
Projects with Industry programs
state vocational rehabilitation programs

DISCHARGE PLAN FROM HOME HEALTH CARE
Before discharge from home health care, the patient should:
• be aware of personal stressors and know effective coping mechanisms
• demonstrate safe transfers
• know signs and symptoms of urinary tract infection, potential skin breakdown, respiratory infection, deep vein thrombosis, contractures, footdrop, wristdrop, and autonomic dysreflexia
• state methods of preventing these health problems and steps to take should they occur
• state a preferred method for dealing with changes in sexual function
• have a Lifeline system in place, if needed
• be able to perform ADLs, ROM exercises, bowel and bladder care, and meal preparation (with the assistance of an aide if the injury is severe)
• have appropriate assistive devices and demonstrate their correct use
• know how to arrange for transportation
• know how to contact available community services and support organizations
• state prescribed dietary and fluid regimen
• have the telephone number of the home health agency for follow-up if needed
• have an aide service arranged if needed (some patients will always require an aide service)
• know the dates and times of doctor appointments
• know emergency department and ambulance service phone numbers.

SELECTED REFERENCES
Carpenito, L. *Handbook of Nursing Diagnosis.* Philadelphia: J.B. Lippincott Co., 1984.
Drayton-Hargrove, S., and Reddy, M. "Rehabilitation and Long-Term Management of the Spinal Cord Injured Adult," *Nursing Clinics of North America* 21(4):599-610, December 1986.
Mathewson, M. "Ascending and Descending Spinal Cord Tracts," *Critical Care Nurse* 5(5):10-14, September-October 1985.
Metcalf, J. "Acute Phase Management of Persons with Spinal Cord Injury: A Nursing Diagnosis Perspective," *Nursing Clinics of North America* 21(4), December 1986.
Snyder, M. *A Guide to Neurological and Neurosurgical Nursing.* New York: John Wiley & Sons, 1983.

NEUROLOGIC SYSTEM

Alzheimer's Disease

DESCRIPTION AND TIME FOCUS

Alzheimer's disease, the fourth leading cause of death in the United States, is a progressive, degenerative neurologic condition whose symptoms result from global degeneration of the cerebral cortex. Characteristic hallmarks of the disease are neurofibrillary tangles in the brain that impair normal neuronal functioning.

The cause of Alzheimer's disease is unknown, and no cure or method to arrest its progression has been discovered. The disease is "diagnosed" after all other conditions with dementia-like symptoms have been ruled out by extensive diagnostic procedures and no other viable cause for the symptoms can be found. A true diagnosis is confirmed only by pathologic findings at autopsy.

Current literature on the disease identifies between three and seven stages. Stage-related symptoms discussed in this care plan, based on a three-stage model, are those most frequently reported and described. The patient may exhibit some or all of these symptoms as the disease progresses and may exhibit other symptoms that reflect a unique response to the disease. Because onset is insidious and the patient may present at any stage, the nurse must develop patient-specific care plans that address his ever-changing needs. Depending on his physical and mental health, age of onset, and amount of health care and support available, the patient can live with this disease for 5 to 20 years.

This clinical plan focuses on home care of the patient with Alzheimer's disease. Nursing care centers on helping the patient and family adjust to the patient's impaired cognitive abilities, providing emotional support to the patient and family, and protecting the patient from injury in the home. The patient-caregiver partnership is an important focus of nursing and other interventions as the disease progresses. The home health care team must anticipate the patient's changing stage-related needs to ensure optimal physical and psychological health, to prevent crises, and to support the family's informed decision for alternative living arrangements, if necessary.

■ Typical home health care length of service for a patient with Alzheimer's disease: varies, depending on the disease's duration; usually begins during the second stage

■ Typical visit frequency: once every 2 weeks for 12 weeks; then readmit for new problems

HEALTH HISTORY FINDINGS

In a health history interview, the patient (or the patient's family) may report many of these findings:

Stage I (Forgetfulness)
• short-term memory loss
• increased use of memory aids
• loss of spontaneity and sense of humor
• social withdrawal
• increased anxiety and irritability
• increased frustration and angry outbursts
• poor concentration and decreased attention span
• impaired judgment
• acalculia (difficulty in performing simple arithmetic calculations)
• altered sleeping habits
• altered eating habits
• decreased or increased libido
• unpredictable mood swings (for example, from melancholia to euphoria)
• weight loss or gain

Stage II (Confusion)
(Diagnosis is often made during this stage)
• increased forgetfulness (names, dates, addresses, appointments)
• dysphasia
• dysphagia (later in this stage)
• visual agnosia
• apraxia
• repetitive speech or actions
• echolalia (repeating what someone has just said)
• wandering
• progressive difficulty with activities of daily living (ADLs)
• suspiciousness or paranoia
• hallucinations or delusions
• incontinence
• catastrophic reactions (unpredictable, exaggerated, or abnormal responses to normal situations and events)

Stage III, or terminal stage (Dementia)
• intensification of previous symptoms
• cessation of talking
• grunting, moaning, or screeching
• impaired mobility
• detachment from environment and people
• total incontinence
• total dependence on others for all functions
• confinement to bed
• myoclonus (involuntary jerking movements that could become seizures of the grand mal type)

Note: A transition takes place between late Stage II and the middle of Stage III: the patient becomes more withdrawn; less aware of his environment and the meaning of relationships and life in general; totally dependent on caregivers for all aspects of functioning; and vulnerable to neglect, physical and emotional abuse, social isolation, sensory deprivation, and complications characteristic of terminally ill, bedridden patients.

PHYSICAL FINDINGS

In a physical examination, the nurse may detect many of the findings below. During the first stage, these are unremarkable unless the patient has an underlying mental or physical problem. The patient's appearance in the early stage usually does not alert an observer to the problem. At the time of diagnosis, which often coincides with early Stage II symptoms, some physical findings begin to emerge. If all diagnostic tests and studies are negative and the behaviors persist, a differential diagnosis of Alzheimer's disease may be made. Physical findings below relate to the second and third stages.

Neurologic

• memory loss (initially short term, progressing to long term by late Stage II or early Stage III)
• ataxia
• apraxia
• visual agnosia
• dysphasia
• dysphagia
• echolalia
• myoclonus and potential for grand mal seizures
• sleep disorder
• anxiety
• reactive depression
• hallucinations or delusions
• paranoia
• aggressive outbursts

Gastrointestinal

• anorexia or voracious appetite
• bowel incontinence or constipation
• malnutrition (from dysphagia or from inability to express hunger or identify food as something to eat)

• consistent weight loss (in third stage, regardless of caloric intake)

Musculoskeletal

• stooped posture and shuffling gait
• joint stiffness and potential for contracture
• potential for injury from falling

Reproductive

• decreased or increased libido
• inappropriate sexual behavior (exhibitionism, masturbation in public, grabbing or fondling others; usually in response to increased stress and anxiety and reduced social inhibitions)

Renal and urinary

• urinary incontinence
• urine retention
• urinary stasis

DIAGNOSTIC STUDIES

The following studies may be performed to evaluate the patient's health status:
• EEG—waves are slower and flatter in dementia, but this is never an independent diagnostic criterion for Alzheimer's disease
• computed tomography (CT) scan—to detect masses, hematomas, hydrocephalus, and cortical degeneration characterized by enlarged cortical sulci and enlarged ventricles; a normal brain may also exhibit cortical degeneration on a CT scan, so signs of cortical degeneration alone do not signify a degenerative dementing illness. Computed tomography is used as an additional diagnostic tool in the absence of any other positive results.

Nursing diagnosis: *Potential for injury related to perceptual-cognitive impairment*

GOAL: To maintain an optimal level of safety

Interventions

1. Work with the caregiver and other family members to promote the patient's safety in the home. Remove potential hazards, such as throw rugs or protruding electrical wires. Keep areas well lit, especially at night. Close doors to rooms not in use, and block stairways and exits, if necessary. Shut off the stove if the patient cannot use it safely. Remove appliances and tools that could cause injury. Keep all chemicals and medicines out of reach. Encourage the family to install grab bars in the bathroom and side rails on the patient's bed. Explain why the patient should refrain from driving.

2. Assess the patient's understanding and judgment of potentially dangerous situations or tasks. Try to eliminate these situations and tasks, if possible.

3. Remove potentially harmful substances, such as medications, plants, pet foods, plastic fruit and vegetable decorations, soaps and candles with fruit or vegetable scents, and objects that look like candy.

Rationales

1. As judgment becomes impaired, the patient may not realize that skills have deteriorated and may be unwilling to give up potentially dangerous activities without assistance and substitution of another activity over which he has some control. Perceptual-motor disturbances may make usual decor, architecture, or furnishings a major source of anxiety for or danger to the patient.

2. The patient may not always be able to tell if a situation or task is becoming too difficult to manage or cope with independently.

3. The patient may mistake these items for food.

Nursing diagnosis: *Altered nutrition: less than body requirements, related to memory loss or malfunctioning hypothalamus*

GOAL: To help the patient achieve and maintain adequate body weight

Interventions	Rationales
1. Assess the patient's previous weight and dietary habits, especially during stress or depression.	1. Decreased food consumption may be characteristic of the patient when depressed or under stress.
2. Assess the patient's functional use of utensils and identification of food as "something to eat."	2. The patient may be hungry but may not understand the concepts of food and hunger or may not remember how to use utensils or know their purpose.
3. Recommend small, frequent, high-calorie meals and snacks and nutritional food and drink supplements (Ensure, Carnation Instant Breakfast Food, milk puddings, ice cream).	3. The patient may find small, frequent meals more appealing than regular portions. A well-balanced, high-calorie diet helps achieve adequate body weight.
4. Encourage nutritious finger foods when possible to permit the patient to feed himself.	4. The patient may be confused by utensils and may resist being fed as long as he can still put his hand to his mouth.
5. Urge the food preparer to try foods of different textures and tastes to stimulate the patient's taste buds.	5. Researchers of Alzheimer's disease have reported changes in taste buds related to cortical degeneration, which may account for the patient's reluctance to eat.
6. Advise the family to avoid elaborate place settings and to have the patient use plate guards.	6. The patient may become confused by a wide selection of utensils, plates, and glasses or by having more than one plate of food before him at one time. Perceptual and spatial problems or apraxia may cause the patient to eat from only one side of the plate or never hit the right spot to lift food from the plate; plate guards can significantly help the patient in coping with this difficulty.

Nursing diagnosis: *Potential fluid volume deficit related to memory loss*

GOAL: To maintain adequate hydration

Interventions	Rationales
1. Establish baseline norms for fluid intake and output and fluid balance.	1. If the patient's past patterns do not explain the current fluid volume deficit, then memory loss is probably the contributing factor.
2. Encourage the patient to drink 8 to 13 8-oz glasses (2 to 3 liters) of fluid daily, and teach him or the caregiver to record intake and output.	2. Inadequate hydration or fluid imbalance can exacerbate dementia symptoms. Drinking plenty of fluids and keeping accurate intake and output records help maintain adequate hydration and promote patient compliance.
3. Assess the patient's skin; mucosa; color, odor, and specific gravity of urine; and body temperature.	3. This assessment establishes a baseline to monitor for changes in dementia symptoms or underlying medical diagnoses.

Nursing diagnosis: *Altered bowel elimination: incontinence, related to cortical degeneration*

GOAL: To achieve and maintain adequate and regular bowel elimination

Interventions	Rationales
1. Assess the patient's present level of bowel functioning. Eliminate the possibility of impaction or stress incontinence, and rule out other disease problems. Observe for such behavior as clutching or picking at the buttocks and anxiety over bowel function.	1. Bowel incontinence, which usually does not occur until the middle of Stage II or later, may not be disease-related. The patient's general health status must be considered.
2. Determine whether the patient can use the toilet independently. Attach a poster to the bathroom door and provide a night-light to assist with orientation.	2. Incontinence may result if the patient forgets to use the toilet and depends on others for help.
3. Monitor and document the patient's bowel movements, noting form, odor, color, and frequency.	3. This helps establish the patient's normal pattern so that changes can be readily identified.
4. Assess the patient's diet to ensure adequate nutrition and hydration. Make sure the diet contains sufficient fiber, such as beans, fruits, and vegetables.	4. Adequate nutrition and hydration contribute to healthy bowel functioning, and increased bulk may stimulate sphincter control.
5. Remind the caregiver to keep the patient clean and dry at all times; recommend adult absorbent briefs if appropriate.	5. These measures reduce the potential for skin complications and infection, minimize odors, and help preserve the patient's dignity.

Nursing diagnosis: *Altered urinary elimination pattern related to cortical degeneration*

GOAL: To achieve and maintain adequate and regular urinary elimination

Interventions	Rationales
1. Assess the patient's present level of urinary elimination. Consider urinary tract infection, stress incontinence, and prostatitis. Rule out underlying causes.	1. Incontinence can occur at any stage of Alzheimer's disease but may not be disease-related. The patient's general health status must be considered.
2. Determine whether the patient can use the toilet independently. Attach a poster to the bathroom door and provide a night-light to assist with orientation.	2. Incontinence may result if the patient forgets to use the toilet and depends on others for help.
3. Monitor and document the patient's urine output, noting color, odor, clarity, and specific gravity. Record his temperature daily.	3. This helps establish the patient's normal pattern so that changes can be readily identified.
4. Remind the caregiver to keep the patient clean and dry at all times; recommend adult absorbent briefs if appropriate.	4. These measures reduce the potential for skin complications and infection, minimize odors, and help preserve the patient's dignity.

Nursing diagnosis: *Activity intolerance related to perceptual-cognitive impairment*

GOAL: To help the patient maintain an optimal level of activity tolerance

Interventions	Rationales
1. Assess the patient's current activity level. Encourage him to express his fears and concerns about participating, and try to dispel them with gentle reassurance. Be	1. From the middle of Stage I until late Stage II, the patient's reluctance to participate in activities usually is the result of depression, fear, or apathy related to de-

alert to behavioral cues that can help you direct him toward meaningful activities he might choose for himself.

mentia. As the patient feels less in control in social situations, he may withdraw from regular activities he has enjoyed with others, which will accentuate perceived losses and exacerbate depressive symptoms. As the disease progresses, the patient becomes less able—physically and especially mentally—to pursue activities independently.

2. Determine which activities the patient has enjoyed in the past, and try to include these in a limited, graduated regimen based on his present mental attitude and willingness to participate. Be alert to sudden or subtle mood changes that could precipitate a catastrophic reaction if the patient becomes taxed or frustrated. Use open-ended activities that do not require completion as a measure of success.

2. Keeping the patient regularly involved and active, even at a minimal level, enhances his self-esteem and may help minimize anxiety, depression, and physical complications. Open-ended activities allow the patient to drop out when he wishes and enable the astute caregiver to suggest a rest period or a different activity.

3. Focus activity around a social situation when possible.

3. Interacting with others can enhance the patient's self-esteem and helps prevent social isolation.

Nursing diagnosis: *Self-care deficit: bathing and hygiene, related to perceptual-cognitive impairment*

GOAL: To meet the patient's bathing and hygiene needs

Interventions

1. Assess the patient's previous bathing routines and preferences, and try to maintain these as much as possible.

Rationales

1. As the disease progresses, the patient may develop a strong resistance to water, removal of clothing, or any attempts at bathing, or he may refuse to shower but may agree to a bath or sponge bath. This behavior can begin in late Stage I and continue until the patient is too unsteady to enter the tub or shower.

2. Establish the degree of assistance required. Divide bathing tasks into manageable subtasks so the patient can assist if he is able and willing. Develop an assessment tool to help the caregiver determine what the patient can still accomplish himself.

2. Involving the patient in his own care enhances his self-esteem and gives him some measure of control over his situation.

3. Help the caregiver determine appropriate and reasonable guidelines for bathing and hygiene.

3. The caregiver may have to reexamine what constitutes proper bathing and hygiene and what he can realistically expect of himself and the patient. For example, although the patient may have showered twice daily before his illness, the caregiver can no longer reasonably expect this to continue.

Nursing diagnosis: *Self-care deficit: dressing and grooming, related to perceptual-cognitive impairment*

GOAL: To ensure appropriate and adequate dressing and grooming

Interventions

1. Assess the patient's current dressing and grooming skills. Have him assist with as many tasks as possible, and urge the caregiver to resist the temptation to complete these tasks if the patient can manage himself.

Rationales

1. The patient may be able to accomplish many dressing and grooming tasks independently or with minimal help but may have learned to let the well-intentioned caregiver do them instead.

2. Establish the degree of assistance required. Divide tasks into manageable subtasks so the patient can assist if he is willing and able. Consider adaptive clothing

2. Involving the patient in his own care enhances his self-esteem and gives him some measure of control over his situation.

(slipover clothes, front fasteners, velcro fasteners, loafer-style shoes) that the patient can manage successfully.

3. Work with the caregiver to determine what he and the patient can accomplish without severely altering the style in which the patient always liked to dress.

3. Looking and feeling well groomed enhances the patient's self-esteem. Accomplishing this requires creativity, imagination, and patience, but many family and professional caregivers succeed.

Nursing diagnosis: *Impaired home maintenance management related to wandering, safety hazards, and lack of environmental consistency*

GOAL: To ensure adequate cleanliness, heating, ventilation, and food supplies in the home

Interventions

1. Determine which household tasks the patient performed before his illness and whether he can still manage them. Work with family members to reallocate these tasks, if necessary.

2. Refer the family to appropriate community resources for assistance with shopping, cleaning, cooking, and other household tasks.

Rationales

1. The patient may no longer be physically or mentally able to perform household tasks. Family members may need support during the transition, but task reallocation can help maintain family integrity and improve their coping skills. (*Note:* If the patient lives alone and cannot manage household tasks safely, a guardian must be designated who can help determine whether the patient can remain with supervision and assistance. Alternate living arrangements may be needed.)

2. Extra support can prevent the family from becoming overtaxed and allows the patient to remain in his home for as long as possible.

Nursing diagnosis: *Sleep pattern disturbance related to alteration in circadian rhythms, possible alteration in neurotransmitters (especially serotonin), malfunctioning reticular activating system, or day-night reversal*

GOAL: To ensure adequate sleep and rest

Interventions

1. Assess the patient's past sleep patterns and present sleeping difficulties.

2. Determine the patient's usual sleeping preferences and habits, such as whether he sleeps alone or with a partner, wears nightclothes or sleeps nude, and uses a hard or soft mattress. Encourage him to resume former preferences and habits he may have forsaken because of the disease.

3. Assess the patient's past and present activity levels. Encourage moderate exercise, and teach the caregiver to monitor and document daily activities, napping, and episodes of insomnia or hypersomnia.

Rationales

1. This assessment helps determine whether the sleep disturbance is a characteristic response to increased stress and anxiety. If so, the patient may have already discovered successful remedies that he can use again.

2. Maintaining usual preferences and habits helps keep parts of the sleep cycle familiar to the patient. A well-intentioned caregiver or family member may have persuaded the patient to alter his routines.

3. Inactivity during the day may induce boredom and napping, which can leave the patient insufficiently tired to fall asleep at night. Persistent insomnia or hypersomnia may exacerbate dementia symptoms, social withdrawal, and isolation. Moderate exercise helps maintain a normal sleep-wake pattern. Careful documentation may identify a sleeping problem that the patient cannot sense or articulate.

4. Work with the family to create a relaxing environment for the patient. Advise them to avoid activities that might overstimulate him, and restrict his intake of food or beverages that contain stimulants, especially before bedtime.

4. A relaxing environment can help reduce the patient's anxiety and stress. Stimulants should be avoided, particularly at night, because the patient may need more time to unwind sufficiently to fall asleep.

5. Encourage the family to remain flexible in allowing the patient to pursue a sleep pattern that is comfortable for him. Explain that the patient may not require 8 hours of uninterrupted nighttime sleep to meet his needs.

5. The patient may develop a sleep pattern that seems abnormal to family members but that becomes normal to one with dementia. For example, he may begin to prefer several sleeping places other than the bed (such as the floor, a couch, or a rocking chair); he also may want to get up in the middle of the night to read, watch television, listen to music, or have a snack. The family may need your support in adjusting to these changes.

Nursing diagnosis: *Altered thought processes related to perceptual-cognitive impairment*

GOAL: To provide opportunities for the patient to interact successfully with others and the environment

Interventions

1. Teach the caregiver and other family members to accept the patient's current cognitive abilities rather than try to restore previous abilities.

2. Work with the caregiver and other family members to reduce external stimuli and distractions for the patient. Involve him in simple tasks, and speak in short, concrete sentences. Avoid topics that require him to think abstractly; instead, focus on what he can recognize or remember.

Rationales

1. The patient's past cognitive skills cannot be restored, and even his current thought processes can alter from one moment to the next. Correcting a mistake or reminding him of the impairment is not helpful. Diverting his attention to a new topic proves more beneficial.

2. These measures keep the patient actively involved in tasks and conversations he can manage successfully, which enhances his self-esteem.

Nursing diagnosis: *Fear related to perceptual-cognitive impairment and anticipatory anxiety*

GOAL: To alleviate the patient's fear by providing him with information and reassurance

Interventions

1. Establish a therapeutic relationship with the patient and caregiver. Assess their attitude toward illness and their knowledge of Alzheimer's disease. Encourage them to ask questions and to express fears or concerns, and try to address these issues with accurate information and gentle reassurance.

2. If the patient cannot identify the cause of his fear, provide unconditional support, trust, and reassurance.

Rationales

1. Misinformation and unresolved fears can severely impair the patient's—and caregiver's—ability to cope with the disease.

2. Unidentified fears may intensify during Stage II. The patient's primary need is to feel safe and unthreatened.

Nursing diagnosis: *Anxiety related to perceptual-cognitive impairment*

GOAL: To alleviate the patient's anxiety

Interventions

1. Assess the patient's current anxiety level (mild, moderate, or severe) and previous coping mechanisms. Suggest other anxiety-reducing measures, such as warm baths, singing, and art or pet therapy.

2. Identify potential anxiety-inducing situations, and work with the caregiver to reduce or eliminate the patient's exposure to them.

3. Consult the doctor about using medication to alleviate the patient's anxiety.

4. Refer the patient and family for psychological counseling if appropriate.

Rationales

1. Some noncognitive methods of dealing with anxiety may still be effective and appropriate for the patient.

2. The patient who experiences anxiety may not always be able to articulate it, identify its cause, or take appropriate action to cope with it effectively.

3. Medical intervention may be necessary if nursing interventions fail to help the anxious patient.

4. Counseling gives the patient and family an opportunity to discuss fears, express grief, come to terms with changing relationships, and plan realistically for the future.

Nursing diagnosis: *Anticipatory grieving related to loss of memory and identity*

GOAL: To help the patient cope successfully with the grieving process

Interventions

1. Establish a therapeutic relationship with the patient. Provide him with accurate information about the diagnosis and course of the disease, using nontechnical language he can understand. Encourage him to ask questions and to express his feelings about anticipated losses.

2. Encourage the patient to meet personal goals and desires while he is able to do so.

Rationales

1. Accurate information helps the patient understand what is happening to him now and enables him to make realistic plans for the future. Sharing his feelings about anticipated losses is a natural part of the grieving process; support and understanding from the nurse during these discussions can help the patient cope with his feelings more effectively.

2. Pursuing unattained goals and desires can give the patient a sense of involvement and control and bring added meaning to his life.

Nursing diagnosis: *Social isolation related to perceptual-cognitive impairment*

GOAL: To promote social interaction as tolerated by the patient

Interventions

1. Assess the patient's reasons for social withdrawal. Try to alleviate his fears and encourage him to socialize, if tolerable, but respect his right to withdraw.

2. Help the patient and family to redefine the patient's socialization needs.

Rationales

1. Social withdrawal may be the patient's response to a real or perceived inability to fit in or to enjoy social situations because of personality changes and increasing memory loss. Increased anxiety and paranoia may accompany social situations and may precipitate social withdrawal.

2. In some situations, social withdrawal may be an appropriate response, allowing the patient to assert control over his environment based on his perceived needs.

3. Identify members of the patient's support network. Explain the nature of the disease, and inform them of possible changes in the patient's behavior and in his socialization needs. Be available to answer questions and provide support.

4. Urge the patient to meet with a spiritual advisor, if appropriate.

3. Friends and neighbors usually want to help but may avoid the patient, primarily because of inadequate knowledge of the disease and uncertainty over how they and the patient will react toward one another.

4. The patient's spiritual advisor can offer much-needed emotional support; the patient may take great comfort from his faith and may want to participate in religious services long after he has lost the ability to hold a conversation or walk unassisted.

Nursing diagnosis: *Impaired verbal communication related to progressive memory loss and impaired cognitive function*

GOAL: To help the patient maintain an optimal level of communication

Interventions

1. Encourage all attempts at verbal communication. Note that the patient may develop new words or symbols—or use a foreign language—to express himself.

2. Educate the caregiver and other family members in basic communication skills, paying particular attention to nonverbal skills. Encourage them to involve him in music and singing, if possible.

Rationales

1. Encouraging verbal communication promotes continued interaction and can enhance self-esteem. As the disease progresses, the patient may invent new words or symbols to convey his thoughts to the nurse or caregiver. A bilingual patient usually reverts to the language he learned first, even if he is fluent in the secondary language and has not used the primary language for many years.

2. As the patient's ability to process verbal information deteriorates, he becomes more sensitive to nonverbal forms of communication. Music and singing also can foster communication and reduce social isolation. Because music is a right hemisphere function and language a left hemisphere function, words set to music are learned and remembered differently from language.

ASSOCIATED CARE PLANS
• Grief and Grieving
• Hospice
• Ineffective Coping
• Malnutrition
• Sex and Sexuality
(See also care plans for related medical disorders)

NETWORKING OF SERVICES
• counseling services
• day care
• respite care
• Meals On Wheels
• support groups
• religious groups
• equipment suppliers (for plate guards, adaptive utensils and cups, grab bars, adaptive clothing, ID bracelet, commode, bed side rails and pads, washable recliner chair, adult absorbent briefs, eggcrate mattress, foam mattress, air bed, water bed, sheepskins and pads, wheelchair)

CARE TEAM INVOLVED
• nurse
• doctor
• patient and family
• social worker
• home health aide
• day care manager
• respite care manager
• support group facilitator
• psychotherapist or counselor
• speech therapist
• physiotherapist
• occupational therapist
• recreational therapist
• religious advisor

IMPLICATIONS FOR HOME CARE
• functional features of the home (change physical environment to minimize patient confusion and hostility)
• pictures on doors and cabinets to identify contents (pictures of objects are remembered longer than words)
• poisonous chemicals and medicines out of reach
• stove switched off if patient cannot use it safely
• main exits from dwelling camouflaged or locked if wandering is a problem
• throw rugs and other obstacles removed
• quiet, nonthreatening environment

PATIENT EDUCATION TOOLS
• literature from support and educational groups
• videotapes and books (available through local Alzheimer's Disease and Related Disorders Association (ADRDA) chapters and support groups, area offices on aging, and divisions of mental health)
• literature from ADRDA, 70 Lake St., Suite 600, Chicago, Ill., 60601. Telephone: 1-800-621-0379

DISCHARGE PLAN FROM HOME HEALTH CARE
During the course of the relationship with the home health care staff, the caregiver should:
• contact the staff if he has questions or concerns
• understand the nature, symptoms, stages, and progression of Alzheimer's disease
• know how to communicate effectively with the patient to reorient him to reality
• learn and practice new skills to cope with stage-related problems or situations as they arise
• know how to recognize his own stress and ways to prevent or reduce it
• learn how and when to ask for help from family, friends, neighbors, and others in the patient's support network
• have telephone numbers of applicable community resources.

SELECTED REFERENCES
Ackerlund, B., and Norber, A. "Group Psychotherapy with Demented Patients," *Geriatric Nursing*, 83-84, March/April 1986.

Cohen, D., and Eisdorfer, C. *Loss of Self.* New York: W.W. Norton & Co., 1986.

Congress of the United States of America, Office of Technology Assessment. *Losing a Million Minds: Confronting the Tragedy of Alzheimer's Disease and Other Dementias.* Washington, D.C.: U.S. Government Printing Office, 1987.

Fox, P.J., and Phil, C. "Alzheimer's Disease: An Historical Overview," *The American Journal of Alzheimer's Care and Related Disorders* 1(4), Fall 1986.

Linderborn, K.M. "The Need to Assess Dementia," *Journal of Gerontological Nursing* 14(1), 1988.

Robinson, B.E. "Dementia: A Three-Pronged Strategy for Primary Care," *Geriatrics* 41(2): 75-86, 1986.

Rogers, C.R. *On Becoming a Person.* Boston: Houghton Miflin Co., 1961.

Shibbal-Champagne, S., and Lipinska-Stachow, D.M. "Alzheimer's Educational/Support Group: Considerations for Success," *Journal of Gerontological Social Work* 9(2), 1986.

Stachow, D.M. *Alzheimer's Disease: A Self-Assessment Learning Module for Nurses.* Manchester, N.H.: St. Anselm College, Department of Continuing Education for Nurses, 1986.

Stachow, D.M., and Sheridan, E.S. "Alzheimer's Disease: A Comprehensive Train-The-Trainers Pilot Project," *Caring*, May 1988.

Williams, L. "The Need for Caring," *Journal of Gerontological Nursing* 12(2), 1986.

NEUROLOGIC SYSTEM

Cerebrovascular Accident

DESCRIPTION AND TIME FOCUS

A cerebrovascular accident (CVA) is the interruption of blood flow to an area of brain tissue, causing ischemia and possibly necrosis in the affected tissue. CVA can be caused by hemorrhage, a thrombus, or an embolus. Signs and symptoms depend on the severity of ischemia and on the brain area affected.

This clinical plan focuses on the patient discharged home from an acute-care hospital or rehabilitation facility after diagnosis and treatment of a CVA. Home care of the CVA patient focuses on rehabilitation to the highest possible level of function and successful adaptation to permanent sensory, perceptual, and motor deficits. The familiarity of the home setting and participation of family members in patient care afford the patient the best possible circumstances for recovery and resumption of his pre-illness life-style.

■ Typical home health care length of service for a patient with CVA: 8 weeks

■ Typical visit frequency: twice weekly for 4 weeks, then once weekly for 4 weeks or until discharge criteria are met

HEALTH HISTORY FINDINGS

In a health history interview, the patient may report many of these findings:
• history of cardiac disease
• history of hypertension
• history of transient ischemic attacks
• tobacco use
• history of diabetes
• oral contraceptive use
• history of sickle cell anemia
• family history of cerebrovascular disease

PHYSICAL FINDINGS

In a physical examination, the nurse may detect many of these findings:

Neurologic
• motor loss

• sensory loss
• visual field deficit
• cognitive loss
• aphasia

Cardiovascular
• hypertension
• dysrhythmias
• heart murmurs indicative of valve dysfunction

Respiratory
• altered respiratory pattern
• diminished breath sounds
• rhonchi in the upper lobes

Gastrointestinal
• dysphagia
• fecal incontinence
• fecal impaction

Musculoskeletal
• hemiparesis
• hemiplegia
• facial muscle droop

Renal and urinary
• urinary incontinence
• urine retention

DIAGNOSTIC STUDIES

The following studies may be performed to evaluate the patient's health status:
• prothrombin time (PT), for patients on anticoagulants—weekly or as ordered, to guide anticoagulant therapy
• computed tomography (CT) scan or magnetic resonance imaging (MRI)—when CVA extension or new CVA is suspected, to detect it and determine its extent

---

Nursing diagnosis: *Altered tissue perfusion: cerebral, related to pathologic alteration in blood flow*

GOAL 1: To maintain adequate, consistent cerebral blood flow

Interventions

1. Monitor the patient's blood pressure in the lying, sitting, and standing positions during each visit, and record the results. Determine normal readings from the hospital chart and doctor's orders; report variations.

Rationales

1. Hypertension and hypotension have profound effects on cerebral perfusion. Wide fluctuations in blood pressure increase the risk of CVA extension.

2. Assess the patient's hydration status and compliance with the medication regimen during each visit. Document findings, using a consistent format.

2. Adequate body fluid volume and consistent drug blood levels help maintain stable cerebral perfusion.

GOAL 2: To ensure early recognition of inadequate cerebral blood flow

Intervention

Assess the patient's neurologic status during each visit, using the same methodology and sequence. Document results precisely.

Rationale

Consistent, precise neurologic assessments are the best nursing indicator of subtle changes in cerebral tissue perfusion.

Nursing diagnosis: *Potential for injury related to loss of neuromuscular control*

GOAL: To ensure a safe home environment for the patient recovering from a CVA

Interventions

1. Evaluate the home setting for safety hazards. Note the placement of phones, width of pathways, height of working areas, and type of furniture.

Rationales

1. After a CVA, the patient frequently moves slowly and awkwardly. Phones must be within easy reach. Lifeline may be necessary if the patient is aphasic. Pathways must be wide enough to accommodate a walker or wheelchair, furniture must accommodate easy transfers, and living areas must be accessible and safe.

2. Evaluate the bathroom, and help the patient and family order equipment such as handrails, elevated toilet seats, and grab bars.

2. The bathroom must be safe and accessible. Accidents in the bathroom can be serious because fixtures and surfaces are hard. A safe, accessible bathroom bolsters the patient's self-esteem by permitting independence when bathing and using the toilet.

Nursing diagnosis: *Impaired physical mobility related to loss of motor function*

GOAL: To prevent deformities and muscle deterioration

Interventions

1. Teach the caregiver positioning methods that prevent contractures, and instruct on how to use such aids as pillows, foam blocks, and braces.

Rationales

1. Contractures develop quickly when paralysis or paresis exists. Caregivers must understand the need for constant attention to this problem and must be proficient in positioning techniques.

2. Teach the caregiver simple range-of-motion (ROM) exercises. Be aware of exercises prescribed by the physical therapist, and monitor the patient's compliance with the home exercise program. Assess ROM during each visit. Report changes in the patient's clinical status to the therapist so adjustments can be made in the patient's home exercise program.

2. The CVA patient with paresis or paralysis will usually require a visiting physical therapist. Although the therapist is primarily responsible for muscle rehabilitation and transfer and ambulation training, the nurse remains responsible for monitoring and helping with the patient's home exercise program.

Nursing diagnosis: *Self-care deficit: bathing and hygiene, dressing and grooming, feeding, or toileting, related to sensory-perceptual and motor deficits*

GOAL: To meet the patient's basic care needs

Interventions

1. Arrange for home health aide service, with visits de-

Rationales

1. Initially, the numerous visits by nurses and therapists

creasing as the patient assumes responsibility for basic care.

and the multiple instruction programs may overwhelm the patient and caregiver. A home health aide can relieve the patient and caregiver during this initial period, allowing them to concentrate on the therapeutic programs.

2. As the patient's independence increases, monitor his ability to perform activities of daily living (ADLs) and help with the program initiated by the occupational therapist. Report changes in the patient's clinical status to the therapist so appropriate adjustments can be made.

2. The occupational therapist is responsible for training the patient to perform ADLs using assistive devices and techniques. The nurse must understand the training program to assist and support the patient's progress.

Nursing diagnosis: *Impaired skin integrity: potential, related to sensory loss and immobility*

GOAL 1: To maintain skin integrity

Interventions

1. Assess skin status during each visit. Pay particular attention to pressure areas and areas of sensory loss. Accurately record all observations, using standard terminology.

Rationales

1. Visual inspection of the skin is a necessity. The patient's limited mobility subjects areas of skin to constant pressure and the risk of tissue breakdown. Sensory impairment can hide the normal discomfort associated with tissue breakdown, or impaired speech may make it impossible to communicate the discomfort to the caregiver.

2. Teach the caregiver how to inspect the skin, with particular attention to skin folds and areas of pressure.

2. The caregiver is in the best position to evaluate day-to-day changes and must be prepared to assume this responsibility when professional services end.

GOAL 2: To help the caregiver recognize and treat skin breakdown

Intervention

Teach the caregiver how to recognize and stage pressure areas. Provide instruction in the use of massage, positioning, nonconstrictive clothing, water cushions, air mattresses, and other pressure-relieving devices. Teach the caregiver the treatment of Stage I pressure areas and the need for medical intervention for more advanced stages.

Rationale

The problem of potential skin breakdown may be permanent, and the caregiver must be able to manage it. The caregiver should know the treatment for simple reddened areas, products that help, and when to seek medical advice.

Nursing diagnosis: *Sensory-perceptual alterations related to damage to specific areas of brain tissue*

GOAL: To accurately identify and assess sensory-perceptual alterations and provide instruction in adaptive measures

Interventions

1. Observe the patient's behavior. Note any tendency of the patient to ignore objects placed to one side or the other. This may indicate a visual field defect or one-sided neglect.

Rationales

1. Visual field defects on the affected side are common. The patient with right hemiplegia often ignores objects on his right side. The opposite is also true. The patient with one-sided neglect is unaware of the affected side of his body.

2. Institute adaptive measures to compensate for visual field defect, and provide instructions for the caregiver. Approach the patient from the unaffected side; encour-

2. Sensory-perceptual alterations may be permanent. Adaptation is possible with the constant and consistent effort of the caregiver and home health staff. All per-

age him to move his head from side to side to receive a full view. Continue to remind the patient of the problem, and encourage the use of the unaffected side.

3. Assess swallowing reflex as the patient swallows a small amount of water. Assess the lungs for evidence of aspiration. Ask the caregiver about the patient's eating habits and ability to swallow thin liquids. If the patient has dysphagia, teach the caregiver a dysphagia diet, proper positioning for eating, and the signs and symptoms of aspiration.

4. Assess the patient's language and communication skills. Ask simple questions and note the appropriateness of the answers. Provide a calm, unhurried environment to reduce the patient's anxiety and frustration.

sons involved must understand the problem and the adaptive techniques to be used.

3. Dysphagia can be a permanent problem. Usually, thin liquids present the greatest problem for the patient with dysphagia. The caregiver must be able to recognize the complications associated with the problem and act appropriately.

4. Aphasia is common after CVA, and the patient's care should include speech therapy. Consult with the speech therapist to determine the best method of communication. Aphasia requires that the caregiver, nurse, patient, and therapist work closely to ensure consistency during the rehabilitation of the patient's communication skills.

Nursing diagnosis: *Altered bowel elimination: incontinence, related to loss of neuromuscular control*

GOAL: To maintain a normal pattern of bowel elimination and impart knowledge of incontinence management to the patient or caregiver

Interventions

1. Teach the patient about the bowel program; establish a time for evacuation, explain physiologic positioning, and discuss dietary factors, such as eating more fruits, vegetables, and fiber and avoiding foods that cause constipation or diarrhea.

2. Explain the physiologic basis of incontinence to the patient and caregiver. Tell the patient to wear protective clothing and to wash the rectal area after each stool to prevent skin breakdown. Avoid referring to "diapers"—instead, call them "adult incontinence pads."

Rationales

1. Establishing a bowel routine can regulate the time of bowel movements and reduce the patient's concern about incontinence. Using dietary aids and fluid intake to soften stool consistency can prevent episodes of diarrhea as well as fecal impactions.

2. Stool incontinence is embarrassing for the patient. His uneasiness will subside when he understands that incontinence is a physiologic problem that can be managed.

ASSOCIATED CARE PLANS
• Grief and Grieving
• Hypertension
• Ineffective Coping
• Neurogenic Bladder

NETWORKING OF SERVICES
• Lifeline
• Meals On Wheels
• durable medical equipment (DME) supplier
• ongoing rehabilitation program
• support group for caregivers

CARE TEAM INVOLVED
• nurse
• doctor
• patient and family
• physical therapist
• occupational therapist

• speech therapist
• medical social worker
• home health aide

IMPLICATIONS FOR HOME CARE
• functional features of the home (stairs, location of bathroom and kitchen)
• safe environment (free of clutter and hazards)
• telephone (communication)
• availability of competent caregiver

PATIENT EDUCATION TOOLS
• literature for each prescribed medication
• American Heart Association literature
• diet information, if applicable

DISCHARGE PLAN FROM HOME HEALTH CARE

Before discharge from home health care, the patient should:
• be neurologically stable
• have underlying disease (for example, hypertension, dysrhythmias) controlled by medication
• be free of complications
• be actively participating in the home programs established by skilled therapists
• be participating in ADLs.

Before discharge, the patient or caregiver should:
• be able to explain applicable dietary restrictions
• know dates of scheduled medical appointments
• have a list of telephone numbers for emergency services, doctor, and home health agency
• have information about support groups and outpatient rehabilitation programs
• have an established system of communication
• know requirements of ongoing care
• know how to use necessary medical equipment
• know availability of transportation services
• know the signs and symptoms of complications and what actions to take.

SELECTED REFERENCES

Birmingham, J. *Home Care Planning Based on DRGs.* Philadelphia: J.B. Lippincott Co., 1986.
Eliopoulos, C. *A Guide to the Nursing of the Aged.* Baltimore: Williams & Wilkins Co., 1987.
Iyer, P., et al. *Nursing Process and Nursing Diagnosis.* Philadelphia: W.B. Saunders Co., 1986.
Scherman, S. *Community Health Nursing Care Plans.* New York: John Wiley & Sons, 1985.
Walsh, J., et al. *Manual of Home Health Care Nursing.* Philadelphia: J.B. Lippincott Co., 1987.

Multiple Sclerosis

DESCRIPTION AND TIME FOCUS

Multiple sclerosis (MS) is a chronic degenerative disease of the central nervous system (CNS) involving disseminated demyelination of CNS white matter. The two major forms of MS are benign, which follows a course of exacerbations and remissions, and malignant, which leads progressively to total incapacitation. About one-quarter of all MS cases involve rapid disease progression; one-quarter involve broadly fluctuating symptoms and modest disability; one-quarter involve transient symptoms and mild disability; and one-quarter involve a subtle form of the disease that causes minimal disability.

Onset typically occurs between ages 20 and 40 and affects women almost twice as often as men. MS alone is not fatal, although respiratory and urinary tract complications resulting from musculoneural dysfunction often cause premature death.

An acute history is the most significant factor in confirming a diagnosis of MS. The history should include:
• one or more episodes suggestive of neurologic impairment and lasting 24 hours or longer
• a remission period of at least 1 month between these episodes
• symptoms unexplained by any other diagnosis.

The MS patient typically waits 2 to 5 years for a confirming diagnosis after a history of intermittent, widely divergent symptoms. Diagnosis of an organic disease may come as a relief to the patient worried about possible mental dysfunction, but it can also cause discouragement by necessitating changes in lifestyle to accommodate a nebulous, chronic, and potentially disabling disease. The emotional and social implications of the diagnosis may hold greater significance to the individual and family confronted with a diagnosis of MS. Thus the patient with MS is a multifaceted challenge to the home health care nurse.

This clinical plan focuses on the patient with a diagnosis of MS in the home setting.

■ Typical home health care length of service for a patient with MS: varies according to the signs and symptoms and the availability of family and community support

■ Typical visit frequency: twice weekly for 4 to 6 weeks to help the patient and family during the initial adjustment period and provide necessary teaching

HEALTH HISTORY FINDINGS

In a health history interview, the patient may report many of these findings:
• excessive fatigue
• transient unilateral blindness or diplopia
• tingling or numbness in limbs, usually bilateral
• loss of balance
• impaired coordination of gait
• clumsiness
• urinary retention, urgency, frequency, or incontinence
• sexual dysfunction
• muscle spasm
• dysarthria
• choking sensation
• shallow breathing
• mood lability

PHYSICAL FINDINGS

In a physical examination, the nurse may detect some or all of these findings:

Neurologic
• Charcot's triad (nystagmus, intention tremors, and slow, monotonous, slurred speech)
• ataxia
• paralysis
• hyperreflexia
• Lhermitte's sign (sensations of sudden, transient, electriclike shocks spreading down the neck and into the extremities precipitated by forward flexion of the neck)
• subtle or overt loss of discriminatory sense in the fingers
• impaired vibration sense and proprioception

Musculoskeletal
• spasticity
• reduced mobility
• contractures (related to immobility)
• pseudoathetosis
• localized peripheral muscle weakness

DIAGNOSTIC STUDIES

The following studies may be performed to evaluate the patient's health status:
• visual evoked potential—at time of diagnosis, to detect delayed response
• computed tomography (CT)—at time of diagnosis, to detect plaques, atrophy, or ventricular enlargement
• cerebrospinal fluid (CSF) electrophoresis—at time of diagnosis, to detect elevated IgG

Nursing diagnosis: *Activity intolerance related to ineffective neuromuscular control*

GOAL 1: To conserve energy for necessary and meaningful tasks

Interventions

1. Have the patient rank his activities by priority. Try to include as many high-priority activities as possible when planning energy conservation measures.

2. Have the patient keep a diary of high and low energy periods, sleep patterns, and daily activities. The patient should also try to identify and record external and internal stressors, such as temperature and humidity changes, emotions, medications, and intervening illnesses (such as cystitis).

3. Work with the patient to develop a trial schedule of activities.

4. Encourage the patient to discuss physical limitations with family members, co-workers, and others who have reason to expect certain standards of performance.

Rationales

1. Compliance with energy conservation measures is more likely when the patient helps establish the goals.

2. Identifying periods of high energy helps the patient maximize energy use. Most MS patients experience extreme weakness when in hot and humid environments. By increasing the patient's internal temperature, fever can cause the same reaction. Increased axon sensitivity may heighten the patient's response to hormones released during emotional expression or in response to medication.

3. Although the nurse can identify mechanisms to maximize the patient's abilities and minimize deficits, these mechanisms can't help until the patient uses them.

4. The patient must understand the degree of disability and honestly acknowledge performance limitations. Otherwise, energy reserves will be depleted as the patient tries to maintain previous levels of achievement. The nurse should provide direction and outline the ramifications of not informing certain individuals, such as the patient's employer.

GOAL 2: To establish appropriate sleep and rest patterns

Interventions

1. Assess the patient's pre-disease sleep patterns, such as usual number of hours required each night and typical times for retiring and waking.

2. Using information from the patient's diary, modify the patient's sleep and rest patterns to compensate for decreased energy levels.

Rationales

1. Previous habits are significant as they remain ingrained in the life-style pattern.

2. Compliance improves when the patient is responsible for establishing a balance of activity and rest and is able to see the advantages.

Nursing diagnosis: *Impaired physical mobility related to incomplete transmission of neural impulses through demyelination*

GOAL 1: To help the patient and family understand MS and specific symptoms

Interventions

1. Be prepared for patient teaching by keeping up-to-date on current diagnostic and treatment methods. Read journals and textbooks; contact the Multiple Sclerosis Society for educational materials; attend education sessions: and communicate with doctors and other members of the health care team.

2. Establish contacts with the Multiple Sclerosis Society to obtain information about self-help groups for family members and educational materials for newly diagnosed patients.

Rationales

1. MS is rarely addressed fully during basic nursing education, and many nurses have had little experience with it. Therefore, the nurse must develop the skills needed to be a qualified resource for the patient and family.

2. The patient and family will continue to live with the disease following nursing intervention and must know how to reach support systems without the nurse's intervention.

3. Review the patient's and family's understanding of MS.

3. Denial is common following the diagnosis of a chronic illness that offers little hope of successful intervention. The nurse can help the patient and family work through the levels of acceptance and live productively despite the disease.

GOAL 2: To develop and implement appropriate treatment plans with the cooperation of the rehabilitation team

Interventions

1. Know the area of responsibility for therapists and counselors specializing in MS, and be prepared to identify the patient's need for these disciplines.

2. Have copies of the treatment plan and health care team recommendations. Encourage the patient and family to follow them.

Rationales

1. MS treatment involves various disciplines during the progress of the disease. The nurse often has more long-term involvement and, therefore, the responsibility for monitoring the patient's progress and symptoms, identifying the need for professional intervention, and intervening appropriately.

2. The nurse must know the recommended treatment to monitor the patient's and family's compliance.

Nursing diagnosis: *Altered patterns of urinary elimination related to decreased motor and sensory nerve transmission*

GOAL: To help the patient maximize bladder control within the limitations of the disease process

Interventions

1. Identify the degree of the patient's dysfunction, and establish a suitable program to maximize the patient's control over urination.

2. Work with the doctor to establish a schedule for testing the patient's urine for bacteria or yeast infections.

3. Instruct the patient to record the frequency and duration of episodes of urinary dysfunction.

4. Ask the patient to record fluid intake.

5. Assess the patient's positioning on the toilet, and suggest ways to maximize bladder evacuation.

Rationales

1. The patient may view incontinence as infantile behavior unacceptable in adults. As a result, he may have difficulty discussing urinary problems and may require extra counseling.

2. Inadequately emptying the bladder increases the patient's risk of urinary tract infection.

3. A diary often identifies causes. Fatigue and poor mobility can prevent the patient from reaching the bathroom in time to void or may eventually reduce the patient's control of the sphincter muscle. A specific schedule for voiding and modifications in the bathroom can help the patient overcome the problem. An occupational therapist can provide constructive advice on widening bathroom doorways for wheelchair entry and on transfer techniques. A portable commode may be appropriate if the patient experiences the urge to void only when the bladder is full.

4. The patient may drink less in the mistaken belief that reduced fluid intake will resolve incontinence. This often causes cystitis, because bacteria flourish in the concentrated urine, and dehydration, which weakens the patient further and leads to an electrolyte imbalance that adversely affects physical balance and cognitive function.

5. The patient may tense abdominal and back muscles to compensate for poor balance and weak back muscles. This can interfere with attempts to relax the external urinary meatus. External pressure techniques can improve the action of weak lower abdominal muscles. Exercises to strengthen and relax abdominal and back muscles, and the use of grab bars for support, can also help resolve the problem.

6. Assess the patient's diet and medications as possible agents of the dysfunction. Implement changes where possible.

6. Some medications, such as muscle relaxants and antihistamines, can affect control of the external sphincter. Digestion of some vegetables and fruits can produce strong alkalines or acids that may irritate the bladder mucosa and urethra.

7. Assess the need for regular or intermittent use of external collection devices.

7. The current trend away from the continuous use of indwelling catheters was prompted by studies linking their use with increased bacterial growth and eventual bladder atrophy. Alternatives are available through pharmacies and medical supply companies.

Nursing diagnosis: *Altered bowel elimination: incontinence or constipation, related to decreased motor and sensory nerve transmission*

GOAL: To help the patient maximize bowel control within the limitations of the disease process

Interventions

1. Have the patient keep a diary, recording the time and frequency of bowel movements, the degree of control, and the amount of difficulty experienced.

2. Assess the patient's mobility and access to the bathroom.

3. Assess the patient's dietary and medication regimen. Modify as needed.

4. Teach the patient the importance of timing defecation to use the gastrocolic reflex.

5. Assess such methods as digital fecal disimpaction and enemas to overcome the lack of muscle response in the rectum, and implement the methods only if needed.

Rationales

1. Defecation depends on effective neuromuscular control of the external sphincter. Constipation or involuntary bowel movements may stem from inadequate stimulation of or control over the nerves governing the anus.

2. The patient may deliberately postpone bowel movements if fatigue or difficult bathroom access are factors. Regular exercise, bathroom modifications that facilitate access and support, and proper posture while defecating help overcome this problem.

3. The patient and food preparer may not understand the role of fiber and fluids. Fiber increases the bulk and stimulates intestinal mucosa to promote peristalsis. The patient may mistakenly believe that fluids are only important in bladder function, overlooking their role as a lubricant as fecal contents pass over the mucosa.

4. Intestinal motility begins when food enters the stomach. This reflex should be an integral consideration when developing a bowel movement schedule.

5. Regular enemas can cause water intoxication; however, a patient lacking control of the anal sphincter retains little fluid. Regular disimpaction can destroy the remaining control in the rectum and should only be used as a last resort.

Nursing diagnosis: *Sexual dysfunction related to decreased stimulation and motor control of the external genitalia*

GOAL 1: To assess the patient's sexual attitudes, abilities, and identified needs

Interventions

1. Introduce questions about sexual activities as part of the general data collection. Consider the patient's level of comfort about sharing this information.

Rationales

1. The patient's sexual history helps define the significance attached to sexual function and attitudes about self and partner and helps identify options for improving the patient's level of performance and satisfaction.

2. Assess medications for side effects, and encourage the patient to discuss concerns with the doctor.

2. Side effects of medications to counteract spasticity can include impaired libido or impotence. For example, dantrolene sodium may impede erection and baclofen may impair ejaculation.

3. Encourage open communication between the patient and partner regarding concerns and the need for adjustments.

3. Sexual dysfunction affects both partners. A cooperative, accepting approach is needed to resolve difficulties.

4. Identify the relationship between the sexual difficulty and other symptoms of MS.

4. Fatigue, muscle spasm, urinary dysfunction, and emotional lability can adversely affect sexual response.

5. Evaluate the patient's need for sex counseling.

5. The reasons for impaired sexual function may be complex and long-standing, requiring the intervention of a psychologist, doctor, or sex counselor. The nurse should recognize personal limitations in knowledge and be willing to make appropriate referrals.

GOAL 2: To evaluate the patient's and partner's understanding and acceptance of limitations imposed by MS on sexual activities

Interventions

1. Review the pathophysiology of MS in accordance with demonstrated symptoms.

Rationales

1. Both partners must understand the reason for decreased sensation or motor response. Because the prognosis for MS is uncertain, they should understand that remission may or may not occur.

2. Suggest alternatives for intercourse, if appropriate.

2. Fatigue is a common symptom of MS; consequently, intercourse may not satisfy the sexual needs of both partners at all times. The patient and partner might want to compromise, replacing intercourse with digital stimulation, caressing established sensitive areas, or masturbation.

3. Help the patient and partner adjust routine sexual behavior to maximize gratification.

3. Weakness and spasticity may necessitate new positions and planning intercourse around medication and activity schedules. A suitable lubricant can improve performance and gratification if hormonal impairment from medication or the disease itself results in dryness of the vaginal mucosa.

GOAL 3: To assess the relationship between the patient's self-image and feelings of sexual attractiveness

Intervention

During discussions with the patient and partner, be alert for indications of difficulty in accepting signs such as impaired gait, facial spasms, or emotional lability. Help the patient and partner understand these changes and the degree to which the patient's actions and responses are affected by the disease.

Rationale

Real or perceived changes in appearance that MS imposes can affect the patient's sexual response. If the patient feels less attractive and others corroborate this feeling, sexual function will probably be affected. Feelings of guilt and anger should be discussed to help the patient accept the illness and adjust to its limitations. Special counseling may be needed.

Nursing diagnosis: *Ineffective breathing pattern related to decreased response of the intercostal and diaphragm muscles*

GOAL: To reduce the risk of lower lobe pneumonia

Interventions

1. Teach the patient diaphragmatic breathing exercises.

Rationales

1. A sedentary life-style decreases respiratory function. If the patient can't perform aerobic activities, regular periods of diaphragmatic breathing should be included in the daily schedule.

2. Teach the patient the signs and symptoms of pulmonary congestion.

2. Patients with decreased muscle action in the chest should know signs and symptoms that require medical attention. Medication or specialized chest therapy may be required.

Nursing diagnosis: *Altered role performance related to physical or cognitive dysfunction*

GOAL: To determine realistic employment goals

Interventions

1. Have the patient itemize the physical aspects of the workplace. Identify activities that will require modification.

2. Help the patient investigate alternative employment opportunities.

3. Examine the financial ramifications and potential changes in the patient's life-style.

Rationales

1. This type of analysis frequently requires the assistance of an occupational therapist. Decisions may seem clear when disabilities are major, such as in quadriplegia. However, modifications in the workplace can enable even extremely disabled patients to return to work. The patient's acceptance of the illness, fear of re-entering an able-bodied work force, or cognitive damage secondary to MS may make the patient unrealistic when assessing the abilities needed to return to work. A social worker can help negotiate the patient's return with the employer, if needed.

2. Job sharing or piecework may be more in line with the patient's energy levels and productivity potential. The homemaker with MS may be able to perform some activities and then have help with other tasks, such as heavy cleaning. If the patient has an overt physical disability and no evidence of remission, job retraining may be needed.

3. MS is usually diagnosed when the patient is between ages 20 and 40, commonly a period of career development. The family may face major changes if the patient's income is a significant portion of the household income. A husband may have to depend on his wife's income. The wife may feel resentful of her new role. The children may have to modify education plans. Social workers and employment counselors can help the family cope with these concerns.

Nursing diagnosis: *Self-care deficit secondary to impaired physical functioning*

GOAL: To maximize the patient's level of independence and dignity

Interventions

1. Identify areas of self-care that the patient can perform independently.

Rationales

1. The patient's ability to resume personal care depends on the degree of physical impairment, attitude, level of family support, and level of cooperation with the nurse. Occasionally, household modifications or medical devices can help. Using a sponge (rather than a cloth), a bath board, or a long-handled brush may help a disabled patient perform personal hygiene independently. Occupational therapists and other specialists can provide helpful advice.

2. Teach the patient energy conservation techniques.

2. Inefficient use of energy reserves can exhaust the patient and cause discouragement. The nurse must observe the ways in which activities are carried out and recommend less taxing methods.

3. Maintain a consistent approach.

3. Copies of all assessments and treatment goals should be accessible to those involved in the patient's care, including the family. Patient care conferences can help ensure a consistent approach by all health care providers working with the patient.

ASSOCIATED CARE PLANS
• Cerebrovascular Accident
• Hospice
• Ineffective Coping
• Pain
• Pneumonia
• Sex and Sexuality
• Spinal Cord Injury
• Urinary Tract Infections

NETWORKING OF SERVICES
• Multiple Sclerosis Society
• home health care services
• durable medical equipment (DME) supplier
• sex therapy counseling
• multiple sclerosis clinic
• outpatient rehabilitation services
• Meals On Wheels
• visiting homemaker services
• employment counseling

CARE TEAM INVOLVED
• nurse
• doctor
• patient and family
• neurologist
• physiatrist
• urologist
• medical social worker
• sex therapist
• occupational therapist
• physical therapist

IMPLICATIONS FOR HOME CARE
• functional features of the home (ramps, stairs, location of bathroom and kitchen)
• telephone (communication)
• equipment (wheelchair, braces, grab bars)

PATIENT EDUCATION TOOLS
• literature for all prescribed medications
• literature about the diagnosis and treatment of MS and necessary adjustments
• literature about bowel and bladder training

• reports from other health care professionals regarding exercise and equipment

DISCHARGE PLAN FROM HOME HEALTH CARE
Before discharge from home health care, the patient should:
• know the symptoms of infection in the lungs and bladder
• understand the importance of reporting symptoms to the doctor
• have a daily schedule for rest, deep breathing, bladder or bowel programs (if needed), and medications
• be responsible for personal care and household management either independently or with the aid of family, friends, or hired help
• have names and phone numbers for the nearest Multiple Sclerosis Society chapter, the home health care agency, and doctors and other health care professionals involved in treatment
• know the appropriate use and maintenance of all equipment
• have a scheduled date to return to work, if feasible.

SELECTED REFERENCES
Liebman, M. *Neuroanatomy Made Easy and Understandable*, 3rd ed. Rockville, Md.: Aspen Publications, 1986.
MS Society of Canada pamphlets:
  Bauer, H.J. *A Manual on Multiple Sclerosis.*
  Dean, G. *The MS Problem.*
  Handling the Handicapped.
  Indicative Abstracts.
  Jurtzke, J. *Some Clues to Diagnosis.*
  Role of Rehabilitation in the Management of Multiple Sclerosis.
  Tarabulcy, E. *Bladder Disturbances in MS and their Management.*
Scheinberg, P. *An Introduction to Diagnosis and Management of Common Neurologic Disorders*, 3rd ed. New York: Raven Press, 1986.

NEUROLOGIC SYSTEM

Brain Tumors

DESCRIPTION AND TIME FOCUS

Brain tumors can be primary cancers or metastatic lesions from another systemic cancer. Brain tumors may affect brain tissue, blood vessels, meninges, cranial nerves, or ductless glands. Symptoms vary according to location and tissue type affected. As the tumor grows, signs of increased intracranial pressure typically appear.

Treatment depends on the tumor type and location. Initial treatment may involve curative or palliative surgery and a tentative plan for follow-up radiation therapy or chemotherapy. Radiation therapy is effective against some types of tumor. Chemotherapy success is limited because many drugs do not cross the blood-brain barrier.

This clinical plan focuses on the patient discharged home from an acute-care hospital after diagnosis and initial treatment of a primary or metastatic brain tumor. Nursing care centers on helping the patient adapt to the disease, understand the treatment options and possible complications, and maintain an acceptable lifestyle as long as possible. The home setting allows the patient and family to participate fully in the nursing process.

■ Typical home health care length of service for the patient with a brain tumor: 6 weeks (this can vary greatly depending on the patient's condition)

■ Typical visit frequency: three visits the first week, two visits weekly for 2 weeks, then one visit weekly for 3 weeks

HEALTH HISTORY FINDINGS

In a health history interview, the patient may report many of these findings:
• previously diagnosed cancer at another site
• sudden onset of headaches
• focal or generalized seizures
• blurred vision
• decreased sensation
• loss of coordination or equilibrium
• anorexia
• nausea and vomiting
• indigestion
• fecal incontinence
• urinary incontinence
• history of gradual mood and behavior changes, periods of drowsiness, and shortened attention span

PHYSICAL FINDINGS

In a physical examination, the nurse may detect many of these findings:

Neurologic (findings depend on tumor location)
• hemiparesis
• aphasia
• altered level of consciousness (LOC)

Integumentary
• thin, friable skin secondary to high-dose steroid therapy

Renal and urinary
• urine retention

General
• edema secondary to high-dose steroid therapy

DIAGNOSTIC STUDIES

The following study may be ordered to evaluate the patient's health status:
• funduscopic examination—twice weekly to monthly to monitor for papilledema

---

Nursing diagnosis: *Sensory-perceptual alterations related to neurologic pathology*

GOAL: To consistently assess neurologic changes and provide timely interventions

Interventions

1. Conduct a thorough neurologic assessment during the initial visit. Check the patient's coordination, vision, sensation, and strength and reflexes in each extremity.

2. Evaluate for signs of increased intracranial pressure during each visit.

Rationales

1. A methodical baseline evaluation makes detecting and verifying changes on subsequent visits possible. The results and techniques used should be accurately documented to ensure consistency in all assessments.

2. Increased intracranial pressure is always a possibility for the patient with a brain tumor. Early detection ensures rapid medical intervention.

Nursing diagnosis: *Potential for injury related to disturbance in mentation and loss of body control*

GOAL: To provide a safe home environment for the patient

Interventions

1. Assess the home for safety hazards, such as stairs and cluttered hallways. Note the room size and fixtures in the bathroom and kitchen. Advise the family on alterations that would improve safety.

2. Inform the caregiver that the patient may develop confusion and loss of judgment. Stress that the patient may need supervision and should avoid potentially harmful activities.

3. Teach the patient and caregiver seizure precautions, such as:
• keeping the patient's environment free of hazardous items that could cause injury during a seizure (such as a coffee table with sharp edges or a glass top)
• maintaining a quiet, calm environment
• installing padded siderails on the patient's bed
• keeping a soft oral airway on hand
• using a rectal thermometer rather than an oral thermometer.

Rationales

1. The patient may experience changes in mentation, coordination, or equilibrium. Hemiparesis may occur. The home must be safe for the patient to have as much freedom as possible. A sleeping area may be needed downstairs. The patient may need grab bars and a bath stool in the bathroom for safety and a measure of independence while bathing and using the toilet.

2. The family may be reluctant to believe that the patient could require 24-hour supervision. An honest approach to the subject and a discussion of the patient's physical condition helps the family prepare for and accept the possibility. If necessary, refer the family to a social worker for additional assistance.

3. Increased intracranial pressure may precipitate seizures in the patient with a brain tumor. The patient and caregiver must be able to respond appropriately.

Nursing diagnosis: *Knowledge deficit related to lack of information about signs and symptoms of complications*

GOAL: To have the patient and caregiver know the signs and symptoms of complications and appropriate responses

Interventions

1. Teach the patient and caregiver about the possible complications associated with the patient's tumor. These may include blurred vision, loss of sensation, loss of bowel or bladder control, hemiparesis, or decreased intellectual function.

2. Teach the patient and caregiver the signs and symptoms of increased intracranial pressure, such as frequent headaches, changes in LOC, or severe vomiting.

Rationales

1. The neurologic complications of a brain tumor depend on the location and size of the mass. As the tumor grows, more brain areas will be affected. The nurse should know the type and location of the tumor and the structures most likely to be affected. The patient and caregiver have more control over their situation when they are aware of potential problems.

2. The skull cannot expand to accommodate a growing tumor. As intracranial pressure increases, the patient will develop associated signs and symptoms that may warrant medical intervention.

Nursing diagnosis: *Altered comfort: pain, related to increased intracranial pressure*

GOAL: To ensure the patient's ability to control the pain associated with the disease process

Interventions

1. Instruct the patient and caregiver on the proper use of prescribed pain medication. Stress that the medication should be taken before pain becomes severe and that the patient should continue to take medication as prescribed to maintain control. Explore their attitudes about the use of medication, and help them understand that pain control is an important part of treatment.

2. Teach the patient relaxation techniques and other techniques to enhance the effect of prescribed medication. Emphasize the need for a quiet environment.

3. Teach the patient and caregiver how to manage adverse drug effects, such as constipation or dry mouth.

Rationales

1. The patient may not know how to use medication appropriately to control pain. He may fear addiction or believe that pain must be severe before the medication is used. Cultural attitudes and the attitudes of others toward the use of pain relievers can also interfere with the patient's use of pain control medications.

2. Supplemental techniques can increase the effect of medication and improve the patient's ability to control pain.

3. The patient may be reluctant to use pain medication because of the potential side effects. The nurse must help the patient and caregiver understand that side effects can be managed.

Nursing diagnosis: *Altered nutrition: less than body requirements, related to anorexia and nausea*

GOAL: To help the patient maintain adequate nutrition to meet metabolic needs

Interventions

1. Assess the patient's baseline nutritional patterns by having him keep a food diary for several days.

2. Explain that consuming adequate nutrients provides energy and helps combat adverse effects of prescribed medications. Stress the need to increase caloric and protein intake.

3. Combat anorexia by advising the patient to consume small, frequent meals; nutritional supplements; and high-protein snack foods, such as cheese cubes and peanut butter and crackers.

4. Teach the patient and caregiver how to manage nausea using medication and relaxation techniques.

Rationales

1. Nutritional teaching is only effective when the patient's eating habits and preferences are considered. A baseline assessment is the first step in developing realistic plans and goals.

2. The patient's tumor may cause a hypermetabolic state. If so, the patient requires additional protein and calories. If the patient is receiving large doses of steroids, adequate food intake can combat steroid side effects in the GI tract.

3. Anorexia may result in part from fatigue when eating. Small meals and snack foods are easy to eat and require minimal energy.

4. Increasing intracranial pressure or steroid therapy can cause nausea, which must be controlled for adequate nutrition to be maintained.

Nursing diagnosis: *Potential for infection related to immunosuppressive effects of disease and medications*

GOAL: To prevent infections

Interventions

1. Teach the patient the importance of avoiding crowds and limiting contact with visitors who may be ill. Teach family members to use masks when necessary to prevent the spread of common respiratory infections to the patient. Stress the need for regular, thorough hand washing—and always before eating.

Rationales

1. The patient's immune system may be compromised by the disease. Steroids to reduce inflammation and edema can contribute to immunosuppression.

2. Teach the patient and caregiver measures to take if the patient has chills, becomes febrile, or has other signs or symptoms of infection.

2. Infections progress quickly in the immunosuppressed patient. Prompt recognition and medical intervention are essential.

Nursing diagnosis: *Disturbance in self-concept: personal identity, related to disease symptoms and treatment*

GOAL: To help the patient maintain self-esteem

Interventions

1. Assess the patient's understanding of his disease and its signs and symptoms. Let the patient make as many decisions as possible, and include the patient in all discussions. Encourage the family to view the signs and symptoms as part of the disease, not part of the patient.

2. Encourage the patient to maintain personal appearance by getting dressed every day, shaving, and performing other grooming activities. A home health aide can help if the patient is too weak or otherwise unable to perform personal care.

Rationales

1. As symptoms increase, the patient may become more frightened and feel unable to control any part of his life. The patient, family, and nurse must cooperate to maintain the patient's participation as long as possible.

2. Treatments may result in hair loss. Steroids may affect skin appearance and cause facial edema and weight gain. Appearance is an important aspect of self-concept. The family and health care team must encourage and assist the patient to maintain good grooming.

Nursing diagnosis: *Impaired home maintenance management related to limitations imposed by the disease process*

GOAL: To promote safe home maintenance by altering the home environment

Interventions

1. Evaluate the patient's support systems, financial needs, equipment needs, and need for community resources. Refer the patient to a social worker if necessary.

2. Evaluate the family's ability to provide 24-hour supervision should it become necessary for the patient's safety.

Rationales

1. Available help can allow the patient to remain at home. The patient may require the nurse's help to obtain the necessary services.

2. The patient may become confused and disoriented. Plans should be made for this possibility before it happens.

ASSOCIATED CARE PLANS
• Grief and Grieving
• Hospice
• Ineffective Coping
• Seizure Disorders

NETWORKING OF SERVICES
• durable medical equipment (DME) supplier
• American Cancer Society
• community transportation services

CARE TEAM INVOLVED
• nurse
• doctor

• patient and family
• neurologist
• oncologist
• home health aide
• medical social worker
• physical therapist
• occupational therapist

IMPLICATIONS FOR HOME CARE
• functional features of the home (stairs, location of furniture, location of bathroom and kitchen)
• telephone (communication)

PATIENT EDUCATION TOOLS

• literature about each medication ordered, including a written dosage schedule and a list of possible adverse effects
• American Cancer Society literature
• list of symptoms that require immediate notification of the doctor
• written information on seizure precautions
• know the dates and times of follow-up appointments, and have transportation arranged
• have a dietary plan that provides adequate nutrition
• know community resources and services offered by the local American Cancer Society.

SELECTED REFERENCES

Birmingham, J.J. *Home Care Planning Based on DRGs.* Philadelphia: J.B. Lippincott Co., 1986.

Eliopoulos, C. *A Guide to the Nursing of the Aged.* Baltimore: Williams & Wilkins Co., 1987.

Groenwald, S.L. *Cancer Nursing Principles and Practice.* Boston: Jones and Bartlett Publishers, 1987.

Iyer, P., et al. *Nursing Process and Nursing Diagnosis.* Philadelphia: W.B. Saunders Co., 1986.

Ozuna, J. "Alterations in Mentation: Nursing Assessment and Intervention," *Journal of Neurosurgical Nursing* 17(1):66-70, February 1985.

Seizure Disorders

DESCRIPTION AND TIME FOCUS
Seizures may be related to metabolic disturbances, nervous system disorders, brain lesions, trauma, or biochemical abnormalities. Idiopathic seizures (epilepsy) result from an abnormality in impulse conduction in the brain. Seizures take many different forms and are classified by type. The nurse must be aware of the exact type of seizures affecting the patient.

This clinical plan focuses on the patient discharged home from an acute-care hospital after diagnosis and initial treatment of a seizure disorder. The patient under discussion has generalized seizures. However, all seizure types require management, and the home setting is an ideal place for the nurse to monitor the patient and provide instruction in the control and management of seizures.

■ Typical home health care length of service for a patient with a newly diagnosed seizure disorder: 4 weeks, or until discharge criteria are met

■ Typical visit frequency: three visits the first week, twice weekly for 2 weeks, then once weekly until discharge criteria are met

HEALTH HISTORY FINDINGS
In a health history interview, the patient may report many of these findings:
• no memory of seizure
• bruising, abrasions, and other minor injuries sustained during the seizure
• drowsiness, confusion, and agitation after seizure

PHYSICAL FINDINGS
Between seizures, physical findings related to the seizure disorder may not exist. When seizures are related to other primary diseases, such as liver or renal failure, brain tumors, or cerebrovascular accident, the physical findings will be those of the underlying disease.

DIAGNOSTIC STUDIES
The following study may be performed to evaluate the patient's health status:
• blood level of anticonvulsant drug—weekly for 4 weeks, then monthly until therapeutic blood drug levels are obtained with minimum side effects

---

Nursing diagnosis: *Potential for injury related to loss of control during seizure activity*

GOAL: To make the patient and caregiver knowledgeable about seizure precautions and injury prevention

Interventions

1. Assess the patient's home for safety hazards, such as stairs and cluttered hallways. Pay particular attention to the bathroom, kitchen, and other rooms often used by the patient.

2. Teach the patient and caregiver about precautions to take during a seizure. Encourage the patient to include friends and relatives in the teaching session. Stress that turning the patient on the side and moving objects away provides the best protection during seizures. Warn against placing padded tongue depressors, spoons, or other implements in the patient's mouth.

3. Explain the appearance and physiology of the patient during a seizure.

4. Teach safety precautions needed during the postseizure period.

Rationales

1. Minimizing potential hazards can promote patient safety and help the patient feel more comfortable in his home. All doors should open outward or fold to prevent the patient from being wedged behind it during a seizure. Door locks should be removed to make sure someone can reach the patient. The patient should take showers, not baths, to prevent the possibility of drowning. The kitchen should be made as safe as possible. Stairs can constitute a hazard if the patient has a seizure there.

2. Seizures are frightening for the patient and family. Simple, accurate instructions promote the patient's safety. Of the many misconceptions about seizures, the most common is that the patient will swallow his tongue. The family and patient must understand that most injuries during seizures occur when someone forces an object into the patient's mouth.

3. Knowing what to expect helps those observing a seizure to overcome fears and take proper actions to prevent injury to the patient.

4. The patient may be lethargic, confused, or belligerent for several hours after a seizure. Close observation by a family member may be needed to ensure patient safety.

5. Discuss with the family the possibility of status epilepticus, describe its appearance, and explain appropriate actions to take.

5. Most seizures are brief. The family should know that a seizure lasting longer than others have may require medical intervention and that they should use emergency medical services.

6. Encourage the patient to order and wear an identification bracelet.

6. An identification bracelet helps promote patient safety. The patient may feel reluctant about making his disorder known, however, and may need encouragement from others to wear the bracelet.

Nursing diagnosis: *Knowledge deficit related to the medication regimen*

GOAL: To make the patient and caregiver knowledgeable about the method of administration, dosage schedule, possible interactions, and adverse effects of all prescribed medications

Interventions

1. Establish a written medication schedule for the patient, and post it in a prominent place.

2. Instruct the patient and caregiver to notify the doctor if the patient experiences any adverse effects from these medications, such as slurred speech and drowsiness.

3. Stress the potential for interactions between anticonvulsants and many prescribed and over-the-counter (OTC) medications. Caution the patient to check with the doctor before taking any drug.

4. Find out if tests have been ordered to determine blood drug levels, and help the patient make arrangements for necessary laboratory work.

Rationales

1. Proper and timely drug administration is crucial to therapeutic blood drug levels and ensures the effectiveness of anticonvulsant therapy.

2. Adverse effects from anticonvulsants are common because of the drugs' narrow therapeutic range and dramatic effect on cerebellar function. If adverse effects occur, the doctor may need to change the medication or adjust the dosage.

3. The patient needs to know that all medications—including OTC medications—can interact with anticonvulsants.

4. These tests help determine whether the therapeutic blood drug levels have been reached.

Nursing diagnosis: *Altered thought processes related to seizure disorder and medication*

GOAL: To have the patient understand potential problems and learn appropriate coping mechanisms

Interventions

1. Explain to the patient that he may experience temporary memory loss and confusion after a seizure.

2. Instruct the patient on adverse medication effects that may affect coordination.

3. Help the patient develop adaptive measures and accept altered thought processes as a condition to be managed constructively.

Rationales

1. A clear understanding of what to expect enables the patient to develop coping mechanisms and alleviates the fear that each seizure causes permanent brain damage.

2. Until therapeutic blood drug levels are reached, the patient may experience adverse medication effects that cause him to question his thought processes. Assure him that this effect is normal and will subside after the dosage has been regulated.

3. A seizure disorder may be permanent. Constructively adapting to the disorder helps the patient maintain a productive life-style.

Nursing diagnosis: *Altered role performance related to activity restrictions imposed by seizure disorder*

GOAL: To help the patient and family adapt to activity restrictions imposed by the seizure disorder

Interventions	Rationales
1. Assess the patient's understanding of activity restrictions associated with a newly diagnosed seizure disorder. For example, the patient may have been instructed to avoid driving cars and operating heavy equipment.	1. The patient needs to understand the need for such restrictions until his seizure disorder can be better evaluated and controlled.
2. Assess the impact of activity restrictions on the patient's life-style and self-concept.	2. The patient's inability to drive may cause hardship for the patient and family. Other restrictions may affect the patient's livelihood or cause him to feel he no longer contributes to the family.
3. Encourage family members to express their concern for the patient's intrinsic value as an individual regardless of imposed limitations.	3. The patient needs the support of loved ones to adjust to activity limitations and to feel like a contributing member of the family.
4. Refer the patient and family to a social worker and support group if necessary. (The Epilepsy Foundation of America is the principal support group for patients with seizure disorders.) Make this referral early in the care process to allow the social worker adequate time to work with all concerned parties.	4. A social worker and support group can help the patient and family understand and cope with activity restrictions.

Nursing diagnosis: *Impaired home maintenance management related to the disease process, activity restrictions, and need for ongoing medical treatment*

GOAL: To provide the assistance and support necessary for the patient to stay at home

Interventions	Rationales
1. Work with the patient to determine changes in the home environment required for safety and comfort.	1. The patient must be involved in decision making to develop a sense of control over his condition.
2. Help the patient evaluate the activities of daily living he can perform himself and those for which he may need assistance.	2. Identifying tasks the patient can perform independently helps maintain his sense of self-worth. Identifying tasks that he may need help with, such as shopping or running errands, promotes patient safety.
3. Evaluate the patient's financial status for problems and make appropriate referrals to agencies that can provide help.	3. Lifelong medical follow-up and medication can create a financial burden for the patient and family. Community resources can offer financial support and guidance.

ASSOCIATED CARE PLANS
- Brain Tumors
- Cerebrovascular Accident
- Chronic Renal Failure
- Cirrhosis
- Ineffective Coping

NETWORKING OF SERVICES
- Lifeline
- Meals On Wheels
- durable medical equipment (DME) supplier
- Epilepsy Foundation of America
- community transportation service

CARE TEAM INVOLVED
• nurse
• doctor
• patient and family
• home health aide
• medical social worker

IMPLICATIONS FOR HOME CARE
• functional features of the home (doors, locks, stairs)
• telephone (communication)
• transportation requirements
• support system of family and friends

PATIENT EDUCATION TOOLS
• written medication schedule
• information for each prescribed medication, including adverse effects and interactions
• Epilepsy Foundation of America literature
• list of actions for family to take in the event of a seizure

DISCHARGE PLAN FROM HOME HEALTH CARE
Before discharge from home health care, the patient and family should:
• explain the basic physiology of a seizure
• understand seizure precautions
• understand activity restrictions
• be complying with the medication regimen
• have telephone numbers for the doctor, home health agency, and emergency medical services posted prominently
• order a medical identification bracelet
• know the dates of appointments with the doctor and laboratory
• have transportation arranged for these appointments.

SELECTED REFERENCES
Adams, R., and Victor, M. *Principles of Neurology*, 3rd ed. New York: McGraw-Hill Book Co., 1985.

Kruse, M. *Nursing the Neurological and Neurotrauma Patient*. Totowa, N.Y.: Rowman and Allanheld, 1986.

Rich, J. "Action Stat: Generalized Motor Seizure," *Nursing 86* 16(4):33, April 1986.

Scheinberg, P. *An Introduction to Diagnosis and Management of Common Neurologic Disorders*, 3rd ed. New York: Raven Press, 1986.

Developmental Disabilities

DESCRIPTION AND TIME FOCUS

The term *developmental disability* covers a variety of conditions, including mental retardation, cerebral palsy, and autism, that present before age 18. According to the Developmental Disabilities Assistance and Bill of Rights Act, a developmental disability results from physical or mental impairment and limits activity in at least three of the following areas: self-care, receptive and expressive language, learning, mobility, self-direction, capacity for independent living, and economic self-sufficiency.

Caring for the developmentally disabled patient is a specialized field for which many nurses, therapists, and ancillary personnel lack experience. In-service programs or continuing education may be needed before staff members can accurately assess and care for the patient.

The home care patient with developmental disabilities may require special nursing considerations. Referral to the home health agency may be unrelated to, but vastly affected by, the disability. The patient may need acute, chronic, or respite care. Important nursing skills include history taking, physical assessment, goal setting, teaching, interdisciplinary case management, and the ability to deliver hands-on care. Less tangible but equally important are love, patience, understanding, and good listening skills.

This clinical plan focuses on the patient at home with a developmental disability.

■ Typical home health care length of stay for a developmentally disabled patient: varies according to the reason for referral

■ Typical visit frequency in uncomplicated situations: once weekly, or once every 2 weeks if other health care providers are involved

HEALTH HISTORY FINDINGS

No typical findings

PHYSICAL FINDINGS

In a physical examination, the nurse may detect many of these findings:

Neurologic
• delays in gross or fine motor skills
• seizure disorders
• tardive dyskinesia

• alterations in reflexes
• visual problems
• hearing loss (associated with cerumen accumulation)

Cardiovascular
• tachycardia or bradycardia
• dysrhythmias
• congenital anomalies

Gastrointestinal
• abnormal weight
• impaired swallowing and chewing
• constipation
• incontinence
• reflux esophagitis
• food allergies
• pica (nutritional or behavioral)

Integumentary
• hypersensitivity or hyposensitivity to heat and cold
• hypersensitivity to sunlight (side effect of some medications, including phenothiazines)
• acne
• perineal rash (caused by infection, incontinence, or inadequate hygiene)
• gum hypertrophy, gingivitis, or dental malformations

Musculoskeletal
• impaired mobility
• muscle weakness, spasticity, rigidity, or contracture
• small stature
• structural malformations, such as scoliosis, kyphosis, or lordosis

Renal and urinary
• urinary tract infections

General
• scars or other sequelae from injuries or self-mutilation
• delayed puberty
• oligomenorrhea or amenorrhea
• history of exposure to hepatitis B virus; more frequent in patients previously institutionalized

DIAGNOSTIC STUDIES

No standard studies

Nursing diagnosis: *Impaired physical mobility related to musculoskeletal defects, weakness, spasticity, or gross motor delays*

GOAL: To maximize the patient's strength and endurance and prevent further disability

Interventions

1. Obtain a thorough assessment of the patient by a physical therapist and clinical nurse specialist.

2. Evaluate the patient's current activity level.

3. Evaluate the patient's ability to communicate activity tolerances.

4. Schedule rest periods throughout the day.

5. Obtain baseline vital signs to assess the patient's cardiac output before, during, and after physical activity.

6. Assess the patient's need for assistive equipment. Consult with physical and occupational therapists as necessary.

Rationales

1. The nurse must be aware of the patient's gait, balance, activity tolerance, and activities that may increase spasticity.

2. Current abilities provide the basis for building strength and endurance. Improvement in these activities encourages the patient to try new ones.

3. The nurse must recognize verbal and nonverbal cues to determine which activities the patient can perform and for how long.

4. Rest improves endurance and reduces spasticity and stress. Limited periods of activity are appropriate for patients with short attention spans.

5. The patient may have undiagnosed cardiac anomalies, tachycardia, bradycardia, or hypertension. Exercise can exacerbate these conditions and adversely affect activity tolerance. Baseline data provide a basis for comparison.

6. A wide range of equipment is available to help with every aspect of mobility and activities of daily living (ADLs). Even if the patient has equipment, his needs may have changed because of growth, debilitation, or acute illness. Many funding sources cover equipment costs, and some agencies offer interest-free loans.

Nursing diagnosis: *Self-care deficit related to physical, cognitive, behavioral, or environmental disabilities*

GOAL 1: To ensure that the patient receives proper nutrition in a safe setting

Interventions

1. Evaluate the patient's ability to feed himself.

2. Evaluate the patient's ability to chew and swallow. Check for dental malformations, tongue thrust, and gag reflex. If necessary, have an occupational therapist assess the patient and develop a nutritional program.

3. Teach the patient and caregiver about proper nutrition and feeding techniques. Observe the patient during mealtime to identify problems and evaluate interventions.

Rationales

1. Patients with poor hand-eye coordination and impaired fine motor skills may require adaptive equipment or assistance to eat.

2. The patient's ability to chew determines whether food must be chopped or pureed. Preparing food in an appropriate form and properly positioning the patient help prevent aspiration. Tongue thrust or gag reflex can make mealtime a battle if the caregiver is untrained in feeding techniques. Using plastic-coated or flexible utensils can prevent damage to the patient's teeth, lips, and gums.

3. Obesity or malnutrition are common and may stem from behavioral problems, lack of knowledge, inactivity, improper feeding techniques, or metabolic disturbances. Written menus that include pictures of appropriate foods, step-by-step feeding techniques, and positioning diagrams can be helpful.

GOAL 2: To promote patient health and social acceptance by improving bathing and personal hygiene routines

Interventions

1. Examine the patient for evidence of inadequate personal hygiene.

2. Establish specific routines for personal hygiene, grooming, and dressing.

3. Consult with an occupational therapist about assistive devices if the patient has physical difficulty performing tasks.

4. Teach the patient and caregiver the signs and symptoms of inadequate hygiene practices.

Rationales

1. Skin and scalp diseases, poor oral hygiene, poor nail care, and perineal rash or infection can easily be overlooked if the patient's history is incomplete or the reason for referral is unrelated to hygiene. The patient may be unaware that signs and symptoms represent treatable problems.

2. The patient is more likely to perform routine activities. Effective routines typically include positive reinforcement for specific tasks.

3. Such devices as an adapted toothbrush handle, dressing stick, or long-handled sponge can provide a simple solution to a serious problem.

4. Patients who can recognize such signs and symptoms as vaginal infection, skin lesions, tooth decay, or ingrown toenails are more likely to seek prompt attention and prevent the problem from worsening.

GOAL 3: To alleviate problems caused by incontinence

Interventions

1. Obtain a medical evaluation or medical records to determine if the cause of incontinence is physiologic, neurologic, behavioral, or developmental.

2. Compile a detailed history of the patient's incontinence. Determine whether it occurs at night; when the patient is fatigued, angry, or upset; with certain medications; or when the patient is in unfamiliar situations or settings.

3. Evaluate the bathroom layout and the patient's ability to unfasten clothing.

4. If necessary, establish a specific toileting program that emphasizes personal hygiene.

Rationales

1. If incontinence results from an underlying disease or structural defect, it may be easily correctable. The etiology of the incontinence affects the focus of planned interventions. In some patients, incontinence is explained by their developmental age.

2. Interventions are most effective when directed toward causative or contributing factors. Asking specific questions and exhibiting sensitivity to the patient's embarrassment about this issue can elicit valuable information.

3. Structural changes, such as widening a doorway or installing grab bars or an elevated toilet seat, may correct the problem. Velcro fasteners are useful for patients with motor impairments.

4. Bowel and bladder training are most effective when they are part of a consistent routine. Training can also improve bowel and bladder muscle tone and voluntary sphincter control. Toileting is preferable to catheterization in most instances (an exception would be neurogenic bladder) because it reduces patient discomfort and risk of urinary tract infections while maintaining the patient's dignity and sense of control.

Nursing diagnosis: *Altered thought processes related to neurologic deficits, medication side effects, aging, isolation, and frustration*

GOAL: To maximize the patient's cognitive abilities

Interventions

1. Determine the patient's ability to understand and process information by reviewing his medical records, collecting appropriate history data from family members and support persons, and directly observing him. If cognitive test results are several years old, consult with the patient's doctor about obtaining a more current evaluation.

2. Identify all prescribed and over-the-counter (OTC) medications used by the patient. Have the caregiver demonstrate the proper method of administration. Observe for adverse effects. Ensure that the patient adheres to the prescribed regimen.

3. If the patient exhibits symptoms of Alzheimer's disease or another form of dementia, arrange for a diagnostic evaluation.

4. Develop an activity routine for the patient that emphasizes increased socialization and uses such techniques as reality orientation.

Rationales

1. The patient may have capabilities not yet discovered. Inappropriate labels and diagnoses are common, especially for older patients. Results from formal cognitive testing sometimes fail to reflect all of a patient's abilities, especially if the test results are several years old. Observations by the nurse, family members, and support persons can sometimes provide more valuable information.

   Conversely, a patient who can perform some tasks may be unable to apply the skills used in those tasks to unfamiliar situations. For example, a patient may have learned to write his name yet may not understand the concept of writing. Helping the patient succeed by establishing realistic, achievable goals is vital in all aspects of care. Current cognitive test results can be useful as a general guide for setting goals and determining teaching methods.

2. Some drug combinations can have potentiating effects, a problem that can occur when prescriptions have been written by more than one doctor. Some medications have a paradoxical effect on neurologically impaired or elderly patients. OTC drugs, such as diet and sleeping aids, may be overlooked when compiling the patient history if the patient doesn't think of them as drugs. For the medication regimen to be effective, the patient or caregiver must not vary the prescribed dosage.

3. Developmentally disabled patients can develop physiologic and psychological disorders. Symptoms of Alzheimer's disease can be misinterpreted when they duplicate symptoms of developmental disability.

4. These activities enhance the patient's self-esteem and can help combat confusion, disorientation, agitation, and depression.

Nursing diagnosis: *Social isolation related to lack of peer group and prejudicial attitudes or stereotypes*

GOAL 1: To increase the patient's social contacts

Interventions

1. Identify local religious groups, special interest groups, and human service agencies that offer activities for disabled patients and their families.

2. Identify the patient's interests, and suggest compatible activities. Be creative in your approach.

Rationales

1. Community resources can significantly decrease the patient's isolation and loneliness while offering encouragement and support to the family.

2. Notifying the patient in advance of an activity that holds interest for him can make his anticipation more pleasurable and less frightening.

3. Be sensitive to the patient's hesitation and fear of meeting new people. Arrange for him to meet a group member or staff person before attending an activity. Introduce him to one new group of people or new place at a time. Gradually increase the time spent in social interaction.

4. Provide positive reinforcement for the patient's efforts to socialize.

5. Anticipate and prepare to handle the patient's regressive behavior.

3. Suddenly thrusting the patient into a strange environment filled with new faces can overwhelm him and be counterproductive. Seeing the outside of a day care center, for example, may be all he can handle on the first visit. Being greeted by a familiar person, such as a staff member, on subsequent visits can enhance his sense of security.

4. Positive reinforcement can motivate the patient to repeat the desirable behavior.

5. Loss of control over a situation, stress, and fear of the unknown may be emotionally overwhelming for the patient. If the patient's language skills are poor, he may attempt to communicate his feelings through such regressive actions as fighting or incontinence. To manage regressive behavior and promote continued social growth, caregivers must view regressive behavior in perspective with the patient's current achievements.

GOAL 2: To help the patient adapt to the community setting

Interventions

1. Assess the patient's previous experiences in the community. Discuss negative reactions to the patient, such as name-calling, rudeness, or frank curiosity, and acknowledge that they would affect anyone's desire to socialize with a nondisabled person. Tell the patient that such reactions reflect a lack of public understanding of disabled individuals and do not indicate dislike of him personally.

2. If necessary, teach the patient the skills needed to function in the community, such as how to shop, handle money, make a phone call, or use public transportation.

3. Stay in touch with the patient and family between visits.

Rationales

1. Success with any patient-related problem is more likely when the nurse approaches the problem from the patient's point of view. Gratuitous statements, such as "I'm sure they meant nothing by it," would undermine the nurse's credibility in this situation. Understanding the motives for behaviors helps prepare the patient to cope with such experiences.

2. To achieve self-sufficiency, the patient must be able to function in the community. Parents often worry about the welfare of the disabled child should they die. Working toward the goal of maximizing the patient's self-sufficiency can help allay these valid family fears.

3. Funding constraints often limit the nurse to one visit a month. A brief phone call or a friendly note to the patient and family can convey a caring attitude and dispel some of the loneliness.

ASSOCIATED CARE PLANS
• Alzheimer's Disease
• Esophagitis
• Gastroenteritis
• Grief and Grieving
• Hepatitis
• Ineffective Coping
• Neurogenic Bladder
• Parkinson's Disease
• Seizure Disorders
• Sex and Sexuality
• Spinal Cord Injury

NETWORKING OF SERVICES
• National Association for Retarded Citizens
• National Easter Seal Society for Crippled Children and Adults

• United Cerebral Palsy Association
• Meals On Wheels
• community action program
• Elder Services agency
• Early Intervention and Head Start programs
• durable medical equipment (DME) supplier
• local consortium for special education
• Health and Human Services, Division of Welfare case workers and prior approval unit (in some areas of the United States)
• third-party insurer's medical case management team
• other disease-specific programs and services. (Check the home health agency reference library for a copy of *The American Association of the University-Affiliated Programs for Persons with Developmental Disabilities.* Write them at 8605 Cameron Street, Silver Spring, Md., 20910, or phone 301-588-8252.)

CARE TEAM INVOLVED
• nurse
• doctor
• patient and family
• nutritionist
• occupational therapist
• physical therapist
• medical social worker
• home health aide
• professional homemaker
• personal care attendant
• school nurse

IMPLICATIONS FOR HOME CARE
• functional features of the home (safe environment, free of barriers, adapted for the patient's needs)
• reliable caregiver
• safe system of medication management
• DME for mobility and ADLs

PATIENT EDUCATION TOOLS
• written feeding programs that include diagrams
• appropriate nutritional information and menus
• written medication schedule
• written toileting program
• teaching materials geared to the developmentally disabled patient, such as anatomic models for sex education
• literature from appropriate national service agencies

DISCHARGE PLAN FROM HOME HEALTH CARE
Before discharge from home health care, the patient should:
• be medically stable
• be in a safe environment
• have a regular schedule of follow-up care by family doctor, neurologist, dentist, podiatrist, and other professionals.

Before discharge from home health care, the patient and primary caregiver should:
• be able to recognize untoward symptoms associated with the patient's diagnosis
• demonstrate an ability to handle seizures appropriately
• demonstrate safe administration of prescribed medications and understand the side effects of prescribed and OTC medications
• understand the principles of proper nutrition
• be able to follow the prescribed diet
• know appropriate feeding techniques
• understand how to use and maintain the patient's DME
• know available community resources and how to contact them
• have a means of transportation
• have a contingency plan for emergencies or for times when the caregiver is unavailable
• have a plan for periodic respite for the caregiver.

SELECTED REFERENCES
Burkhart, J., et al. "Obesity of Mentally Retarded Individuals: Prevalence, Characteristics, and Intervention," *American Journal of Mental Deficiency* 90(3):303-12, November 1985.

Howell, M.C. "Old Age in the Retarded: A New Program," *Journal of the American Geriatric Society* 34(1):71-72, January 1986.

Kessler, J.W. *Psychopathology of Childhood*, 2nd ed. Englewood Cliffs, N.J.: Prentice-Hall, 1988.

Orduna, A., and Vinal, D. "Community Assessment: Services for the Physically Handicapped," *Journal of Community Health Nursing* 3(2):99-107, 1986.

Remis, R., et al. "Hepatitis B Infection in a Day School for Mentally Retarded Students: Transmission from Students to Staff," *American Journal of Public Health* 77(9):1183-86, September 1987.

Rowitz, L. "Multiprofessional Perspectives on Prevention," *Mental Retardation* 24(1):1-3, February 1986.

Sigman, M., ed. *Children with Emotional Disorders and Developmental Disabilities: Assessment and Treatment.* New York: Grune & Stratton, 1985.

Williams, C., et al. "Hepatitis B Virus Transmission in a Public School: Effects on Mentally Retarded HBsAg Carrier Students," *American Journal of Public Health* 77(4):476-78, April 1987.

GASTROINTESTINAL SYSTEM

Gastrointestinal Cancer

DESCRIPTION AND TIME FOCUS
Cancer of gastrointestinal (GI) tract organs— esophagus, stomach, liver, and pancreas—often is far advanced before significant clinical findings appear and diagnosis is established. Morbidity and mortality statistics reveal a dismal prognosis; the combined 5-year survival rate is less than 7 percent. Often, a patient decides to forego treatment and looks to health care providers for empathetic and respectful terminal care.

Treatment modalities for GI cancer include surgery (often radical), radiation therapy, and chemotherapy. The effectiveness of these treatments varies with cancer location:
• Localized liver cancer can be safely and effectively treated with surgery when cirrhosis is not a complicating factor. Radiation therapy may provide limited symptom palliation but fails to improve survival. Chemotherapy is not effective.
• Esophageal cancer usually is diagnosed only after metastasis has occurred and surgery is no longer an option. A patient who cannot ingest food after palliative radiation therapy or chemotherapy will need a gastrostomy or jejunostomy feeding tube.
• Surgery rarely is effective in treating pancreatic cancer. Radiation therapy may decrease pain. Chemotherapy does little to arrest tumor growth.
• Symptoms of stomach cancer rarely appear until long after surgery could be helpful. Radiation therapy is not effective, but chemotherapy may palliate symptoms.

This clinical plan focuses on the patient discharged home from a hospital or an outpatient setting after diagnosis and treatment of GI cancer. Nursing care should maximize the patient's resources and enjoyment of life within the limits imposed by the disease. The home provides an excellent environment for the nurse to help the patient and family develop and implement rehabilitative or terminal care goals.

■ Typical home health care length of service for a patient with GI cancer: variable, depending on the patient's symptoms, prognosis, and response to teaching
■ Typical visit frequency: variable

HEALTH HISTORY FINDINGS
In a health history interview, the patient may report many of these findings:

Esophageal cancer
• smoking
• excessive alcohol use
• rapid, significant weight loss
• vague substernal pain
• dysphagia
• early satiety

Stomach cancer
• history of pernicious anemia or achlorhydria
• anorexia
• early satiety
• recurrent indigestion or heartburn
• rapid, significant weight loss
• weakness and fatigue
• episodic nausea and vomiting
• melena
• vertigo and syncope

Liver cancer
• occupational exposure to vinyl chloride
• long-term use of anabolic steroids
• history of cirrhosis or hepatitis
• excessive alcohol use
• weakness, fatigue, and malaise
• rapid, significant weight loss
• anorexia
• episodic nausea and vomiting
• dull abdominal pain
• dyspnea (from pressure of tumor)

Pancreatic cancer
• history of diabetes or chronic pancreatitis
• smoking
• excessive alcohol use
• vague upper abdominal pain
• episodic nausea and vomiting
• recurrent indigestion and heartburn
• anorexia
• rapid, significant weight loss
• weakness
• early satiety
• pruritus

PHYSICAL FINDINGS
During physical examination, the nurse may detect many of these findings:

Esophageal cancer
• Gastrointestinal
  □ hepatomegaly
  □ increased salivation
  □ red, swollen, sometimes bleeding gingivae
  □ hoarseness
• Integumentary
  □ poor skin turgor

- General
  - ☐ cachexia
  - ☐ emaciation
  - ☐ low-grade fever

Stomach cancer
- Gastrointestinal
  - ☐ abdominal ascites
  - ☐ palpable abdominal mass
- Integumentary
  - ☐ pallor
  - ☐ yellowish skin and sclera
- General
  - ☐ cachexia
  - ☐ enlarged left supraclavicular, left axillary, and umbilical lymph nodes

Liver cancer
- Gastrointestinal
  - ☐ abdominal ascites
  - ☐ hepatomegaly
  - ☐ abdominal tenderness
- Integumentary
  - ☐ yellowish skin and sclera
  - ☐ ecchymoses
  - ☐ purpura

- General
  - ☐ cachexia
  - ☐ peripheral edema
  - ☐ fever

Pancreatic cancer
- Gastrointestinal
  - ☐ abdominal ascites
  - ☐ abdominal tenderness
  - ☐ hepatomegaly
  - ☐ splenomegaly
  - ☐ gallbladder enlargement
  - ☐ dark urine and pale stools
- Integumentary
  - ☐ yellowish skin and sclera
  - ☐ superficial thrombophlebitis
- General
  - ☐ cachexia
  - ☐ peripheral edema
  - ☐ enlarged supraclavicular lymph nodes
  - ☐ anxiety and agitation

DIAGNOSTIC STUDIES
The following study may be performed to evaluate the patient's health status:
- guaiac testing of stool: weekly, to detect occult GI bleeding

---

Nursing diagnosis: *Altered nutrition: less than body requirements, related to effects of cancer or cancer treatment*

GOAL 1: To assess the patient's dietary intake

Interventions

1. Obtain a recent dietary history from the patient or caregiver. Include a 24-hour dietary history and a list of foods that the patient can tolerate and ones that cause him discomfort or that he finds unappealing.

2. On your first visit, measure the patient's height and weight and compare results to his pre-illness weight and to the norms on a standard height and weight chart. On each subsequent visit, measure the patient's weight and compare results to his previous weight.

3. Assess the patient's ability to ingest food by checking his oral cavity for caries, signs of gum disease, missing teeth, and poorly fitting dentures; by evaluating his ability to swallow; and, if appropriate, by evaluating feeding tube function.

4. Assess the patient for nausea or vomiting. Note the typical pattern and frequency of episodes; the relationship of episodes to meals, specific foods, pain, and activity; and whether symptoms are relieved by medication or other treatments.

Rationales

1. These baseline data help the nurse plan dietary interventions.

2. These data allow the nurse to compare the patient's current weight with previous weight and with desirable norms as a way to assess adequacy of dietary intake.

3. In order to maintain proper nutrition, the patient must be able to properly chew and swallow food or, if necessary, use a feeding tube.

4. Nausea and vomiting prevent the absorption of needed nutrients and also may discourage the patient from eating.

GOAL 2: To ensure the patient's intake of a tolerable high-calorie, high-protein diet

Interventions

1. Encourage the patient to rest for 15 to 30 minutes before each meal.

2. Teach the patient and caregiver methods to help minimize abdominal pain, nausea, and vomiting during meals, such as keeping the eating environment pleasant, clean, and odor-free; playing soft, relaxing music; and keeping mealtime conversation upbeat.

3. Instruct the patient or caregiver to perform oral hygiene before each meal.

4. Teach the patient and caregiver some essentials of nutrition and about methods of improving the patient's nutritional intake. Explain that the patient should:
• eat small, frequent meals and snacks of well-liked and tolerated foods
• avoid fried, greasy, and very hot or very cold foods
• drink adequate amounts of fluid between meals
• increase protein intake by adding powdered milk to such foods as soups, sauces, gravies, puddings, custards, or regular milk; using grated cheese and scrambled eggs whenever possible; and by using liquid protein supplements or instant breakfast products
• increase caloric intake by adding sugar, honey, jelly, syrup, and whipped toppings to foods when possible; providing high-calorie foods, such as pie, cake, cookies, donuts, and danish; and by keeping snacks within the patient's reach.

5. If appropriate, teach the caregiver how to administer gastrostomy tube feedings. Explain that the food can be a commercial product or regular food prepared in a blender. Teach the caregiver to:
• remove the tube clamp and aspirate for residual stomach contents
• return residual contents to the tube
• wait 2 hours and try again if residual contents are more than 100 ml
• contact the nurse if the residual contents remain high after 2 hours
• position the patient in high Fowler's or sitting position and attach the syringe or feeding tube to the gastrostomy tube
• flush the tube with 50 ml water (more if specifically ordered)
• pour room temperature feeding into the bag or syringe and administer a typical 200 to 500 ml feeding over 30 minutes by gravity or with a feeding pump
• flush the tube with at least 50 ml of water
• detach the syringe or feeding tube, bag, and clamp and wash components with mild soap and warm water.

6. Refer the patient to a nutritionist or dietitian if necessary.

Rationales

1. The patient will tolerate food better when rested and relaxed before eating.

2. The patient can better tolerate food when pain and the threat of nausea or vomiting are minimized.

3. When the patient's mouth is clean, he may find that foods taste better and his appetite increases.

4. The patient is likely to eat more when desirable, high-quality foods are readily available. Because maintaining a high total caloric intake is paramount, the patient should be encouraged to eat as much as possible, even though this may mean including foods that are not highly nutritional.

5. The caregiver must know how to safely administer tube feedings to prevent complications.

6. Professional counsel can help if the patient and caregiver are unable to implement a plan for proper nutrition.

Nursing diagnosis: *Fluid volume deficit related to the effects of cancer or cancer treatment*

GOAL: To maintain normal fluid and electrolyte balance and prevent dehydration

Interventions	Rationales
1. Teach the patient or caregiver how to monitor and record fluid intake and output.	1. An accurate intake and output record is needed to evaluate the patient's hydration status.
2. Assess the patient's skin turgor.	2. Poor skin turgor can indicate dehydration.
3. Assess the patient for dysphagia.	3. The patient's upper GI tract must be intact and functioning to enable adequate fluid ingestion.
4. Encourage the patient to drink 1½ to 2 liters of fluid daily, if tolerated.	4. This is the minimum daily fluid intake needed to maintain adequate hydration.
5. Teach the patient to drink fluids high in electrolytes— such as Gatorade, clear fruit juice, or carbonated beverages—during episodes of nausea or vomiting.	5. These fluids replace electrolytes lost through vomiting.
6. Teach the caregiver to administer antiemetics before and after the patient undergoes chemotherapy or radiation therapy.	6. Antiemetics minimize the nausea and vomiting associated with these treatments.

Nursing diagnosis: *Activity intolerance related to weakness associated with the disease process, treatment modality, or anorexia*

GOAL: To maintain or improve the patient's activity tolerance

Interventions	Rationales
1. Schedule daily rest periods and naps for the patient, as needed. Start with a schedule of resting before meals: 11 a.m. until noon and 4 p.m. until 5 p.m. Add rest periods whenever the patient is fatigued.	1. Resting conserves oxygen and increases the patient's energy level during meals, which may help him eat.
2. Schedule regular exercise for the patient, as his condition permits. For example, have the patient walk as far as he can tolerate three or more times each day— outdoors when possible.	2. Regular exercise, such as walking, improves the patient's cardiovascular, respiratory, musculoskeletal, and mental status.
3. Arrange for the patient to receive appropriate durable medical equipment (DME), such as a walker, wheelchair, or hospital bed.	3. Durable medical equipment can increase the patient's potential for activity.
4. Arrange for the services of a home health aide if needed.	4. A home health aide can help minimize the patient's energy expenditures.
5. As possible, schedule treatments at times when the patient feels most rested.	5. Treatments often cause fatigue. Scheduling treatments when the patient has maximum energy minimizes the likelihood of severe fatigue.

ASSOCIATED CARE PLANS
• Grief and Grieving
• Hospice Care
• Ineffective Coping
• Malnutrition
• Pain
• Smoking Cessation
• Substance Abuse

NETWORKING OF SERVICES
• American Cancer Society
• Cancer Response System
• hospice
• National Cancer Institute
• Comprehensive Cancer Center Network
• civic organizations
• state and local departments of health and social services

- Lifeline
- Meals On Wheels
- DME supplier

CARE TEAM INVOLVED
- nurse
- doctor
- patient and family
- medical social worker
- nutritionist
- clergy
- speech therapist
- occupational therapist
- physical therapist

IMPLICATIONS FOR HOME CARE
- functional features of the home (stairs, location of bathroom and kitchen)
- telephone (communication)

PATIENT EDUCATION TOOLS
- information on how to record fluid intake and output and weight
- information on gastrostomy tube use and safety measures
- information on feeding pump use and safety measures
- American Cancer Society literature

DISCHARGE PLAN FROM HOME HEALTH CARE
Before discharge from home health care, the patient should:
- understand and implement necessary dietary changes and restrictions
- know how to accurately monitor intake and output
- know how to prevent dehydration during episodes of nausea and vomiting
- be participating in a program of regular exercise
- know dates of follow-up doctor appointments
- have the telephone number of the home health agency for follow-up, as needed
- have the telephone number of the emergency department and ambulance service
- have the Lifeline system in place, if appropriate
- be participating in a smoking cessation program, if necessary
- be participating in an alcohol rehabilitation program, if necessary.

SELECTED REFERENCES
Brown, M., Kiss, M., Outlaw, E., and Viamontes, C., eds. *Standards of Oncology Nursing Practice*. New York: John Wiley & Sons, 1985.
Caine, R., and Bufalino, P., eds. *Nursing Care Planning Guides for Adults*. Baltimore: Williams & Wilkins, 1987.
DeMeester, T., and Levin, B., eds. *Cancer of the Esophagus*. Orlando: Grune & Stratton, 1985.
McNally, J., Stair, J., and Somerville, E., eds. *Guidelines for Cancer Nursing Practice*. Orlando: Grune & Stratton, 1985.
Preece, P., Cuschieri, A., and Wellwood, J., eds. *Cancer of the Stomach*. Orlando: Grune & Stratton, 1986.
Siegel, M. *The Cancer Patient's Handbook*. New York: Walker and Company, 1986.
Silverberg, E., Lubera, J., and Garfinkle, L. *Cancer Statistics, 1987/Cancer Clusters*. New York: American Cancer Society, 1987.

GASTROINTESTINAL SYSTEM

Esophagitis

DESCRIPTION AND TIME FOCUS
Esophagitis, an acute or chronic inflammation of the esophageal mucosa, usually is related to an incompetent cardiac sphincter of the stomach. The inflammation produces burning pain that can radiate to the throat and jaw, arms, and back. The patient also may experience recurrent belching, gastroesophageal reflux, and dysphagia from esophageal spasm or edema.

This clinical plan focuses on the patient discharged home after hospitalization for treatment of esophagitis. Patient care centers on the management of dysphagia and gastric reflux. The home health nurse should work with the patient and caregiver to develop a care plan that accommodates the patient's life-style at home.

■ Typical home health care length of service for a patient with uncomplicated esophagitis: 3 weeks

■ Typical visit frequency: Two visits the first week, then weekly visits for 2 weeks

HEALTH HISTORY FINDINGS
In a health history interview, the patient may report many of these findings:
- gastroesophageal reflux
- dysphagia
- heartburn
- weight loss
- exposure to chemical or physical irritants
- smoking
- excessive alcohol use
- history of achalasia
- history of hiatal hernia
- history of gastric or duodenal surgery
- prolonged nasogastric intubation
- chronically poor nutrition

PHYSICAL FINDINGS
In a physical examination, the nurse may detect many of these findings:

Gastrointestinal
- possible melena or hematemesis

Respiratory
- difficulty coughing and removing secretions

General
- weight loss

DIAGNOSTIC STUDIES
The following studies may be performed to evaluate the patient's health status:
- hemoglobin and hematocrit—usually 1 week after hospital discharge, to detect anemia
- serum electrolytes—usually 1 week after discharge, to detect electrolyte imbalances

---

Nursing diagnosis: *Impaired swallowing related to mechanical impairment of the esophagus*

GOAL: To reduce the risk of aspiration and facilitate adequate nutrition

Interventions

1. Assess the patient's ability to swallow; check the cough, gag, and swallow reflexes.

2. Have the patient sit upright with the head flexed slightly forward while eating.

3. Start the patient's food intake with pureed solids and progress gradually to a standard soft diet.

4. Gradually introduce liquids as the patient demonstrates an ability to swallow solids.

5. Encourage the patient to eat small, frequent meals rather than fewer large ones.

6. Encourage the patient to relax and eat slowly.

Rationales

1. This assessment will indicate whether the patient can eat safely. An impaired cough or gag reflex hinders the patient's ability to move secretions to the front of the mouth, which increases the risk of aspiration.

2. Upright positioning allows gravity to aid movement of food down the esophagus. Flexing the neck closes the trachea and reduces the risk of aspiration.

3. The patient will find that solids are easier to swallow than liquids.

4. The ability to swallow decreases the risk of aspiration.

5. Excessive food intake at one sitting can overdistend the stomach and aggravate gastroesophageal reflux.

6. Bolting food increases the risk of aspiration.

7. Have the patient remain in an upright position for 10 to 15 minutes after eating.

7. Maintaining an upright position after eating helps prevent gastroesophageal reflux.

8. Instruct the patient to carefully measure and record body weight weekly.

8. This record will indicate whether the patient is gaining, maintaining, or losing weight.

Nursing diagnosis: *Altered comfort: pain, related to gastric mucosal inflammation and gastroesophageal reflux*

GOAL: To eliminate or minimize inflammation and gastroesophageal reflux

Interventions

1. Teach the patient the importance of remaining in an upright position before, during, and after meals.

2. Teach the patient to avoid eating for 3 hours before bedtime and to sleep with the head elevated.

3. Instruct the patient to avoid spicy foods, citrus juice, coffee, alcohol, and very hot and very cold liquids.

4. Encourage a patient who smokes tobacco to stop.

5. Stress the need to avoid bending, lifting heavy objects, straining during bowel movements, and wearing constrictive clothing.

6. Encourage the patient to take antacids as prescribed.

Rationales

1. Recumbent positioning before, during, and after eating increases intra-abdominal pressure and can aggravate gastroesophageal reflux.

2. These measures can help prevent gastroesophageal reflux during sleep.

3. These foods and liquids can cause physical irritation of the esophageal and stomach lining, which can lead to increased pain.

4. Smoking stimulates increased gastric secretion, which may exacerbate inflammation.

5. These activities decrease esophageal pressure and increase intra-abdominal pressure, which can precipitate gastroesophageal reflux.

6. Antacids increase the pH of stomach contents, which reduces the acidity of gastric juice and minimizes pain and damage to the esophageal mucosa from gastroesophageal reflux.

ASSOCIATED CARE PLANS
• Hiatal Hernia
• Malnutrition
• Pain
• Substance Abuse

NETWORKING OF SERVICES
• durable medical equipment supplier (if patient requires a foam wedge or hospital bed to maintain head elevation during sleep)
• Meals On Wheels

CARE TEAM INVOLVED
• nurse
• patient and family
• nutritionist
• doctor
• homemaker

IMPLICATIONS FOR HOME CARE
• pleasant, relaxed environment that promotes relaxation during eating
• hospital bed to maintain head elevation (foam wedge if condition is temporary)
• adequate kitchen equipment for special diet
• telephone for communication

PATIENT EDUCATION TOOLS
• instructions for proper positioning while eating
• list of foods allowed and foods to avoid
• literature about each prescribed medication, including dosage schedule, interactions, and possible adverse effects

DISCHARGE PLAN FROM HOME HEALTH CARE
Before discharge from home health care, the patient should:

• demonstrate the proper position for eating
• list appropriate foods for the prescribed diet
• know the name, dosage schedule, and adverse effects of each prescribed medication
• explain the importance of eating small, frequent meals
• have the telephone number of the home health agency.

SELECTED REFERENCES

Birmingham, J. *Home Care Planning Based on DRGs: Functional Health Pattern Model*. Philadelphia: Fleschner Publishing Co., 1986.

Carpenito, L. *Nursing Diagnosis: Application to Clinical Practice*, 2nd ed. Philadelphia: J. B. Lippincott Co., 1987.

Hufler, D. "Helping Your Dysphagic Patient Eat," *RN* 50(9):36-38, September 1987.

Loustau, A., and Lee, K. "Dealing with the Dangers of Dysphagia," *Nursing85* 15(2):47-50, February 1985.

Robinson, C., et al. *Normal and Therapeutic Nutrition*, 17th ed. New York: Macmillan Publishing Co., 1986.

Tucker, S., et al. *Patient Care Standards: Nursing Process, Diagnosis and Outcomes*, 4th ed. St. Louis: C.V. Mosby Co., 1988.

Gastroenteritis

DESCRIPTION AND TIME FOCUS
Gastroenteritis is an acute inflammation of the stomach and intestinal mucosa characterized by diarrhea, nausea and vomiting, and abdominal cramping. It has many possible causes, including infection from bacterial, viral, parasitic, or amebic organisms; ingestion of irritating food or drink; and adverse drug reactions.

This clinical plan focuses on the patient discharged home after hospitalization for treatment of gastroenteritis. Patient care centers on relieving symptoms. The home health nurse also must instruct the patient and family in proper techniques for handwashing and food preparation to prevent or limit the spread of infection.

■ Typical home health care length of service for a patient with uncomplicated gastroenteritis: 3 weeks

■ Typical visit frequency: two visits the first week, then one visit weekly for 2 weeks

HEALTH HISTORY FINDINGS
In a health history interview, the patient may report many of these findings:
• intermittent diarrhea
• episodic nausea and vomiting
• abdominal cramping
• history of infection or allergy
• foreign travel within the past year
• chronically poor nutrition
• recent ingestion of contaminated food

PHYSICAL FINDINGS
In a physical examination, the nurse may detect many of these findings:

Gastrointestinal
• hyperactive bowel sounds

Integumentary
• poor skin turgor
• dry mucous membranes
• excoriated buttocks

Renal and urinary
• decreased urine output

General
• debilitated condition
• unexplained weight loss of more than 10 pounds

DIAGNOSTIC STUDIES
The following studies may be ordered to evaluate the patient's health status:
• stool specimen analysis—as needed, to determine type of infection and check for occult blood
• complete blood count (CBC) with differential—as needed, to detect elevated white cell count with infection or elevated hematocrit with dehydration
• serum electrolyte levels—as needed, to check for electrolyte imbalance

---

Nursing diagnosis: *Altered bowel elimination patterns: diarrhea, related to infection or irritating substance in the bowel*

GOAL: To promote passage of formed stools and decreased frequency of bowel movements

Interventions

1. Assess the frequency and consistency of the patient's bowel movements.

2. Encourage the patient to use prescribed antidiarrheal medications, and explain how such medications work.

3. Ensure that the patient takes prescribed anti-infective medications as ordered.

4. Instruct the patient in dietary modifications: fasting until diarrhea subsides (usually for about 12 hours); then clear liquids, progressing to a low-residue diet; and finally a regular diet when stools return to normal.

Rationales

1. This assessment establishes a baseline for determining the patient's progress toward the goal.

2. Antidiarrheal medications help control diarrhea either by decreasing intestinal motility and peristaltic movements or by increasing intestinal absorption of water.

3. Anti-infective medications may be prescribed to destroy the causative agent.

4. The patient will better tolerate a diet that advances gradually. The patient should return to this regimen if symptoms recur.

5. Instruct the patient to avoid milk products.

5. Milk products contain lactose, which aggravates diarrhea.

6. Instruct the patient to perform frequent oral hygiene while fasting.

6. Fasting causes oral mucosal dryness, which can lead to mucosal breakdown and possible infection.

7. Teach the patient measures to prevent anal excoriation, such as cleansing the perianal area thoroughly with mild soap and water after each bowel movement, drying the area completely after cleansing, applying emollient or cream to the area after drying, and using "Tucks" or a similar product to relieve burning and itching.

7. These measures promote comfort and healing and help prevent skin beakdown and possible infection.

Nursing diagnosis: *Fluid volume deficit related to fluid loss from vomiting and diarrhea*

GOAL: To restore normal fluid balance, as evidenced by adequate urine output, good skin turgor, and moist mucous membranes

Interventions

1. Assess the patient's fluid intake, urine output, skin turgor, and mucous membrane hydration.

2. Teach the patient measures to control nausea and vomiting, such as a modified diet and use of antiemetics.

3. Implement a plan to control diarrhea. Promote compliance with diet and medication regimens, and minimize odors by performing meticulous skin care, changing linens regularly, and using a room deodorizer.

4. Encourage the patient to drink 1½ to 2 liters of fluid daily, including oral electrolyte solutions as appropriate.

5. Instruct the patient to measure and record body weight weekly.

Rationales

1. This assessment establishes a baseline for determining the patient's progress toward the goal.

2. Controlling vomiting will enable restoration of fluid balance.

3. Controlling diarrhea minimizes fluid loss through the bowel.

4. Lost fluids and electrolytes must be replenished for restoration of proper hydration and electrolyte balance.

5. Such a record helps track restoration, maintenance, or loss of body weight and the progress of rehydration.

Nursing diagnosis: *Potential for infection related to improper handwashing and food handling*

GOAL: To prevent recurrence or spread of gastroenteritis

Interventions

1. Teach the patient the proper technique for washing hands, and instruct the patient to wash hands thoroughly after using the toilet and before handling food.

2. Teach the patient and caregiver proper methods of food storage and preparation.

3. Instruct the patient to avoid drinking or eating raw (unpasteurized) dairy products.

Rationales

1. These measures reduce the chance of fecal contamination of food.

2. Proper food storage and cooking methods help prevent bacterial contamination of food.

3. Raw dairy products may be high in pathogenic bacteria.

ASSOCIATED CARE PLANS
• Intermittent I.V. Therapy
• Malnutrition
• Substance Abuse

NETWORKING OF SERVICES
• Meals On Wheels

CARE TEAM INVOLVED
• nurse
• patient and family
• nutritionist
• social worker
• physical therapist
• occupational therapist
• doctor

IMPLICATIONS FOR HOME CARE
• functional features of the home (clean food preparation and storage areas, clean and readily accessible bathroom)
• support for patient in meal preparation and light housekeeping
• telephone (communication)

PATIENT EDUCATION TOOLS
• list of diet progression
• list of foods to avoid
• literature for each prescribed medication
• instructions for proper food storage and preparation

DISCHARGE PLAN FROM HOME HEALTH CARE
Before discharge from home health care, the patient should:
• demonstrate a return to normal bowel habits
• return to normal fluid balance
• understand the connection between bacterial contamination and gastroenteritis and the need for cleanliness to minimize contamination
• demonstrate proper hand-washing technique
• describe proper food storage and preparation measures
• verbalize required dietary changes.

SELECTED REFERENCES
Birmingham, J. *Home Care Planning Based on DRGs: Functional Health Pattern Model*. Philadelphia: Fleschner Publishing Co., 1986.
Carpenito, L. *Nursing Diagnosis: Application to Clinical Practice*, 2nd ed. Philadelphia: J. B. Lippincott Co., 1987.
Maresca, J., and Stringari, S. "Assessment and Management of Acute Diarrheal Illness in Adults," *Nurse Practitioner* 11(11):15-28, November 1986.
Robinson, C., et al. *Normal and Therapeutic Nutrition*, 17th ed. New York: Macmillan Publishing Co., 1986.
Sleisenger, M., and Fordtran, J. *Gastrointestinal Disease: Pathophysiology, Diagnosis, and Management*, 3rd ed. Philadelphia: W.B. Saunders Co., 1983.
Tucker, S., et al. *Patient Care Standards: Nursing Process, Diagnosis and Outcomes*, 4th ed. St. Louis: C.V. Mosby Co., 1988.

GASTROINTESTINAL SYSTEM

Herniorrhaphy

DESCRIPTION AND TIME FOCUS

A hernia is the protrusion of an organ, tissue, or structure through the wall of the cavity that normally contains it. Most hernias occur when increased intra-abdominal pressure from coughing or straining forces a structure against a congenital or acquired weakness in a portion of the abdominal musculature.

Herniorrhaphy, the surgery of choice for inguinal and other abdominal hernias, returns the protruding intestine to the abdominal cavity and repairs the abdominal wall defect. Herniorrhaphy is usually an elective procedure that can be done quickly and produces few complications.

This clinical plan focuses on the patient discharged home after undergoing herniorrhaphy. Care for this patient focuses on promoting comfort and healing and monitoring for signs of wound infection and other complications.

■ Typical home health care length of service for a patient with uncomplicated recovery from herniorrhaphy: 2 weeks
■ Typical visit frequency: once or twice weekly

HEALTH HISTORY FINDINGS

In a health history interview, the patient may report one or more of these findings:
• abdominal pain or discomfort
• decreased urination
• constipation

PHYSICAL FINDINGS

In a physical examination, the nurse may detect many of these findings:

Gastrointestinal
• abdominal distention
• decreased or absent bowel sounds

Respiratory
• dyspnea
• crackles

Reproductive (male)
• scrotal swelling

General
• fever
• restlessness
• signs of wound infection

DIAGNOSTIC STUDIES

None applicable to home care.

Nursing diagnosis: *Ineffective breathing pattern related to postoperative pain and inactivity*

GOAL: To promote adequate respiratory function and prevent respiratory complications

Interventions

1. Administer prescribed pain medication as ordered.

2. Teach the patient deep-breathing and coughing exercises and explain their importance. If necessary, give prescribed pain medication approximately 20 minutes before the patient performs these exercises.

3. Teach the patient how to splint the surgical incision site with a pillow or the hands while performing deep-breathing and coughing exercises and when coughing, sneezing, or laughing.

4. Monitor the patient for signs and symptoms of pulmonary complications, such as dyspnea, fever, crackles, and increased restlessness. Report any such signs and symptoms to the doctor immediately.

Rationales

1. Pain control is vital for a patient who has undergone abdominal surgery, who may restrict respiratory effort in an attempt to avoid pain. By facilitating deep breathing, pain relief helps reduce the risk of respiratory complications.

2. These exercises help the patient achieve full lung expansion and clear secretions from respiratory passages.

3. Splinting helps diminish abdominal movement and relieves associated discomfort, enabling greater respiratory effort.

4. Early detection and reporting of such signs and symptoms facilitate prompt intervention to prevent complications.

5. Encourage the patient to walk as soon as the doctor permits. Until that time, have the patient change position every 2 hours.

5. Early ambulation helps reduce the risk of post-operative pulmonary complications by promoting full lung expansion and clearing of secretions.

Nursing diagnosis: *Altered bowel elimination: constipation, related to decreased intestinal peristalsis secondary to abdominal surgery*

GOAL: To restore normal peristaltic action and prevent constipation

Interventions

1. Monitor the return of normal bowel function by:
• assessing bowel sounds at each visit
• instructing the patient or a family member to keep a written record of bowel movements for the first 3 days after discharge from the hospital
• assessing for continued abdominal distention at each visit.

2. Encourage the patient to drink 2½ liters of fluids daily and to eat a normal, high-fiber diet, unless contraindicated.

3. Administer a stool softener or an enema if the patient fails to have a bowel movement within 3 days or within whatever time is normal for the patient.

4. Encourage the patient to walk as soon as possible after surgery.

Rationales

1. Avoiding postoperative constipation decreases the risk of bowel obstruction and enhances the patient's recovery from surgery.

2. Adequate fluid intake helps soften the stool, and a high-fiber diet promotes the return of normal peristalsis—both of which help prevent constipation.

3. Stool softeners and enemas help stimulate peristalsis and resumption of normal bowel activity after surgery.

4. Early ambulation promotes return of normal peristalsis.

Nursing diagnosis: *Altered urinary elimination patterns related to effects of surgery*

GOAL: To prevent or relieve urine retention

Interventions

1. Teach the patient to keep an accurate fluid intake and output record; assess this record on each visit.

2. Teach the patient methods to promote urination, such as walking before attempting to void, standing to void (for a male patient), running tap water, applying warm water to the perineum, performing Crede's maneuver, and ensuring privacy.

3. Instruct the patient to void whenever the urge strikes and not to delay urination, even if urination is painful or difficult.

Rationales

1. An accurate fluid intake and output record facilitates early detection of complications, such as urine retention and fluid and electrolyte imbalance.

2. These measures can help relax the bladder sphincter and promote voiding, precluding the need for catheterization to relieve urine retention.

3. Delaying urination can cause bladder distention and create additional strain on the incision line. It also can cause pooling of urine in the bladder, which may lead to urinary tract infection.

Nursing diagnosis: *Potential for infection related to surgery*

GOAL: To prevent infection and promote healing of the surgical incision

Interventions

1. Each visit, assess the patient for signs and symptoms of wound infection, evisceration, and dehiscence,

Rationales

1. Early detection of wound infection enables prompt intervention, such as antibiotic therapy, to prevent fur-

such as fever persisting for more than 3 days after surgery and increased redness, pain, edema, and drainage at the incision site. Teach the patient and family to recognize and promptly report any of these signs and symptoms.

ther complications, such as dehiscence and evisceration.

2. Teach the patient and family about the need for adequate nutrition and fluid intake during the healing process.

2. Sufficient intake of protein, calories, vitamins and minerals, and fluids is essential to proper wound healing.

3. Teach the patient and family proper aseptic wound care and dressing techniques. (A home health aide may be needed to perform dressing changes if no one in the family can master this technique.)

3. Proper technique can decrease the risk of complications, such as infection from bacterial contamination and impaired circulation from too-tightly applied dressings.

Nursing diagnosis: *Knowledge deficit of self-care measures related to recovery from herniorrhaphy*

GOAL: To provide the patient and family with necessary information to enhance postoperative recovery

Interventions

1. Explain to a male patient that scrotal swelling and discomfort may occur 24 to 48 hours after surgery. Instruct the patient to take analgesics as necessary, apply an ice pack to the scrotal area intermittently to help reduce swelling, and wear an athletic supporter to provide scrotal support.

2. Reinforce the doctor's instructions on activity restrictions and resumption of normal activities. Doctors generally recommend limited activity for 5 to 7 days after herniorrhaphy and avoidance of heavy lifting for 6 to 8 weeks after herniorrhaphy.

3. Teach the patient proper body mechanics and lifting techniques to use after activity restrictions are lifted.

Rationales

1. A well-informed patient is better prepared to effectively cope with problems. Analgesics, ice packs, and scrotal support can help relieve pain and discomfort.

2. Activity restrictions promote healing and help prevent complications.

3. Using proper body mechanics and lifting techniques helps reduce the risk of reinjury.

ASSOCIATED CARE PLANS
• Ineffective Coping
• Pain

NETWORKING OF SERVICES
• Meals On Wheels
• pharmacy

CARE TEAM INVOLVED
• nurse
• patient and family
• home health aide
• doctor

IMPLICATIONS FOR HOME CARE
• telephone (communication)
• safe home environment

PATIENT EDUCATION TOOLS
• written instructions on surgical wound care
• literature on prescribed pain medications, including dosage schedules, possible interactions, and adverse effects

DISCHARGE PLAN FROM HOME HEALTH CARE
Before discharge from home health care, the patient should:
• understand physical limitations and activity restrictions during recovery and know when to resume normal activity
• know the signs and symptoms of complications and understand the need to report them promptly
• know the dates and times of scheduled follow-up doctor appointments
• have the telephone number of the home health agency.

SELECTED REFERENCES

Brunner, L., and Suddarth, D. *Textbook of Medical-Surgical Nursing*, 6th ed. Philadelphia: J.B. Lippincott Co., 1988.

Brunner, L., and Suddarth, D. *The Lippincott Manual of Nursing Practice*, 4th ed. Philadelphia: J.B. Lippincott Co., 1986.

Deters, G. "Managing Complications After Abdominal Surgery," *RN*(3):27-30, March 1987.

Jacobs, M., and Geels, W. *Signs and Symptoms in Nursing: Interpretation and Management*. Philadelphia: J.B. Lippincott Co., 1985.

Krause, M., and Mahan, K. *Food, Nutrition, and Diet Therapy: A Textbook of Nutritional Care*, 7th ed. Philadelphia: J.B. Lippincott Co., 1984.

GASTROINTESTINAL SYSTEM
Hiatal Hernia

DESCRIPTION AND TIME FOCUS
Hiatal hernia occurs when a portion of the stomach protrudes through the diaphragmatic opening (the esophageal hiatus) into the chest cavity. Two basic types of hiatal hernia can develop. In a *sliding* hernia, the most common type, both the stomach and the gastroesophageal junction pass through the esophageal hiatus. In a *rolling* hernia, a section of the fundus and greater curvature of the stomach protrudes through the esophageal hiatus, forming a pouch next to the esophagus.

Usually, hiatal hernia results from enlargement and loosening of the esophageal hiatus caused by congenital weakness, trauma, or a general loss of muscle tone. In such a state, any increase in intra-abdominal pressure (as from pregnancy, abdominal tumor, straining from heavy lifting, constrictive clothing, Valsalva's maneuver, coughing, bending, or obesity) can push the stomach through the enlarged esophageal hiatus.

Symptoms typically do not occur until the lower esophageal sphincter malfunctions. Normally, this sphincter is contracted; however, certain substances—such as alcohol, irritating foods, and tobacco smoke—can affect its operation. When this sphincter relaxes, gastroesophageal reflux occurs.

Possible complications of hiatal hernia include esophagitis, hemorrhage from erosion, stenosis, ulceration of herniated stomach, strangulation of the hernia, and regurgitation with tracheal aspiration. Surgery may be required if herniation progresses or if interventions fail to control the problem.

This clinical plan focuses on the patient at home who has been diagnosed as having hiatal hernia. Care centers on relieving symptoms and preventing or managing complications.

■ Typical home health care length of service for a patient with hiatal hernia: 2 weeks or longer, until symptoms are well controlled

■ Typical visit frequency: once or twice weekly for 2 weeks or until symptoms are controlled

HEALTH HISTORY FINDINGS
In a health history interview, the patient may report many of these findings:
• gradually developing dysphagia relieved only by drinking liquids while swallowing food
• feelings of abdominal fullness
• increased lower chest pain on smoking or on drinking citrus juices, alcohol, or very hot or cold liquids
• frequent belching
• recurring heartburn
• gastroesophageal reflux that feels "hot" or "bitter"
• episodic nausea and vomiting
• unexplained weight loss
• lower chest pain on bending, lifting, coughing, or defecating
• nocturnal cough relieved by antacids or liquids
• chronically poor nutrition
• history of prolonged bedrest

PHYSICAL FINDINGS
In a physical examination, the nurse may detect many of these findings:

Gastrointestinal
• ascites

Respiratory
• signs of respiratory infection (associated with aspiration of gastroesophageal reflux)

Integumentary
• poor skin turgor

General
• obesity

DIAGNOSTIC STUDIES
The following study may be performed to evaluate the patient's health status:
• guaiac testing of stool: periodically, to rule out GI bleeding from esophagitis

---

Nursing diagnosis: *Altered comfort: pain, related to dysphagia and gastroesophageal reflux*

GOAL: To prevent or minimize pain or discomfort from dysphagia and gastroesophageal reflux

Interventions

1. Encourage the patient to eat small, frequent meals rather than fewer large ones.

Rationales

1. Ingestion of large meals increases intra-abdominal pressure, which can aggravate gastroesophageal reflux.

2. Recommend that the patient maintain a low-fat diet.

2. Fatty foods stimulate the release of cholecystokinin, which relaxes the lower esophageal sphincter and increases the chance of reflux.

3. Instruct the patient to avoid spicy foods, alcoholic beverages, chocolate, coffee, and soft drinks containing caffeine.

3. These foods cause the lower esophageal sphincter to relax and increase the likelihood of reflux.

4. Tell the patient to eat slowly, chew food thoroughly, and drink water with meals.

4. These actions soften foods, making them easier to swallow.

5. Instruct the patient to sit upright while eating, to avoid eating for several hours before bedtime, and to avoid lying down for at least 2 hours after meals.

5. These actions enable the action of gravity to help prevent gastroesophageal reflux.

6. Teach the patient methods of preventing constipation, such as eating high-fiber foods and drinking plenty of fluids.

6. Constipation can cause the patient to strain during bowel movements, which increases intra-abdominal pressure and the chance of reflux.

7. If the patient is overweight, recommend safe methods of weight reduction.

7. Obesity increases intra-abdominal pressure.

8. If the patient smokes cigarettes, encourage him to stop. Refer the patient to a smoking cessation class if necessary.

8. Smoking causes the lower esophageal sphincter to relax and increases the likelihood of reflux.

9. Instruct the patient to avoid wearing constrictive clothing and undergarments.

9. Constrictive clothing can increase intra-abdominal pressure.

10. Place blocks under the patient's bed to elevate the head of the bed 6 to 10 inches.

10. Elevating the head of the bed uses gravity to reduce the likelihood of reflux.

11. Ensure that the patient is complying with the prescribed medication regimen, which may include antacids, stool softeners, and histamine$_2$-receptor antagonists (such as cimetidine).

11. Antacids neutralize stomach acids and minimize esophageal irritation when reflux occurs. Stool softeners minimize straining on defecation and help prevent increased intra-abdominal pressure. Histamine$_2$-receptor antagonists decrease the production of hydrochloric acid in the stomach, thus reducing esophageal irritation from reflux.

Nursing diagnosis: *Knowledge deficit related to the nature, possible complications, and management of hiatal hernia*

GOAL: To provide the patient with complete and accurate information about the nature, possible complications, and management of hiatal hernia

Interventions

1. Explain to the patient that hiatal hernia is a chronic disorder, but that proper care can control symptoms and help prevent complications.

2. Review with the patient possible complications of hiatal hernia, such as esophagitis, hemorrhage from erosion, stenosis, ulceration of herniated stomach, strangulation of the hernia, and regurgitation with tracheal aspiration, and the signs and symptoms that may point to such complications, such as increased pain, hematemesis, and progressively severe dysphagia. Stress the importance of promptly reporting these signs and symptoms to the doctor.

Rationales

1. A patient with a chronic disorder must become involved in the care regimen to prevent worsening of symptoms and complications. A well-informed patient is more apt to comply with the care regimen.

2. Complications of hiatal hernia may prove serious and require medical attention. For example, strangulation of the herniated stomach portion can result in gangrene; it requires immediate surgery.

3. Teach the patient the purpose, proper use, and possible adverse effects of all prescribed medications.

3. The patient's knowledge of the purpose, proper use, and possible adverse effects of medications tends to improve compliance with the prescribed medication regimen.

4. Help the patient identify sources of stress in his daily life.

4. Stress increases the production of hydrochloric acid in the stomach, which can exacerbate symptoms related to gastroesophageal reflux.

5. Instruct the patient in stress management techniques, such as exercising regularly, eating nutritious foods, expressing feelings and concerns, getting adequate rest and sleep, and using support systems.

5. Exercise reduces tension, improves muscle tone and posture, controls weight, and promotes relaxation. A proper diet provides the energy needed for effective coping and gives the patient a sense of well-being. Expressing concerns gives the patient a chance to review and resolve issues and facilitates coping. Rest and sleep refresh the body and promote physical and mental relaxation, which enhances coping ability. Adequate support systems, such as family, friends, and church or community groups, can help the patient effectively manage stress.

ASSOCIATED CARE PLANS
• Esophagitis
• Gastroenteritis
• Ineffective Coping
• Smoking Cessation
• Substance Abuse

NETWORKING OF SERVICES
• Meals On Wheels

CARE TEAM INVOLVED
• nurse
• doctor
• patient and family
• social worker

IMPLICATIONS FOR HOME CARE
• functional features of the home (adequate food preparation facilities)
• telephone (communication)
• support person or group

PATIENT EDUCATION TOOLS
• list of dietary recommendations and restrictions
• literature on safe, effective weight loss methods
• literature on smoking cessation methods
• list of prescribed medications and their actions, dosage schedules, and adverse effects
• list of signs and symptoms of possible complications to watch for and report

DISCHARGE PLAN FROM HOME HEALTH CARE
Before discharge from home health care, the patient should:
• understand that the disorder is chronic but can be controlled by proper self-care
• list the effects, dosage schedules, and adverse effects

of all prescribed medications
• understand necessary dietary restrictions and modifications
• understand the importance of losing weight, if necessary, and have a plan for doing so
• recognize the need to quit smoking, if necessary, and have a plan for doing so
• know to sit while eating and for several hours after meals
• know to elevate the head of the bed to prevent reflux
• understand the importance of preventing constipation to eliminate straining during bowel movements and know techniques to prevent or control constipation
• understand the need to avoid lifting heavy objects and bending at the waist
• recognize how stress exacerbates symptoms and be familiar with stress-reduction techniques.

SELECTED REFERENCES
Doenges, M., and Jefferies, M. *Nursing Care Plans*. Philadelphia: F.A. Davis, 1984.
Hufler, D. "Helping Your Dysphagic Patient Eat," *RN* 50(9):36-38, September 1987.
Paternal, E. "A High-Tech Approach to a GI Problem," *RN* (6):44, June 1985.
Robinson, C., and Lawler, M. *Normal and Therapeutic Nutrition*, 17th ed. New York: Macmillan Publishing Co., 1986.
Robinson, M. "Management of Reflux Esophageal Disease," *American Journal of Medicine* 77(5B):106-10, November 1984.
Sweet, K. "Hiatal Hernia," *Nursing83*, 13(12):39-45, December 1983.
Tucker, S., et al. *Patient Care Standards*. St. Louis: C.V. Mosby, 1988.

GASTROINTESTINAL SYSTEM
Colostomy

DESCRIPTION AND TIME FOCUS
Colostomy involves surgical resection of diseased or damaged colonic segments and creation of an opening (stoma) on the outer abdominal wall to allow elimination of feces. The feces, in the form of a semisolid effluent, exits the stoma and is collected in an external pouch. Colostomy is performed when normal intestinal function is no longer possible, as a result of bowel disease or injury. Bowel problems possibly requiring colostomy include colorectal cancer, bowel perforation, colitis, and irritable bowel syndrome. Types of colostomy include end colostomy, double-barreled colostomy, and loop colostomy. Colostomy may be temporary or permanent.

This clinical plan focuses on the patient discharged home after hospitalization for creation of a permanent colostomy. The home provides an ideal recovery setting for this patient. The nurse can assess the patient's progress and provide self-care education in an environment in which the patient feels comfortable and secure.

■ Typical home health care length of service for a patient with a new colostomy: 6 weeks

■ Typical visit frequency: three visits weekly for 2 weeks, two visits weekly for 2 weeks, then one visit weekly for 2 weeks

HEALTH HISTORY FINDINGS
In a health history interview, the patient may report many of these findings:

- recent weight loss
- anorexia
- change in amount or character of fecal effluent
- bloated sensation
- increased flatus

PHYSICAL FINDINGS
In a physical examination, the nurse may detect many of these findings:

Gastrointestinal
- passage of watery effluent through ostomy stoma
- hematochezia
- mucus discharge from stoma
- rectal polyps

Respiratory
- shallow respirations (secondary to pain)
- atelectasis (secondary to inactivity)

Integumentary
- poor skin turgor
- redness and irritation around the ostomy site

Musculoskeletal
- poor muscle tone (secondary to inactivity)

DIAGNOSTIC STUDIES
None applicable

Nursing diagnosis: *Altered bowel elimination related to colostomy*

GOAL: To detect abnormal colostomy discharge and to teach the patient to recognize abnormal colostomy discharge and respond appropriately

Interventions

1. Assess discharged effluent for amount, color, consistency, and frequency.

2. Teach the patient to watch for and report excessively watery effluent, constipation, abnormal stool color, bloody effluent, or the absence of effluent.

Rationales

1. After a colostomy, effluent may be watery, mucoid, and frequent. As healing and adjustment take place, effluent should become brown, semi-soft, less frequent, and more regular.

2. After colostomy, the patient must learn new bowel habits and be aware of possible abnormalities. Because the patient has less bowel to absorb fluid, diarrhea can quickly lead to dehydration. Constipation may require increased fluid intake or possibly colostomy irrigation. Bleeding or the absence of effluent may require medical intervention.

Nursing diagnosis: *Knowledge deficit related to unfamiliarity with colostomy management*

GOAL 1: To teach the patient how to change the ostomy pouch and appliance

Interventions

1. Assess the patient's hospital records to determine the size and appearance of the stoma at the time of discharge, the type and size of appliance used, and the patient's response to care. If possible, consult with the patient's stomal therapist.

2. Store ostomy supplies and equipment in a place convenient for the patient. Let the patient decide where colostomy care will take place.

3. Perform a pouch change while the patient observes. Explain each step while performing the procedure.

4. Gradually transfer responsibility for pouch changing to the patient. Start by having the patient inspect the stoma during each change.

5. Perform the first appliance change slowly; explain each step as you do it. On subsequent changes, use the same technique consistently.

6. Gradually transfer responsibility for appliance change to the patient. Start by letting the patient prepare the materials. Suggest that the patient write down the procedure to use as guide.

7. After teaching is completed, periodically observe while the patient performs the entire pouch and appliance change procedure.

Rationales

1. The patient may have difficulty accepting a colostomy. Self-care instruction often starts in the hospital; transition to home care should be smooth.

2. The patient may regain a sense of control by making decisions about personal care; this sense of control will encourage the patient to participate more fully in colostomy care.

3. A pouch change is the easiest facet of care to learn. Observing the patient's response to this procedure will help in planning additional teaching.

4. The patient may find learning to perform colostomy care easier and less threatening when the procedure is broken down into discrete steps.

5. Technique consistency prevents confusion and helps the patient become familiar with the steps of the procedure.

6. Transferring responsibility one step at a time lets the patient become confident with one task before moving on to the next. Writing down the procedure reinforces learning, promotes a sense of control, and demonstrates the patient's understanding.

7. Occasional observation allows the nurse to detect incorrect techniques and make corrections.

GOAL 2: To teach the patient to care for the stoma and surrounding skin and to watch for and report stomal complications

Interventions

1. Teach the patient how to inspect and care for the stoma and surrounding skin.

2. Teach the patient the signs of stomal complications, such as a change in color or a break in the tissue. Explain the importance of promptly reporting such signs to the home health agency or doctor.

Rationales

1. Stoma and skin irritation often result from fecal contamination of skin or a hypersensitivity reaction to appliance adhesives. Because the patient will be responsible for skin care as long as the colostomy exists, teaching efforts in this area will have long-term benefits to the patient.

2. A change in the color of the stoma may indicate loss of blood supply and requires rapid assessment and intervention. Breaks in stomal tissue can provide a route for infection.

Nursing diagnosis: *Activity intolerance related to loss of muscle tone or postoperative restrictions*

GOAL: To maximize the patient's activity tolerance within the limits of postoperative restrictions

Interventions	Rationales
1. Assess the patient's activity tolerance during each visit. Watch for such indications of intolerance as fatigue, dyspnea, rapid respirations, or a reluctance to walk.	1. Activity tolerance varies among colostomy patients. Ongoing assessment will help the nurse plan a realistic activity program for the patient and alter the program as the patient's activity tolerance increases.
2. Observe for and explain possible complications of limited activity, such as respiratory or circulatory problems.	2. Normal activity is restricted after surgery, placing the patient at risk for complications of immobility, such as atelectasis and phlebitis.
3. Assess the patient's compliance with any prescribed activity restrictions. Explain the importance of not lifting or carrying heavy loads.	3. A patient who has undergone major surgery must comply with all routine postoperative restrictions.
4. Evaluate the patient's home for obstacles to activities of daily living (ADLs). Help the patient and family make necessary adjustments.	4. Such factors as a significant distance between the patient's bedroom and bathroom and the presence of stairs may represent obstacles for the patient returning from the hospital.
5. With the patient's help, plan to gradually increase activity each day. Suggest that the patient conserve energy by separating tasks usually performed together, such as bathing and dressing, into individual tasks performed at different times during the day—for example, dressing in the morning and bathing in the evening. If necessary, arrange for a home health aide to assist the patient with ADLs.	5. Gradually increasing activity improves the patient's endurance and muscle tone. Spacing ADLs throughout the day helps the patient conserve energy and feel more productive.

Nursing diagnosis: *Impaired home maintenance management related to patient recuperation*

GOAL: To facilitate safe home maintenance by adapting the home environment

Interventions	Rationales
1. Evaluate the patient's home for overall safety, location of telephones, need for stair climbing, and accessibility of bathroom and kitchen. Suggest necessary modifications.	1. The home may have to be adapted to accommodate the patient's ability to perform ADLs. A safe and convenient home environment can increase the patient's independence.
2. Evaluate the patient's need for financial assistance, equipment, and community resources. Refer the patient to a social worker if necessary.	2. The patient may need financial assistance and help with such tasks as meal preparation, transportation, and obtaining equipment and supplies. A social worker can help the patient contact social service agencies, which may be able to provide needed assistance to help the patient remain at home.

Nursing diagnosis: *Altered self-concept related to loss of control over fecal elimination, flatus, and odor*

Goal: To promote a positive self-image by enhancing the patient's sense of control

Interventions	Rationales
1. Encourage the patient to ask questions and express feelings about the colostomy and self-care. Answer the	1. When home and faced with the prospect of dealing with a colostomy every day, the patient's anger may

patient's questions as honestly and completely as possible and maintain a calm, matter-of-fact attitude.

2. Help the patient choose comfortable and functional clothing.

3. Assure the patient that the ostomy need not interfere with an active life-style, including sexual activity and most occupations. If possible, enlist the aid of a local ostomates group.

4. Instruct the patient in measures to control flatus through the stoma: avoiding gas-producing foods, such as cabbage, legumes, fresh yeast, cauliflower, onions, and carbonated beverages; consuming gas-inhibiting foods, such as yogurt and cranberry juice; and avoiding activities that increase air swallowing, such as smoking, mouth-breathing, and talking while eating.

5. Teach the patient odor-control measures: avoiding odor-producing foods, such as eggs, fish, asparagus, mushrooms, onions, and garlic; eating odor-inhibiting foods, such as spinach, lettuce, parsley, yogurt, and cranberry juice; and using a pouch deodorant—either a commercial product or baking soda or powdered charcoal.

peak. The nurse must help the patient deal with emotions.

2. The patient may worry that the ostomy pouch is noticeable; appropriate clothing can help alleviate this concern.

3. Such assurance and the support of other ostomates can help the patient regain a positive self-image.

4. These measures may help control flatus and give the patient a greater sense of control over bowel function.

5. These measures can reduce embarrassing odor and give the patient a greater sense of control and self-confidence.

ASSOCIATED CARE PLANS
• Ineffective Coping
• Pain
• Sex and Sexuality

NETWORKING OF SERVICES
• durable medical equipment supplier
• Meals On Wheels
• ostomates support group

CARE TEAM INVOLVED
• nurse
• doctor
• patient and family
• medical social worker
• home health aide
• enterostomal therapist
• clinical dietitian

IMPLICATIONS FOR HOME CARE
• functional features of the home (stairs, location of bathroom and kitchen)
• telephone (communication)
• financial resources to purchase ostomy supplies

PATIENT EDUCATION TOOLS
• written instructions for pouch and appliance changing technique
• list of signs of ostomy complications that must be reported to the doctor

DISCHARGE PLAN FROM HOME HEALTH CARE
Before discharge from home health care, the patient should:
• demonstrate how to change the ostomy pouch and appliance
• demonstrate how to perform peristomal skin care
• understand suggested diet modifications
• understand the need to increase activity gradually
• have the phone numbers of the home health agency, doctor, and ambulance service prominently posted
• know about available community resources and support groups
• know the times and dates of follow-up doctor appointments and have transportation available
• understand the signs of possible complications and the need to report these promptly
• have a list of sources of ostomy supplies and equipment.

SELECTED REFERENCES

Birmingham, J. *Home Care Planning Based on DRGs*. Philadelphia: J.B. Lippincott Co., 1986.

Broadwell, D., and Jackson, B. *Principles of Ostomy Care*. St. Louis: C.V. Mosby Co., 1982.

Eliopoulos, C. *A Guide to the Nursing of the Aged*. Baltimore: Williams & Wilkins Co., 1987.

Groenwald, S. *Cancer Nursing Principles and Practice*. Boston: Jones and Barlett Publishers, 1987.

Iyer, P., Taptich, B., and Bernocchi-Losey, D. *Nursing Process and Nursing Diagnosis*. Philadelphia: W.B. Saunders Co., 1986.

Hepatitis

DESCRIPTION AND TIME FOCUS

Hepatitis is an inflammatory process in the liver characterized by liver cell destruction, necrosis, and autolysis, leading to anorexia, jaundice, and hepatomegaly. Viral hepatitis is caused by type A (infectious), B (serum), or non-A, non-B virus. Nonviral hepatitis (toxic or drug-induced) is caused by exposure to certain chemicals or drugs.

This clinical plan focuses on the patient discharged home from an acute-care hospital after diagnosis, management, and treatment of hepatitis or on the patient cared for in the home without hospitalization. Care centers on strengthening the patient's body to withstand the infection, relieving symptoms, and making the patient comfortable. The patient's home provides an excellent environment for healing and allows the nurse to monitor the patient for such complications as dehydration, hepatic coma, or neurologic complications and to provide patient and family teaching.

■ Typical home health care length of service for a patient with hepatitis: 4 weeks

■ Typical visit frequency: twice weekly

HEALTH HISTORY FINDINGS

In a health history interview, the patient may report many of these findings:
• pain over liver
• abdominal tenderness
• dyspnea on exertion
• pruritus
• joint pain
• anorexia
• headache
• fatigue
• history of I.V. drug use
• history of alcohol abuse
• history of blood transfusions
• ingestion of contaminated food, water, or milk

PHYSICAL FINDINGS

In a physical examination, the nurse may detect many of these findings:

Gastrointestinal
• bleeding gums
• hepatomegaly
• splenomegaly
• nausea and vomiting
• rectal bleeding
• diarrhea
• tarry stools
• clay-colored stools
• flatulence
• bile obstruction

Respiratory
• shallow respirations
• pharyngitis
• cough

Integumentary
• ecchymosis
• urticaria
• yellowish skin and sclera
• poor skin turgor
• dry mucous membranes
• enlarged lymph nodes
• pruritus

Renal and urinary
• decreased urinary output
• dark urine
• blood in urine

General
• fever (100° to 101° F.)
• abdominal pain in right upper quadrant
• moderate weight loss

DIAGNOSTIC STUDIES

The following studies may be performed to evaluate the patient's health status:
• anti-HAV antibody—presence of anti-HAV confirms diagnosis of type A hepatitis
• hepatitis B surface antigen—during incubation and first 3 weeks of acute infection; after 3 weeks, may get false-negative results; presence of hepatitis B surface antigen (HBsA) and hepatitis B antibodies (antibodies HBs) confirms a diagnosis of type B hepatitis
• liver enzymes: aspartate aminotransferase (AST, formerly SGOT), lactic dehydrogenase (LDH), alanine aminotransferase (ALT, formerly SGPT), alkaline phosphates—every 3 days for 1 to 2 weeks, then decrease to once weekly until normal
• serum bilirubin—usually once each week, then decrease to once every 2 weeks until normal
• prothrombin time (PT)—usually once each week, then decrease to once every 2 weeks until normal

Nursing diagnosis: *Potential for infection related to contact with others*

GOAL: To prevent the spread of the hepatitis virus

Interventions

1. Teach the patient methods of preventing disease dissemination, such as not donating blood, using a condom during sexual activity, covering cuts and oozing sores, and not sharing items that may be contaminated with blood or body fluids, such as razors and toothbrushes.

2. Instruct the patient to inform doctors, dentists, nurses, and other health-care personnel of his hepatitis status.

3. Ask the patient to name anyone with whom he has come into recent contact. Encourage the family and others having close contact to see a doctor for hepatitis testing and prophylaxis.

4. Instruct the patient to dispose of tissues, menstrual pads, and tampons in closed paper bags for burning. Containers should be well marked.

Rationales

1. The virus is transmitted parenterally in blood, serum, or plasma. Hepatitis patients can become chronic carriers, capable of spreading the disease indefinitely.

2. When health-care personnel know of the disease, they can take protective measures.

3. An injection of gamma globulin is 80% to 90% effective in preventing type A hepatitis in contacts. The injection should be given to high-risk contacts as soon as possible after exposure and certainly within 2 weeks after jaundice appears in the patient. Immunoglobulin contains low titers of antibody against hepatitis B, which probably transmits some passive protection. A combination of hepatitis B vaccine and hepatitis B immune globulin currently offers the best protection after exposure to hepatitis B.

4. The virus is in the patient's bloodstream and can be transmitted on menstrual pads and tampons. The virus has also been found in saliva, semen, urine, bile, tears, vaginal secretions, and breast milk.

Nursing diagnosis: *Altered nutrition: less than body requirements related to nausea, vomiting, or anorexia*

GOAL: To maintain adequate hydration and nutrition and to prevent nausea and vomiting

Interventions

1. Administer antiemetics (such as trimethobenzamide or benzquinamide) or corticosteroids, as ordered.

2. Instruct the patient to eat small, frequent meals throughout the day, or suggest a large breakfast if anorexia worsens later in the day. Encourage well-balanced meals that include the patient's food preferences.

3. Recommend that the patient maintain a diet high in protein and carbohydrates.

4. Advise the patient to eat in a sitting position.

5. Assess the patient's intake and output.

Rationales

1. Antiemetics help control nausea and vomiting, allowing the patient to eat to maintain nutritional status. Corticosteroids may be given for severe hepatitis to stimulate appetite and decrease itching and inflammation.

2. Small, frequent meals are usually better tolerated and less likely to exacerbate nausea. Well-balanced meals that include some of the patient's favorite foods promote adequate nutrition while stimulating appetite.

3. The body requires increased amounts of protein to repair and rebuild liver tissue. Carbohydrates provide glycogens and additional calories.

4. A sitting position decreases abdominal tenderness and feelings of fullness.

5. Fluid balance can be assessed by comparing the volume of fluid ingested to the volume of urine.

6. Encourage the patient to use a mouthwash before meals.

6. A mouthwash can remove unpleasant tastes that inhibit appetite.

7. Encourage the patient to drink at least 3 liters of fluid daily. Offer fruit juice, chipped ice, and soft drinks.

7. Adequate fluid intake reduces the risk of dehydration, which can lead to hepatic coma. Fruit juice, chipped ice, and soft drinks help maintain adequate hydration without inducing vomiting.

Nursing diagnosis: *Knowledge deficit related to the disease process and treatment*

GOAL: To teach the patient and family about the nature of hepatitis and its treatment

Interventions

1. Explain the pathophysiology of hepatitis and the specifics of treatment to the patient and family. Tell them how the disease was contracted, and review medications to be used, their purpose, and adverse effects. Explain that disease management consists largely of treating symptoms and supporting the patient during convalescence.

2. Encourage the patient and family to express fears and other feelings they may have concerning the disease or treatment.

Rationales

1. The patient and family probably lack knowledge about hepatitis. Treatment success depends on their understanding of the situation and their willingness to adhere to the treatment regimen.

2. For a therapeutic plan to be effective, the nurse must understand how the patient and family view the disease and clarify misconceptions they may have about treatment. The nurse can encourage discussion by generating a warm, caring, honest, and reassuring attitude.

Nursing diagnosis: *Activity intolerance related to fatigue and weakness resulting from decreased liver metabolism*

GOAL: To increase the patient's activity tolerance

Interventions

1. Have the patient maintain bed rest for 2 to 3 weeks before increasing activity.

2. Plan adequate rest periods during the patient's waking hours. Have the patient nap at least 2 hours daily.

3. Evaluate the patient's sleep patterns to facilitate rest.

4. Assess the patient for clammy skin, dizziness, and dyspnea, and have him report all dyspneic episodes.

5. Teach the patient relaxation techniques, such as music therapy, watching television, reading, or working with his hands.

Rationales

1. Rest limits the demands made on the body and increases the blood supply to the liver, giving the liver an opportunity to regenerate and repair itself.

2. Adequate rest increases endurance, which in turn improves activity tolerance.

3. Poor sleep patterns increase fatigue. Sleep promotes healing of injured tissue.

4. Clammy skin, dizziness, and dyspnea are signs and symptoms of increased fatigue. When the patient experiences few or no episodes of dyspnea on exertion, his normal functions are returning.

5. Noninvasive relaxation techniques help reduce stress and foster feelings of calm and well-being.

Nursing diagnosis: *Altered comfort: pain, related to liver enlargement and pruritus*

Goal: To alleviate pain

Interventions	Rationales
1. Bathe or sponge the patient's skin with tepid water and then apply oil-based lotion at least once daily.	1. These actions soothe the skin and help relieve itching.
2. Help the patient get to sleep by providing a back rub, offering a warm beverage, or suggesting a more comfortable sleeping position.	2. Many sleep medications are toxic to the liver; restlessness must be alleviated by nursing interventions.

ASSOCIATED CARE PLANS
• Chronic Congestive Heart Failure
• Chronic Renal Failure
• Grief and Grieving
• Hepatitis
• Hospice Care
• Ineffective Coping
• Malnutrition

NETWORKING OF SERVICES
• Council on Aging
• Medicaid-sponsored community care, if patient is eligible
• Meals On Wheels
• American Liver Foundation, 998 Pompton Avenue, Cedar Grove, N.J., 07009, 1-800-223-0179

CARE TEAM INVOLVED
• nurse
• doctor
• patient and family
• medical social worker
• nursing assistants

IMPLICATIONS FOR HOME CARE
• telephone (communication)
• functional features of the home

PATIENT EDUCATION TOOLS
• literature for each prescribed medication, including dosage, interactions, and possible adverse effects
• written dietary instructions
• literature about hepatitis

DISCHARGE PLAN FROM HOME HEALTH CARE
Before discharge from home health care, the patient should:
• understand necessary activity restrictions
• demonstrate proper personal hygiene
• know to avoid alcohol for at least 1 year
• understand necessary dietary modifications

• know not to donate blood
• know the signs and symptoms of recurrence and understand the importance of immediately reporting them
• understand the importance of avoiding persons with infections, especially upper respiratory infections
• know the dates and times of scheduled doctor or laboratory appointments
• know the dosage, interactions, and adverse effects of each prescribed medication
• know to check with the doctor before using over-the-counter medications
• have the telephone number of the home health agency for follow-up, if needed.

SELECTED REFERENCES
Merck Manual of Diagnosis and Therapy. Rahway, N.J.: Merck & Co., 1987.
Professional Guide to Diseases, 3rd ed. Springhouse, Pa.: Springhouse Corporation, 1989.
Tucker, S. *Patient Care Standards*, 4th ed. St. Louis: C.V. Mosby Co., 1989.
"Update on Heptatitis B Prevention," *Morbidity and Mortality Weekly Report* 36(23):1-4, July 19, 1987.
Vargo, J. "Viral Hepatitis: How to Protect Patients and Yourself," *RN* 47(7):22-29, July 1984 .

GASTROINTESTINAL SYSTEM

Cirrhosis

DESCRIPTION AND TIME FOCUS

Cirrhosis is a chronic hepatic disorder characterized by progressive fibrosis of liver tissue. Widespread fibrosis eventually obstructs hepatic blood flow and leads to tissue necrosis, which results in irreversible liver damage. Cirrhosis occurs twice as often in men than in women; alcoholics are especially susceptible. Mortality is high—in fact, cirrhosis trails only cardiovascular disease and cancer as a cause of death in persons ages 45 to 65.

This clinical plan focuses on the patient who has been discharged home from an acute care setting after diagnosis and treatment of cirrhosis that has resulted in some degree of irreversible liver damage. Patient care focuses on maintaining liver function for as long as possible, preventing infection and other complications, and helping the patient cope with life-style adjustments.

■ Typical home health care length of service for a patient with cirrhosis: 6 weeks

■ Typical visit frequency: twice weekly for 3 weeks, then once weekly for 3 weeks

HEALTH HISTORY FINDINGS

In a health history interview, the patient may report many of these findings:
• weakness and fatigue
• nausea
• hematemesis
• diarrhea or constipation
• hematochezia
• chronic dyspepsia
• chronic gastritis
• anorexia
• amenorrhea and possibly decreased fertility in females
• alcoholism
• history of malnutrition
• history of significant exposure to carbon tetrachloride, phosphorus, or other chemicals
• previous infection with hepatitis virus
• history of I.V. drug abuse

PHYSICAL FINDINGS

In a physical examination, the nurse may detect many of these findings:

Gastrointestinal
• ascites
• hepatomegaly
• decreased bowel sounds
• splenomegaly

Respiratory
• dyspnea on exertion
• orthopnea

Neurologic
• confusion
• disorientation
• asterixis

Integumentary
• thin skin
• yellowish skin and sclera
• xanthomas
• spider nevi
• massive dependent edema or anasarca

Musculoskeletal
• muscle wasting in legs

Reproductive
• signs of hypogonadism and possibly feminization in males

Renal and urinary
• oliguria
• dark amber urine
• hematuria

Hematologic
• easy bruising
• bleeding gums

DIAGNOSTIC STUDIES

The following studies may be performed to evaluate the patient's health status:
• serum bilirubin—to evaluate liver function
• aspartate aminotransferase (AST, formerly SGOT), alanine aminotransferase (ALT, formerly SGPT), lactic dehydrogenase (LDH)—to monitor disease progress and prognosis
• serum albumin—to evaluate liver function
• prothrombin time (PT)—to evaluate clotting factors
• complete blood count (CBC)—to detect anemia, thrombocytopenia, or leukopenia
• plasma glucose—to evaluate liver function
• serum ammonia—to monitor disease progress and detect developing complications
Note: These studies typically are performed weekly until results reflect adequate function.

Nursing diagnosis: *Potential for injury: GI hemorrhage, related to altered clotting factors secondary to liver disease*

Goal: To reduce the risk of GI hemorrhage

Interventions

1. Instruct the patient to use an electric razor and to avoid aspirin, vigorous toothbrushing, straining during bowel movements, and foods that irritate the gastric mucosa—such as excessively salty or spicy foods.

2. Obtain baseline laboratory data from the patient's chart and maintain a copy of all laboratory records.

3. Assess the patient for indications of GI bleeding, such as tarry stools, hematemesis, tachycardia, decreased blood pressure, pallor, and pale mucous membranes.

4. Teach the patient and caregiver the signs and symptoms of GI hemorrhage, such as tarry stools and hematemesis, and instruct them to immediately report any such signs or symptoms.

Rationales

1. Clotting factor deficiency makes major and occult GI hemorrhage a constant concern. The patient must realize that these strict precautions are necessary to prevent GI bleeding.

2. Laboratory results provide a complete picture of the patient's anemia and clotting factor status.

3. A systematic assessment during each visit will alert the nurse to subtle changes in the patient's condition and enable prompt intervention to prevent serious problems.

4. GI hemorrhage can progress rapidly from onset to a life-threatening condition. The patient or caregiver must take immediate action if such signs and symptoms develop.

Nursing diagnosis: *Fluid volume deficit related to changes in serum osmolarity or osmolality or to electrolyte imbalance*

Goal: To stabilize intravascular fluid volume and minimize edema

Interventions

1. Each visit, assess the patient's weight, abdominal girth, and degree of dependent edema. Assess for urinary or cardiovascular signs and symptoms of reduced vascular volume.

2. Obtain baseline data (weight, degree of edema, abdominal girth) from the patient's hospital chart.

3. Teach the patient about the proper use of prescribed diuretics, weight monitoring, and fluid restrictions. Explain the rationales for these interventions.

Rationales

1. Liver dysfunction promotes the movement of fluid from the vascular bed to the tissue spaces (third-space shifting). An increase in edema may indicate low vascular volume.

2. Baseline data are essential to detecting variances that require intervention.

3. The patient may have trouble understanding that edema indicates fluid volume loss. This understanding may improve compliance with treatment.

Nursing diagnosis: *Ineffective breathing patterns related to massive ascites*

GOAL: To promote adequate ventilation

Interventions

1. Monitor the patient's lung sounds during each visit. Immediately report any indication of respiratory infection, atelectasis, or pulmonary edema, such as dyspnea, chest pain, wheezing, and productive cough.

Rationales

1. Massive ascites alters breathing patterns, resulting in shallow respiration and increasing the risk of infection or atelectasis. The massive shift of fluid and electrolytes may cause congestive heart failure or pulmonary edema.

2. Teach the patient to enhance ventilation by assuming comfortable positions, such as lying with the head and shoulders elevated 45 degrees, lying on one side, or sitting in a reclining chair rather than a straight-back chair.

2. Massive ascites elevates the diaphragm and inhibits lung expansion. These positions reduce diaphragmatic pressure, which allows better lung expansion and enhanced gas exchange.

3. Teach the patient how to conserve energy and minimize dyspnea during activities of daily living (ADLs). Also teach the patient slow, deep-breathing techniques.

3. Conserving energy and using breathing techniques reduces the patient's oxygen demand, thereby minimizing dyspnea and promoting independence.

Nursing diagnosis: *Altered nutrition: less than body requirements, related to anorexia, nausea, and problems with dietary compliance*

GOAL: To ensure adequate nutrition within prescribed dietary restrictions

Interventions

1. Instruct the patient to eat small, frequent meals, rest before and after eating, and use prescribed antiemetic medications appropriately. Encourage the caregiver to create a pleasant, relaxed eating environment for the patient.

2. When teaching the patient and caregiver about prescribed diet modifications, take into consideration the patient's usual dietary habits and favorite foods and any limitations imposed by poor food storage and meal preparation facilities. Allow appropriate choices and options to decrease the patient's resistance to necessary dietary modifications.

Rationales

1. Resting before meals, maintaining a pleasant eating environment, and eating small portions can help stimulate appetite. Antiemetic medications decrease nausea and may increase the patient's ability and desire to eat.

2. Taking into account the patient's food preferences and the household's facilities for food storage and preparation helps the nurse plan an effective and workable diet regimen. Involving the patient in diet planning tends to improve patient compliance with diet modifications.

Nursing diagnosis: *Potential for impaired tissue integrity related to edema, limited mobility, and poor tissue turgor*

GOAL: To maintain skin integrity

Interventions

1. Each visit, thoroughly assess the patient's skin and document any abnormalities, such as redness or pressure ulcers.

2. Teach the patient and caregiver preventive skin care: keeping skin dry, avoiding prolonged pressure on an area, and thoroughly examining the skin daily, paying particular attention to the perirectal area.

3. Teach the patient and caregiver the signs of skin breakdown and when to notify the nurse or doctor of such signs.

Rationales

1. Patients with cirrhosis are at risk for skin breakdown resulting from edema, limited mobility, and poor nutrition. Detailed documentation of changes and abnormalities enables effective interventions.

2. Prevention of skin breakdown is the best treatment, and requires constant attention. The perirectal area is especially prone to breakdown in patients with cirrhosis.

3. The potential for skin breakdown is a problem that will persist after the patient no longer is a client of the home care agency. The patient and caregiver must assume responsibility for detecting and reporting significant skin problems.

Nursing diagnosis: *Disturbed self-concept: body image, related to rapid physical changes associated with cirrhosis*

GOAL: To promote the patient's acceptance of his altered body image

Intervention	Rationale
Teach the patient about the physical changes associated with cirrhosis, such as ascites, jaundice, weight loss, edema, and bleeding tendencies. Encourage the patient to express emotions, especially anger, about radical changes. Suggest ways to adapt, such as changes in clothing and footwear.	Ascites, muscle wasting, anasarca, and jaundice significantly alter the patient's appearance and serve as constant reminders of the disease process. An understanding of these changes and an accepting attitude can ease the patient's adjustment.

Nursing diagnosis: *Impaired home maintenance management related to chronic progressive disease*

Goal: To provide a safe, comfortable environment with adequate support systems

Interventions	Rationales
1. Assess the patient's home for safety, comfort, and convenience. Recommend changes to promote energy conservation, such as use of a bedside commode, an overbed table, and grab bars in the bathroom.	1. Patients with cirrhosis have limited endurance and require areas for resting, eating, and bathing in close proximity on one floor.
2. Evaluate the patient's need for durable medical equipment (DME), such as a hospital bed, bedside commode, or home oxygen, if ordered. Help the patient arrange for delivery of necessary equipment.	2. Specific equipment may be needed to help the patient conserve energy and to ensure patient safety.
3. Evaluate the patient's need for support systems—such as Alcoholics Anonymous (AA), church groups, or hospice care—and financial assistance. Refer the patient to a medical social worker or appropriate social service agencies as needed.	3. Cirrhosis is a chronic and debilitating disease. Additional support can relieve the patient's anxiety concerning household tasks.
4. Evaluate the caregiver's need for support and provide referrals as necessary.	4. During the course of the disease, the caregiver's role becomes more demanding. Assistance and support helps the caregiver maintain effective patient care.

ASSOCIATED CARE PLANS
- Chronic Congestive Heart Failure
- Chronic Renal Failure
- Grief and Grieving
- Hepatitis
- Hospice Care
- Ineffective Coping
- Malnutrition

NETWORKING OF SERVICES
- Lifeline
- DME supplier
- local AA chapter
- respiratory therapy, if oxygen is ordered
- hospice

CARE TEAM INVOLVED
- nurse
- doctor
- patient and family
- medical social worker
- home health aide
- dietitian

IMPLICATIONS FOR HOME CARE
- functional features of the home (location of kitchen and bathroom)
- telephone (communication)

PATIENT EDUCATION TOOLS
• literature about the disease process
• nutritional and dietary guidelines
• list of support groups for alcoholics
• information on energy conservation measures
• list of the signs and symptoms of complications

DISCHARGE PLAN FROM HOME HEALTH CARE
Before discharge from home health care, the patient should:
• understand the dosage schedule and adverse effects of each prescribed medication
• be maintaining a desirable weight with minimal daily variance
• have no active bleeding
• know about major complications, the signs and symptoms of complications, and appropriate responses
• understand skin care, dyspnea management, and energy conservation measures
• understand dietary restrictions and necessary meal planning adjustments
• have emergency phone numbers conveniently posted
• know the dates and times of scheduled follow-up doctor and laboratory appointments
• have phone numbers of applicable community service organizations
• demonstrate effective coping with the chronic nature of the disease.

SELECTED REFERENCES
Birmingham, J. *Home Care Planning Based on DRGs.* Philadelphia: J.B. Lippincott Co., 1986.
Eliopoulos, C. *A Guide to the Nursing of the Aged.* Baltimore: Williams & Wilkens Co., 1987.
Iyer, P., Taptich, B., and Bernocchi-Losey, D. *Nursing Process and Nursing Diagnosis.* Philadelphia: W.B. Saunders Co., 1986.
Larocca, F., ed. *Eating Disorders.* San Francisco: Jassey-Bass Inc., 1986.
Thompson, J., et al. *Clinical Nursing.* St. Louis: C.V. Mosby Co., 1986.
Walsh, J., Persons, C., and Wieck, L. *Manual of Home Health Care Nursing.* Philadelphia: J.B. Lippincott Co., 1987.

INTEGUMENTARY SYSTEM

Psoriasis

DESCRIPTION AND TIME FOCUS
Psoriasis is a chronic, noninfectious, inflammatory, abnormal skin condition resulting from hyperplasia of the keratinocytes in the skin's epidermal layer. Onset usually occurs early in adulthood, although it can occur at any age.

Although the cause of psoriasis is not known, genetic factors may influence mitosis and the rate of cell proliferation, causing skin replacement at an excessive rate. Epidermal turnover time—the time required for a cell to move from the basal layer of the epidermis to the surface—is reduced from 28 days to 3 or 4 days because of increased mitotic activity in the basal cell layer. Skin thickening may not be uniform, and desquamation may be inconsistent. Scaling occurs as the proliferating cells die and flake off.

This clinical plan focuses on home care of the patient with psoriasis. The condition requires ongoing, aggressive treatment of topical therapy to clear psoriatic lesions. Systemic therapy usually is reserved for severe cases that resist topical therapy. Care centers on keeping psoriasis in remission. Effective treatment can minimize the disease's long-term psychosocial effects. The nurse teaches the patient about the disease and treatment regimen and monitors the patient's compliance.

■ Typical home health care length of service for a patient with psoriasis: varies from 1 to 4 weeks

■ Typical visit frequency: initially, once or twice weekly, then once weekly until discharge

HEALTH HISTORY FINDINGS
In a health history interview, the patient may report many of these findings:

• family history of psoriasis or psoriatic arthritis
• bilaterally symmetrical lesions on knees, elbows, sacrum, scalp, ears, eyebrows, forehead, gluteal cleft, nails, or trunk

PHYSICAL FINDINGS
In a physical examination, the nurse may detect many of these findings:

Integumentary
• ichthyosis
• red, elevated, well-marginated plaques and papules
• silvery-white scale on plaques and papules
• lesion scaling
• Koebner's phenomenon
• erythema or fissuring in intergluteal area
• fingernail or toenail abnormalities (pitting, scaling, subungual keratotic material, ridging and furrowing, alteration in nail transparency, onycholysis, nail destruction)

Musculoskeletal
• psoriatic arthritis in distal interphalangeal joints
• juxta-articular bone destruction

DIAGNOSTIC STUDIES
The following study may be performed to evaluate the patient's health status:
• complete blood count (CBC) with differential—initially to monitor for signs of infection

---

Nursing diagnosis: *Impaired skin integrity related to skin lesions and other changes in skin condition associated with psoriasis*

GOAL: To maintain the patient's skin integrity

Interventions

1. Assess the patient's life-style. Identify activities or habits that may increase the risk of skin impairment.

2. Explain psoriasis to the patient, emphasizing remission and exacerbation patterns.

3. Monitor the patient's skin status during each visit. Inspect and palpate the patient's skin at regular intervals,

Rationales

1. Psoriatic plaques are covered with a thick, silvery scale. The skin beneath is thinly stretched and easily injured.

2. For no known reason, the condition can improve or worsen at any time. Knowledge of psoriasis and its recurring patterns helps the patient cope more effectively with the disease.

3. Psoriatic lesions on the soles and palms may develop into deep, painful vesicular and pustular fissures.

paying particular attention to the patient's soles and palms to identify fissure sites, which can be particularly painful. Teach the patient protective measures, such as wearing sturdy, well-fitting shoes and comfortable, loose-fitting clothes.

4. Teach the patient all aspects of the treatment regimen, such as application of topical agents and occlusive dressings and the importance of balneotherapy. Encourage patient compliance.

4. Topical agents, occlusive dressings, and balneotherapy can be effective in treating psoriasis if used appropriately. Teaching should be tailored to the severity of the disease and to the patient's readiness to learn.

5. Assess the patient's eating habits. Teach him the importance of maintaining a balanced and nutritious diet that includes appropriate foods from the four basic food groups, and emphasize the need for protein and carbohydrate consumption.

5. A balanced diet promotes healing. Protein and carbohydrates help the body maintain a positive nitrogen balance to protect skin integrity.

Nursing diagnosis: *Potential for infection related to skin lesions and other changes in skin condition associated with psoriasis*

GOAL: To prevent skin infection

Interventions

1. Monitor the patient's skin status, inspecting and palpating the skin regularly.

2. Teach the patient health promotion activities, such as proper skin cleaning, lubricating the skin with emollients when it feels dry, and protecting the hands with gloves when engaging in manual work.

Rationales

1. Psoriatic lesions and fissures may become infected.

2. Abraded skin can become a point of entry for microorganisms.

Nursing diagnosis: *Potential for injury related to etiologic factors that exacerbate psoriasis*

GOAL: To prevent injury to the skin by reducing or eliminating exacerbating factors

Interventions

1. Assess the patient's exposure to sunlight and humidity. Instruct him to avoid direct exposure to sunlight or to wear sunscreen, a broad-brimmed hat, long sleeves, and cotton gloves when outdoors.

2. Assess the patient's home environment, behavior patterns, and life-style for exacerbation risks. Suggest ways that the patient can minimize exacerbations, such as through guided imagery or biofeedback. Provide primary prevention health teaching.

Rationales

1. Excessive exposure to sunlight and humidity can aggravate psoriasis. Patients residing in areas with strong sunlight should take the precautions mentioned here.

2. Conditions, habits, and activities with the potential to irritate and injure the patient's skin should be modified or avoided because they can exacerbate the disease.

Nursing diagnosis: *Altered comfort: pain related to psoriatic lesions or itching*

GOAL: To alleviate the patient's discomfort

Interventions

1. Identify the patient's degree of discomfort.

Rationales

1. Discomfort can vary, depending on the location and extent of psoriatic lesions. The patient may experience pain from fissures, infection, or psoriatic arthritis. Itching may or may not occur.

2. Tell the patient to avoid strenuous exercise, hot baths, and sunbathing. Advise him to keep his skin well lubricated, and suggest that he keep his nails cut short and that he wear gloves when sleeping.

2. Strenuous exercise, hot baths, and sunbathing can cause pressure, pain, or itching. Well-lubricated skin eases the patient's discomfort. Keeping nails cut short and wearing gloves at night help prevent scratching, which can lead to infection.

Nursing diagnosis: *Powerlessness related to implications of long-term psoriasis care*

GOAL: To enhance the patient's confidence in being able to render effective self-care

Interventions

1. Observe the patient for listlessness, apathy, or depression. Encourage the patient to participate in all care activities, particularly in making decisions.

2. Teach assertiveness skills to help the patient identify and express personal needs and desires. Provide positive reinforcement when he participates in disease management.

Rationales

1. Psoriasis is a chronic condition with no known cure. Complying with the therapeutic regimen can be physically, financially, and psychologically draining. In severe cases, the disease and treatment can seem overwhelming. Involving the patient in care activities and decision making can lessen the feeling that the disease has taken control of his life.

2. Passive and dependent behaviors can intensify feelings of loss of control. Encouraging the patient's participation in disease management and providing positive reinforcement promote feelings of control.

Nursing diagnosis: *Disturbance in self-concept: body image, related to the disease*

GOAL: To enhance the patient's self-esteem and self-confidence

Interventions

1. Encourage the patient to express positive and negative feelings, especially those related to psoriasis and its effect on his appearance.

2. Touch the patient when appropriate and without appearing uncomfortable or distressed. Teach family members about psoriasis, emphasizing that it is not contagious, and encourage them to touch the patient when such contact is appropriate.

3. Encourage the patient to participate in normal social activities, and provide him with ongoing emotional support.

Rationales

1. Skin appearance and texture can influence body image, sexuality, roles, and relationships. The patient's self-esteem may be closely linked to physical appearance. Psoriasis can cause disfigurement, and the patient may feel that his appearance is revolting or that he is unclean. Discussion gives the nurse opportunities to reassure the patient and point out positive aspects of his appearance and personality.

2. Physical contact communicates acceptance. The patient and family may mistakenly believe that lesions can contaminate others or that the disease is contagious. The patient occasionally may experience some form of rejection, such as meeting an individual who appears to be shocked by the patient's appearance or who seems to fear contact. Individuals typically isolate themselves when they feel repulsive and rejected. Teaching family members about the disease helps them feel comfortable with the patient.

3. A patient with psoriasis may attempt to change his life-style, activities, and manner of dress to hide lesions and avoid social contacts. Receiving emotional support and participating in social activities can improve the patient's self-image.

Nursing diagnosis: *Anxiety related to emotional strain created by psoriasis*

GOAL: To alleviate the patient's anxiety

Interventions	Rationales
1. Encourage the patient to express his concerns or fears related to psoriasis.	1. Stress or anxiety related to psoriasis can exacerbate the condition. Having the patient discuss concerns and fears helps the nurse identify and correct misconceptions that may be contributing to stress or anxiety.
2. Help the patient identify sources of stress.	2. Emotions influence circulation and hormone production, which affect integumentary processes. Stress may contribute to reduced nutritional intake, poor skin health and appearance, poor hygiene, noncompliance with prescribed therapeutic regimens, or substance abuse.
3. Teach the patient stress management skills and strategies and relaxation techniques. Review his ability to use these skills and techniques.	3. Stress management and relaxation help the patient diffuse emotional tension and alleviate psoriatic symptoms.

Nursing diagnosis: *Hopelessness related to implications of long-term psoriasis care*

GOAL: To alleviate the patient's hopelessness and enhance his self-image

Interventions	Rationales
1. Encourage the patient to maintain existing personal, social, and occupational relationships.	1. Skin disfigurement often generates anxiety and causes the patient to withdraw from established relationships. Anxiety is especially intense for a patient who highly values physical appearance. The patient may also withdraw as he becomes focused on the disease and its treatment.
2. Encourage the patient to participate in support group social activities, such as day-care psoriatic programs or National Psoriasis Foundation programs.	2. Group activities facilitate networking and the establishment of peer support from other psoriatic patients.
3. Monitor the patient's psychological status and interpersonal relationships. Encourage him to discuss fears, anger, despair, and feelings of failure. Refer him to a mental health professional if needed.	3. Visible psoriatic lesions may inhibit interpersonal relationships. Role and relationship changes can lead to changes in the patient's emotional response and personality. Exacerbation and remission cycles may cause him to feel a loss of control. Depression or suicidal ideation may follow, and prompt intervention is essential.

Nursing diagnosis: *Impaired home maintenance management related to the therapeutic regimen*

GOAL: To facilitate the patient's independent management of the prescribed regimen

Interventions

1. Teach the patient the prescribed therapeutic regimen. Break instruction into manageable segments, progress from simple to complex concepts, and demonstrate procedures whenever possible. Encourage him to ask questions and perform a return demonstration. Provide positive reinforcement for appropriate behaviors.

2. Teach the patient health promotion activities. Emphasize methods of limiting sunlight exposure, preventing localized skin trauma, and coping with emotional crises. With the patient's help, develop an achievable treatment plan.

Rationales

1. Patients with psoriasis require careful instruction to adequately manage long-term therapeutic skin care. Effective teaching provides the patient with an understanding of the relationship between the disease process and the corresponding treatment. Return demonstrations promote patient competence, self-confidence, and self-esteem. Positive reinforcement of appropriate patient self-care behaviors promotes their continuance.

2. Health promoting behaviors help keep psoriasis in remission and reduce exacerbations. A convenient, achievable treatment plan, developed with the patient's participation, encourages independence and compliance.

ASSOCIATED CARE PLANS
- Grief and Grieving
- Ineffective Coping
- Osteoarthritis
- Sex and Sexuality

NETWORKING OF SERVICES
- National Psoriasis Foundation
- local psoriasis care program
- community support services, such as mental health centers, social service agencies, or health care facilities

CARE TEAM INVOLVED
- nurse
- doctor
- patient and family
- friends
- social worker
- psychologist
- therapist
- members of peer groups

IMPLICATIONS FOR HOME CARE
- ongoing praise, reminders, and reassurance
- primary prevention (adequate nutrition, exercise, and rest)
- illness (can precipitate lesions or initiate an exacerbation)
- psychosocial and physical concerns
- family participation in patient education
- assertiveness techniques
- relaxation or guided imagery techniques

PATIENT EDUCATION TOOLS
- National Psoriasis Foundation literature
- local psoriasis day-care programs
- support groups
- stress management publications
- information about relaxation techniques
- literature about each prescribed medication

DISCHARGE PLAN FROM HOME HEALTH CARE
Before discharge from home health care, the patient should:
- know all aspects of the therapeutic regimen (the correct amount of topical medication to use; how, when, and where to apply it; desired and adverse effects; use of gloves; dressing protocols)
- understand that the therapeutic regimen must be continued, even if skin lesions heal and psoriasis goes into remission
- identify and begin to eliminate sources of stress that may exacerbate psoriasis
- identify and avoid environmental etiologies that may exacerbate psoriasis
- identify and use private and community resources to facilitate stress reduction and psoriatic disease prevention
- understand and use appropriate health promotion activities
- understand and use appropriate self-care techniques
- know conditions that require the immediate notification of the nurse or doctor
- understand and adapt to the disease process
- have a plan for ongoing medical supervision.

SELECTED REFERENCES

Brunner, L.S., and Suddarth, D.S. *Textbook of Medical-Surgical Nursing,* 6th ed. Philadelphia: J.B. Lippincott Co., 1988.

Bullock, B.L., and Rosendahl, P.B. *Pathophysiology: Adaptations and Alterations in Function.* Boston: Little, Brown & Co., 1984.

Gordon, M. *Manual of Nursing Diagnoses: 1986-1987.* New York: McGraw-Hill Book Co., 1987.

Heckel, P. "The Unshared Disease," *Nursing81,* 49-51, June 1981.

Howe, J., et al. *The Handbook of Nursing.* New York: John Wiley & Sons, 1984.

Kneisl, C.R., and Ames, S.A.W. *Adult Health Nursing: A Biopsychosocial Approach.* Reading, Mass.: Addison-Wesley Publishing Co., 1986.

Rodman, G.P., and Schumacher, H.R., eds. *Primer on the Rheumatic Disease,* 8th ed. Atlanta: Arthritis Foundation, 1983.

Rosen, T., et al. *The Nurse's Atlas of Dermatology.* Boston: Little, Brown & Co., 1983.

Thompson, J., et al. *Clinical Nursing.* St. Louis: C.V. Mosby Co., 1985.

Wyngaarden, J.B., and Smith, L.H. *Cecil Textbook of Medicine,* 17th ed., Vol. 2. Philadelphia: W.B. Saunders Co., 1985.

INTEGUMENTARY SYSTEM

Cellulitis

DESCRIPTION AND TIME FOCUS

Cellulitis is an inflammation of the upper layers of the dermis and the subcutaneous tissue but may involve deeper areas and spread into connective tissue. The condition usually is caused by streptococcal or staphylococcal infection. Organisms invade through a break in the skin or through the lymphatics from infection elsewhere in the body. The legs are the most common infection sites. The patient with cellulitis can be treated in the home, with or without a stay in the hospital.

This clinical plan focuses on the patient discharged home from an acute-care hospital after diagnosis and treatment of cellulitis.

■ Typical home health care length of service for a patient with cellulitis: 4 weeks

■ Typical visit frequency: if the patient is on I.V. therapy, three times daily until the patient or caregiver demonstrates an ability to follow the care plan, then two or three times weekly; for other patients, two or three times weekly

HEALTH HISTORY FINDINGS

In a health history interview, the patient may report many of these findings:
• recent injury, puncture wound, infection, or stasis ulcer
• malaise
• underlying medical condition predisposing the patient to injury or infection (for example, peripheral vascular disease or diabetes mellitus)

PHYSICAL FINDINGS

In a physical examination, the nurse may detect many of these findings:

Integumentary
• fever
• localized erythema, tenderness, edema, warmth, maceration, or exudate
• localized vesicles and abscesses
• regional lymph node enlargement
• pain in and near affected area
• peau d'orange

Cardiovascular
• tachycardia
• fatigue

Respiratory
• rapid respirations

Neurologic
• irritability

Gastrointestinal
• anorexia

Musculoskeletal
• reduced range of motion (ROM) or use of affected body parts

General
• malnourishment (related to underlying medical condition or aging)

DIAGNOSTIC STUDIES

The following study may be performed to evaluate the patient's health status:
• white blood cell (WBC) count—after completion of antibiotic therapy; normal range is 4,100 to 10,900/mcl

---

Nursing diagnosis: *Impaired skin integrity related to inflammation secondary to bacterial infection*

GOAL 1: To help the patient achieve and maintain adequate skin integrity

Interventions

1. Assess overall skin integrity for color, moisture, temperature, cleanliness, and turgor.

2. Assess involved areas for redness, streaks, tenderness, edema, warmth, maceration, vesicles, abscesses, exudate, and regional enlargement of lymph nodes.

Rationales

1. Assessment provides baseline data to develop the care plan and to detect potential problems quickly.

2. This assessment establishes the baseline data for evaluating healing progress.

3. Measure the degree of swelling and note the extent of redness in the affected body part; compare the findings with those from an unaffected part.

3. Measurement and comparison help the nurse evaluate treatment progress in reducing redness and edema.

4. Assess the patient's vital signs at each visit.

4. Increased pulse, respirations, and body temperature may indicate infection.

5. Assess the ROM of the involved body part.

5. Tenderness and edema may limit movement.

6. Assess the patient for anorexia, fatigue, malaise, and irritability.

6. Infection may cause these manifestations.

7. Assess the patient's nutritional status.

7. Malnourishment can delay healing.

8. Encourage the patient to consume 2,000 to 3,000 calories daily, including at least 65 g of protein, and to drink 2 to 3 liters of fluid daily, unless contraindicated. Consult with a dietitian, if necessary, for expert advice on managing the patient's nutritional problems.

8. Proper nutrition and hydration promote healing.

9. Assess the affected part for complications, such as thrombophlebitis superinfection and osteomyelitis.

9. Assessment facilitates the prompt detection and treatment of complications that can exacerbate the patient's condition.

10. Monitor the patient's WBC count, as ordered.

10. A WBC count reflects the patient's response to the prescribed treatment; the normal range is 4,100 to 10,900/mcl.

GOAL 2: To promote compliance with the prescribed plan of care

Interventions

1. Teach the patient the importance of elevating and supporting the affected body part.

Rationales

1. Elevating the affected part promotes venous return and decreases edema. Supportive positioning protects against strain and spasm of the involved muscles.

2. Encourage the patient to comply with activity restrictions. Schedule necessary activity of the affected part to coincide with peak effectiveness of analgesics or anti-inflammatory agents.

2. Timing activity with peak medication action decreases discomfort while allowing necessary mobility.

3. Tell the patient to change position every 2 hours while awake.

3. Changing position increases circulation to the affected body part and prevents skin breakdown.

4. Use a bed cradle, as needed.

4. A bed cradle reduces skin irritation caused by bed linens.

5. Encourage the patient to use pressure-relieving equipment, such as sheepskin, a trapeze bar, heel pads, or a special mattress.

5. These devices help mimimize the shearing force that occurs when underlying tissue moves in the opposite direction of the skin surface. Such movement, common during transfers between bed and chair or when the patient changes positions, can stretch and tear capillaries, leading to tissue destruction.

6. Teach the patient the importance of lifting, not pulling, the affected body part.

6. Lifting minimizes the shearing force.

7. Teach the patient and caregiver to wash their hands before performing any treatments (such as warm soaks or dressing changes), to avoid touching inflamed areas, to separate adjoining skin surfaces with gauze, to use sterile technique when changing dressings, to dispose of contaminated dressings safely, and to wash contaminated bed linens in hot water.

7. These procedures prevent contamination and the spread of microorganisms.

8. Teach the patient and caregiver to wash the affected body part with mild soap or a warm saline solution and then rinse thoroughly.

8. Gentle washing rids the affected part of skin debris and exudate, which promotes healing.

9. Teach the patient and caregiver how to perform ordered treatments, such as warm soaks.

9. Effective patient teaching improves compliance with established procedures.

10. Teach the patient and caregiver the importance of gently massaging healthy skin around the inflamed area (while not touching the inflamed area itself).

10. Massage promotes circulation and healing.

11. Teach the patient deep breathing exercises.

11. Deep breathing promotes oxygenation, which enhances healing.

Nursing diagnosis: *Impaired physical mobility related to reduced ROM of affected body part*

GOAL: To optimize the patient's physical mobility

Interventions

1. Assess the patient's ability to perform activities of daily living (ADLs) and his ROM in the affected part.

2. Assess the patient's respiratory status for signs and symptoms of pneumonia, such as coughing, sputum production, dyspnea, and crackles.

3. Teach the patient the importance of observing activity restrictions, such as elevating and supporting the affected part to reduce swelling.

4. Tell the patient to ask for assistance when attempting a transfer or walking.

5. Place items the patient is likely to need (such as a handbell, lamp, snack, or radio) within easy reach of his bed or chair.

6. Teach the patient how to use necessary medical equipment, such as a walker, cane, or wheelchair.

7. Refer the patient to a physical therapist when appropriate.

Rationales

1. Initial assessment establishes a baseline for developing the nursing care plan and evaluating the patient's progress.

2. Assessment facilitates early detection and treatment of pulmonary complications secondary to cellulitis.

3. Compliance with the prescribed management plan improves when the patient understands the underlying rationale.

4. Assistance minimizes the patient's risk of falling.

5. Having needed items nearby promotes safety and allows the patient to signal the caregiver.

6. Proper instruction promotes safety and minimizes the patient's risk of falling.

7. A physical therapist provides expert advice about managing problems associated with impaired mobility.

Nursing diagnosis: *Knowledge deficit related to the disease process and wound care after injury*

GOAL: To teach the patient measures to prevent cellulitis

Interventions

1. Assess the patient's ability to learn by verifying his ability to see, hear, and read, observing his manual dexterity, assessing his motivation, and considering his cultural influences.

2. Assess the patient's knowledge of the disease process and wound care after injury.

Rationales

1. Assessment provides a baseline for developing the nursing care plan.

2. A knowledge assessment provides baseline data for developing a teaching plan.

3. Establish mutually acceptable goals.

3. Involving the patient in setting goals fosters learning and promotes compliance.

4. Conduct teaching in a quiet room without distractions. Include the patient's family in teaching sessions when possible.

4. A quiet, distraction-free atmosphere enhances learning. Involving family members improves their understanding and the patient's compliance.

5. Teach the patient and family the factors that can precipitate cellulitis (such as puncture wounds and infections), the patient's personal risk factors (such as stress, ulcers, and immunosuppression), wound care after injury, early signs and symptoms of cellulitis, and the importance of seeking medical advice promptly.

5. Providing the patient and family with an understanding of the disease process and requisite treatments improves compliance and promotes healing.

6. Provide clear, thorough explanations in language the patient can understand. Vary the delivery of information; speak, read, provide written information, and demonstrate procedures. Encourage questions.

6. A carefully planned presentation facilitates retention. Questions enhance learning by focusing the discussion on points the patient does not understand or may not believe.

ASSOCIATED CARE PLANS
• Intermittent I.V. Therapy
• Osteomyelitis
• Pain
• Pneumonia
• Thrombophlebitis

NETWORKING OF SERVICES
• Meals On Wheels
• durable medical equipment supplier

CARE TEAM INVOLVED
• nurse
• doctor
• dietitian
• physical therapist
• medical social worker

IMPLICATIONS FOR HOME CARE
• functional features of the home (activity regulation and infection control)
• telephone (communication)

PATIENT EDUCATION TOOLS
• literature for each medication ordered
• written instructions for wound care
• guidelines for physical therapy

DISCHARGE PLAN FROM HOME HEALTH CARE
Before discharge from home health care, the patient should:
• show evidence of healing
• know the name, method of administration, dosage, action, and adverse effects of each prescribed medication
• comply with the plan of care
• recognize signs of healing
• have the telephone number of the home health agency for follow-up care, as needed
• know the date of follow-up doctor or laboratory appointments
• have a satisfactory level of physical mobility

• know factors contributing to cellulitis development
• know personal risk factors of cellulitis
• know proper wound care
• know the early clinical manifestations of cellulitis
• know the importance of seeking medical attention promptly.

SELECTED REFERENCES
Brunner, L.S., et al. *Textbook of Medical-Surgical Nursing,* 6th ed. Philadelphia: J.B. Lippincott Co., 1988.
Doenges, M.E., et al. *Nursing Care Plans: Nursing Diagnoses in Planning Patient Care.* Philadelphia: F.A. Davis Co., 1984.
Fitzpatrick, T.B., et al. *Dermatology in General Medicine,* 3rd ed. New York: McGraw-Hill Book Co., 1987.
Gulanick, M., et al., eds. *Nursing Care Plans: Nursing Diagnosis and Intervention.* Michael Reese Hospital and Medical Center. St. Louis: C.V. Mosby Co., 1986.
Lewis, S.M., and Collier, I.C. *Medical-Surgical Nursing: Assessment and Management of Clinical Problems,* 2nd ed. New York: McGraw-Hill Book Co., 1987.
Luckman, J., and Sorensen, K.C. *Medical-Surgical Nursing: A Pathophysiological Approach,* 3rd ed. Philadelphia: W.B. Saunders Co., 1987.
Meislin, H.W. "Pathogen Identification of Abscesses and Cellulitis." *Annals of Emergency Medicine* 15(3): 329-32, 1986.
Patrick, M.L., et al. *Medical-Surgical Nursing: Pathophysiological Concepts.* Philadelphia: J.B. Lippincott Co., 1986.
Skidmore-Roth, L., and Jaffe, M. *Medical-Surgical Nursing Care Plans: Nursing Diagnosis and Interventions.* East Norwalk, Conn.: Appleton & Lange, 1986.
Sundberg, M.C. *Fundamentals of Nursing with Clinical Procedures,* 2nd ed. Boston: Jones and Bartlett, 1989.
Taylor, C., et al. *Fundamentals of Nursing: The Art and Science of Nursing Care.* Philadelphia: J.B. Lippincott Co., 1989.

MUSCULOSKELETAL SYSTEM
Total Knee Replacement

DESCRIPTION AND TIME FOCUS
Total knee replacement usually is performed to reduce pain and improve mobility for a patient with arthritis or one who has had unsuccessful reconstructive surgery. The patient usually is over age 60 and may have concurrent chronic illnesses that can affect recovery.

Many types of knee prostheses are available. Although nursing care is essentially the same for all, the nurse should become familiar with the patient's prosthesis type. The nurse also must know the patient's weight-bearing status at the time of the first visit. The patient with a cemented knee replacement is usually on partial weight bearing initially, progressing to full weight bearing in 4 to 6 weeks. A patient with a cementless knee replacement usually is on non-weight bearing or touch-toe weight bearing for 4 to 6 weeks.

This clinical plan focuses on the patient discharged home from an acute-care facility after total knee replacement. Nursing care includes assessing home safety, monitoring for complications, and providing instruction that promotes an uncomplicated recovery and allows the patient to resume a normal life-style.

■ Typical home health care length of service for a patient with a total knee replacement: 2 weeks

■ Typical visit frequency: twice the first week and once the second week

HEALTH HISTORY FINDINGS
In a health history interview, the patient may report many of these findings:

• physical limitations
• pain
• unsteady gait
• steroid use
• concurrent diagnosis of arthritis

PHYSICAL FINDINGS
In a physical examination, the nurse may detect many of these findings:

Musculoskeletal
• limited range of motion (ROM) in the affected knee (75 to 90 degrees of flexion, usually 10 degrees short of full extension)

Cardiovascular
• mild pretibial pitting
• pedal edema in the affected leg

Integumentary
• incision over the affected knee
• mild redness and warmth in area of incision

DIAGNOSTIC STUDIES
The following study may be performed to evaluate the patient's health status:
• knee X-ray—4 weeks after hospital discharge to monitor healing progress and to determine whether patient is ready for full weight bearing

---

Nursing diagnosis: *Impaired tissue integrity related to surgical incision*

GOAL: To promote complete and uneventful healing of the incision

Interventions

1. Assess the incision for drainage, redness, increased warmth, edema, or dehiscence.

2. Teach the patient and caregiver to care properly for the incision. Explain the signs and symptoms of infection (redness, edema, drainage, foul odor, fever, chills, bleeding, tenderness, and sloughing of tissue) and the need to report these to the doctor and nurse.

Rationales

1. If the patient is elderly, skin turgor and healing ability may be decreased. Steroids, commonly used to treat arthritis, inhibit healing and increase the risk of infection. The knee has little subcutaneous tissue; consequently, inordinate tension on the incision during flexion and extension increases the risk of edge separation.

2. Infection requires prompt medical attention. The patient and caregiver must understand routine incision care and recognize signs and symptoms of infection.

Nursing diagnosis: *Potential for infection related to invasive surgical procedure*

GOAL: To prevent joint space infection

Interventions

1. Teach the patient and caregiver the signs and symptoms of joint space infection (edema, redness, severe pain, fever).

2. Assess wound status at each visit, and teach the patient and caregiver to keep the wound clean and dry.

Rationales

1. Joint space infection may occur after medical follow-up is completed. The patient and caregiver must recognize this problem and seek medical attention quickly.

2. Regular assessment and proper care of the wound site help prevent infection.

Nursing diagnosis: *Altered tissue perfusion related to limited mobility*

GOAL: To maintain adequate tissue perfusion

Interventions

1. Schedule alternating periods of rest and activity to promote circulation.

2. Collaborate with the physical therapist to teach the patient appropriate exercises. Provide assistance as needed.

Rationales

1. Long periods without a position change can contribute to venous stasis and thromboembolism development.

2. Exercises prescribed for orthopedic recovery also improve the patient's circulation.

Nursing diagnosis: *Ineffective breathing pattern related to limited mobility*

GOAL: To maintain normal ventilation with adequate lung expansion

Interventions

1. Assess the patient's lung sounds for evidence of lower lobe atelectasis.

2. Teach the patient deep-breathing techniques or the proper use of an incentive spirometer.

Rationales

1. An elderly patient may have shallow respiration patterns because of limited physical activity. Shallow respirations can lead to atelectasis.

2. These measures help prevent atelectasis and the pooling of secretions.

Nursing diagnosis: *Knowledge deficit related to necessary safety measures*

GOAL: To promote the patient's safety during healing

Interventions

1. Inform the patient of ROM restrictions and their significance. Tell him to avoid kneeling on the affected knee or pivoting on the affected leg.

2. Assess the patient's home for potential safety hazards (such as width of pathways; height of chairs, bed, and toilet seat; and access to tub or shower).

Rationales

1. These restrictions facilitate proper alignment during healing and promote safety.

2. The affected knee has a limited ROM. Home furnishings may require modification or replacement so the patient can comfortably perform activities within ROM limitations.

3. Assist the patient in making inexpensive home alterations. Suggest that he use firm cushions, platforms, or blocks to raise the height of chairs and the bed. Advise him to order an elevated toilet seat, if needed. Arrange the living area so he can avoid stairs and narrow hallways. Remove all throw rugs, and warn him not to hold on to furniture that moves easily.

3. These measures help ensure the patient's safety and promote compliance with ROM activities and restrictions.

ASSOCIATED CARE PLANS
• Osteoarthritis
• Osteomyelitis
• Pain

NETWORKING OF SERVICES
• Meals On Wheels
• durable medical equipment supplier
• Lifeline

CARE TEAM INVOLVED
• nurse
• doctor
• patient and family
• physical therapist
• home health aide

IMPLICATIONS FOR HOME CARE
• functional features of the home (raised toilet seat, access to bathroom and shower)
• telephone (communication)

PATIENT EDUCATION TOOLS
• home safety measures
• written list of precautions
• written home exercise program

DISCHARGE PLAN FROM HOME HEALTH CARE
Before discharge from home health care, the patient should:
• know the signs and symptoms of incision or joint space infection
• be free of circulatory and respiratory complications
• understand routine care of the incision and surrounding skin
• modify the home for safety and compliance with ROM restrictions
• post phone numbers for the doctor, nurse, and home health agency in a prominent place
• know the dates of follow-up doctor appointments.

SELECTED REFERENCES
Crownshield, R. "An Overview of Prosthetic Materials for Fixation," *Clinical Orthopaedics and Related Research* 235:166, October 1988.
Eliopoulos, C. *A Guide to the Nursing of the Aged.* Baltimore: Williams & Wilkins Co., 1987.
Iyer, P., et al. *Nursing Process and Nursing Diagnosis.* Philadelphia: W.B. Saunders Co., 1986.
Scherman, S. *Community Health Nursing Care Plans.* John Wiley & Sons, 1985.
Stearns, H.C. "Principles of Lower Extremity Fracture Management," in *Assessment and Fracture Management of the Lower Extremities* (NAON monograph), October 1984.
Walsh, J., et al. *Manual of Home Health Care Nursing.* Philadelphia: J.B. Lippincott Co., 1987.

MUSCULOSKELETAL SYSTEM

Total Hip Replacement

DESCRIPTION AND TIME FOCUS

Total hip replacement usually is performed to relieve pain and improve mobility for a patient with arthritis or severe femoral neck fracture or for one who has had unsuccessful reconstructive surgery. The patient usually is over age 60 and may have concurrent chronic illnesses that can affect recovery.

The nurse should know the patient's weight-bearing status at the time of the first visit. A patient with cemented hip replacement usually is on partial weight bearing initially, progressing to full weight bearing in 4 to 6 weeks. A patient with cementless hip replacement usually is on non-weight bearing or touch-toe weight bearing for 4 to 6 weeks.

This clinical plan focuses on the patient discharged home from an acute-care facility after a total hip replacement. Nursing care includes assessing home safety, monitoring for complications, and providing instruction that promotes an uncomplicated recovery and allows the patient to resume a normal life-style.

■ Typical home health care length of service for uncomplicated total hip replacement: 2 weeks

■ Typical visit frequency: twice the first week and once the second week

HEALTH HISTORY FINDINGS

In a health history interview, the patient may report many of these findings:
• obesity
• concurrent health problem and treatment
• history of steroid use (severe arthritis)
• osteoporosis
• chronic pain

PHYSICAL FINDINGS

In a physical examination, the nurse may detect many of these findings:

Musculoskeletal
• limited range of motion (ROM) in affected hip (no more than 90 degrees flexion, 45 degrees abduction, neutral rotation)

Cardiovascular
• mild pretibial pitting
• pedal edema in affected leg

Integumentary
• incision on affected hip
• mild redness and warmth in area of incision

DIAGNOSTIC STUDIES

The following study may be performed to evaluate the patient's health status:
• hip X-ray—2 to 4 weeks after hospital discharge to monitor healing progress and to determine whether the patient is ready for full weight bearing

---

Nursing diagnosis: *Impaired tissue integrity related to surgical incision*

GOAL: To promote complete and uneventful healing of the incision

Interventions

1. Assess the incision for drainage, redness, increased warmth, edema, or dehiscence.

2. Teach the patient and caregiver to care properly for the incision. Explain the signs and symptoms of infection (redness, edema, foul odor, drainage, pain, elevated temperature) and the need to report these to the doctor and nurse.

Rationales

1. If the patient is elderly, skin turgor and healing ability may be reduced. Steroids, commonly used to treat arthritis, inhibit healing and increase the risk of infection.

2. Infection requires prompt medical attention. The patient and caregiver must understand routine incision care and recognize signs and symptoms of infection.

Nursing diagnosis: *Potential for infection related to invasive surgical procedure*

GOAL: To prevent joint space infection

Intervention

Teach the patient and caregiver the signs and symptoms of joint space infection (edema, redness, severe pain, fever).

Rationale

Joint space infection may occur after medical follow-up is completed. The patient and caregiver must recognize this problem and seek medical attention quickly.

Nursing diagnosis: *Altered tissue perfusion related to limited mobility*

GOAL: To maintain adequate tissue perfusion

Interventions

1. Schedule alternating periods of rest and activity to promote circulation.

2. Collaborate with the physical therapist to teach the patient appropriate exercises. Provide assistance as needed.

Rationales

1. Long periods without a position change can contribute to venous stasis and thromboembolism development.

2. Exercises prescribed for orthopedic recovery also improve the patient's circulation.

Nursing diagnosis: *Ineffective breathing pattern related to limited mobility*

GOAL: To maintain normal ventilation with adequate lung expansion

Interventions

1. Assess the patient's lung sounds for evidence of lower lobe atelectasis.

2. Teach the patient deep-breathing techniques or the proper use of an incentive spirometer.

Rationales

1. An elderly patient may have shallow respiration patterns because of limited physical activity. Shallow respirations can lead to atelectasis.

2. These methods help prevent atelectasis and the pooling of secretions.

Nursing diagnosis: *Knowledge deficit related to necessary safety measures*

GOAL: To promote the patient's safety during healing

Interventions

1. Inform the patient of ROM restrictions and their significance. Tell him to maintain neutral rotation and to avoid crossing his legs, pivoting on the affected leg, sleeping on the affected side, and bending to put on shoes or socks.

2. Teach the patient and caregiver the signs and symptoms of hip dislocation (severe hip pain, affected leg shortened, external rotation of affected hip, inability to bear weight on affected leg).

3. Assess the patient's home for potential safety hazards (such as width of pathways; height of chairs, bed, and toilet seat; and access to tub or shower).

4. Assist the patient in making inexpensive home alterations. Suggest that he use firm cushions, platforms, or blocks to raise the height of chairs and the bed. Advise him to order an elevated toilet seat, if needed. Arrange the living area so he can avoid stairs and narrow hallways. Remove all throw rugs, and warn him not to hold on to furniture that moves easily.

Rationales

1. These restrictions facilitate proper alignment during healing, prevent dislocation, and promote safety.

2. The patient and caregiver must know these signs and symptoms so they can notify the doctor and home health agency if dislocation occurs. Risk is greatest during the first 2 to 4 weeks at home.

3. Hip flexion after a replacement is limited to 90 degrees. Home furnishings may require modification or replacement so the patient can comfortably perform activities within ROM limitations.

4. These measures help ensure the patient's safety and promote compliance with ROM activities and restrictions.

ASSOCIATED CARE PLANS
- Osteoarthritis
- Pain
- Thrombophlebitis

NETWORKING OF SERVICES
- Meals On Wheels
- durable medical equipment supplier
- Lifeline
- transportation

CARE TEAM INVOLVED
- nurse
- doctor
- patient and family
- physical therapist
- home health aide
- rehabilitation nurse

IMPLICATIONS FOR HOME CARE
- functional features of the home (raised toilet seat, access to bathroom)
- telephone (communication)

PATIENT EDUCATION TOOLS
- home safety measures
- list of precautions
- written home exercise program

DISCHARGE PLAN FROM HOME HEALTH CARE
Before discharge from home health care, the patient should:
- know the signs and symptoms of incision or joint space infection
- be free of circulatory and respiratory complications
- understand routine care of the incision and surrounding skin
- know actual and ordered weight-bearing status
- know mobility and ROM limitations
- modify the home for safety and compliance with ROM restrictions
- post telephone numbers for the doctor, nurse, and home health agency by the phone
- know the dates of follow-up doctor appointments.

SELECTED REFERENCES
Carlson, D.C., and Robinson, H.J. "Surgical Approaches for Primary Total Hip Arthroplasty," *Clinical Orthopaedics and Related Research* 222:161, September 1987.

Eliopoulos, C. *A Guide to the Nursing of the Aged.* Baltimore: Williams & Wilkins Co., 1987.

Harper, A. "Initial Assessment and Management of Femoral Neck Fractures in the Elderly," *Orthopaedic Nursing* 4:55, May/June 1985.

Iyer, P., et al. *Nursing Process and Nursing Diagnosis.* Philadelphia: W.B. Saunders Co., 1986.

Scherman, S. *Community Health Nursing Care Plans.* John Wiley & Sons, 1985.

Thompson, J., et al. *Clinical Nursing.* St. Louis: C.V. Mosby Co., 1986.

Walsh, J., et al. *Manual of Home Health Care Nursing.* Philadelphia: J.B. Lippincott Co., 1987.

MUSCULOSKELETAL SYSTEM

Amputation

DESCRIPTION AND TIME FOCUS
Amputation is the surgical removal of a diseased portion of the body, representing for the patient a combined loss of the body part and its associated functions and feeling. Amputation may be unilateral or bilateral. Above-knee, below-knee, and upper-extremity amputations are performed and can involve a closed, open, or guillotine method. After amputation, the patient may experience phantom limb syndrome, a phenomenon in which the patient feels sensation or pain in the missing limb. The mechanism of phantom limb pain is unknown, and no cure exists.

This clinical plan focuses on the patient discharged home from an acute-care facility after amputation but before fitting for a definitive prosthesis. Nursing care should be individualized to address his needs, type of amputation, underlying diseases, and potential for rehabilitation. The nurse must assess his self-care abilities, knowledge, and attitudes and help him understand health problems and treatments.

■ Typical home health care length of service for a patient with uncomplicated amputation: 4 to 8 weeks

■ Typical visit frequency: three visits the first week, then twice weekly for 3 weeks, then once weekly for 4 weeks

HEALTH HISTORY FINDINGS
In a health history interview, the patient may report many of these findings:
• history of peripheral vascular disease
• diabetes
• history of cigarette smoking
• obesity
• familial pattern of limb loss
• recurrent limb ulcerations

PHYSICAL FINDINGS
In a physical examination, the nurse may detect many of these findings:

Musculoskeletal
• decreased ambulation
• limited movement of limb or appendage
• pain
• contracture

Cardiovascular
• hypertension or hypotension
• palpable peripheral pulse
• intermittent claudication
• dependent edema
• capillary refill time greater than 3 seconds

Neurologic
• phantom limb sensation, pain
• neuroma

Integumentary
• nonhealing wound
• shiny skin
• skin cool to touch
• stump edema
• hematoma
• cyanosis
• necrosis
• hemorrhage (rare)
• palpable mass
• calluses
• rash
• blisters
• stasis ulcer
• thickened nails

Endocrine
• glucose intolerance
• diabetes

DIAGNOSTIC STUDIES
The following studies may be performed to evaluate the patient's health status:
• glucose tolerance test (if diabetic)—weekly until stable, then monthly
• prothrombin time (if taking anticoagulants)—weekly until stable, then decrease according to amount of medication and doctor's orders

---

Nursing diagnosis: *Self-care deficit related to lower limb amputation*

GOAL 1: To maintain the patient's current abilities, prevent complications, restore function, and promote self-care

Interventions

1. Assess the patient's endurance, balance, and coordination (for example, his ability to stand, pivot, and transfer from the bed to the wheelchair); also evaluate his desire to perform self-care activities.

Rationales

1. The patient's ability and desire to perform self-care activities influence his rehabilitation.

2. Institute range-of-motion (ROM) exercises for all limbs.

2. The patient must maintain full use of other limbs to retain optimal functioning. ROM exercises help maintain joint mobility and prevent muscle atrophy and contracture.

3. Have the patient alternate periods of activity and rest.

3. The patient needs to participate in activities, but undue fatigue from excessive activity or insufficient rest may cause stress, which increases blood pressure, pulse rate, and cardiac work load.

4. Institute a plan of simple exercises the patient can perform safely, and teach him the importance of maintaining proper posture.

4. Simple exercises and proper posture, combined with ROM exercises, further promote joint mobility while helping to prevent muscle atrophy and contracture.

5. Refer the patient to a physical therapist.

5. The physical therapist institutes exercises specifically designed to prepare the patient for prosthesis use. These exercises promote normal joint alignment, compensate for changes in balance resulting from the amputation, and help prevent edema.

GOAL 2: To promote a well-formed, mature stump that can bear weight

Interventions

1. Wrap the stump with a compression bandage.

2. Teach the patient and family to apply the compression bandage in a figure-eight pattern and to extend the bandage well above the joint proximal to the surgical site.

3. Advise the patient to keep a compression wrap on the stump until a permanent prosthesis is fitted, and to wrap the stump each night for an additional 3 to 4 weeks after he begins wearing the prosthesis.

4. Apply additional stump socks as the stump shrinks.

5. Encourage the patient with a temporary prosthesis to gradually increase weight bearing on the stump, but warn him never to place his full weight on the stump before healing is complete.

Rationales

1. A compression bandage promotes stump shrinkage, controls edema, and molds the stump for a prosthesis.

2. Improperly applied dressings slip off after a few hours and must be reapplied. The patient may have difficulty applying dressings alone and may need a family member's help.

3. Stump edema may develop at any time and, without appropriate dressing, can make the stump asymmetrical.

4. Failure to add stump socks as the stump shrinks could result in a loose, poorly-fitting socket shortly after prosthesis fitting.

5. Although gradually increasing the stump's weight-bearing ability is desirable, placing full weight on the stump should be delayed until total healing has occurred. Tissue healing takes 4 to 8 weeks, depending on the patient; obtaining a permanent prosthesis usually takes 3 to 4 months.

GOAL 3: To promote safety and prevent injuries

Interventions

1. Instruct the patient and family to install side rails on the patient's bed, and explain why the rails are necessary.

2. Advise the patient to use caution when transferring (for example, from the bed to a chair) to prevent abrasions or bruises.

3. Inspect all equipment for safety; be sure it is in good repair and suitable for home use.

Rationales

1. Because of the amputation and lack of sensation, the patient may be unable to sense the edge of the bed or prevent an unexpected fall.

2. The other limb is at risk for amputation if the cause for surgery was a circulatory disorder or a neuropathy. Injuries increase this risk; if circulation or sensation is impaired, uncontrolled infection may result.

3. Equipment problems, such as uneven legs, lost tips, poor brakes, and loose screws, increase the risk for injuries.

4. Urge the family to remove all loose, small rugs.

4. Loose, small rugs can slide easily and cause falls and accidents.

5. Adjust all equipment to wheelchair height to facilitate safe, easy transfers.

5. Self-care independence depends on the patient's ability to move freely. Having all equipment at wheelchair height improves freedom of movement.

6. Advise the patient with a unilateral amputation to select shoes with low heels, rubber soles, and adequate support.

6. Good walking shoes with rubber soles minimize the risk of a fall.

7. Palpate pulses in the remaining leg.

7. Most leg amputations result from vascular disease; the remaining leg may experience similar compromised circulation.

Nursing diagnosis: *Potential for infection related to impaired skin integrity*

GOAL: To prevent infection and promote skin integrity

Interventions

1. Assess the incision site for healing, sutures, and signs and symptoms of infection, such as edema, redness, and exudate.

2. Assess changes in skin temperature, color, or appearance. Teach the patient to examine the limb regularly during dressing changes or before exercising.

3. Assess for hemorrhage, hematoma, edema, and necrosis.

4. Teach the patient and caregiver to wash the stump with soap and water, rinse and dry it thoroughly, and expose it to the air for 20 minutes after washing. Be sure the patient or caregiver can provide thorough skin care, and explain that such care is essential not just during healing but for the rest of the patient's life.

5. Teach the patient the importance of frequent position changes. Be sure he knows how to do this whether he's lying in bed or sitting in a wheelchair.

6. Caution the patient and caregiver never to apply powders, oils, or alcohol to the stump.

Rationales

1. The patient must have a well-healed stump with adequate skin integrity for prosthesis use.

2. Changes may indicate infection or other complications. Early detection facilitates prompt intervention and treatment.

3. Blood vessel necrosis can cause hemorrhage. Hematomas can delay healing and provide a medium for bacterial growth. Prothesis fitting is contraindicated when edema is present. Skin edge necrosis more than ½" wide may require surgical revision.

4. Proper skin care is the most important aspect of stump care.

5. Decubitus ulcers result from pressure on skin caused by spending prolonged periods in one position.

6. These products can prevent healing and increase the risk of infection.

Nursing diagnosis: *Altered comfort related to phantom limb pain*

GOAL: To minimize episodes of phantom limb pain

Interventions

1. Assess the patient's perception of phantom limb pain using the seven variables: "Where is the pain? How long have you had it? How long does it last? How often do you experience it? What makes it better or worse? Do you have recurrent episodes? How would you describe the pain?"

Rationales

1. Having the patient describe such aspects of pain as location, onset, intensity, frequency, and duration may provide the nurse with useful clues in treating the pain.

2. Reassure the patient that many amputees experience the same phenomenon.

2. Phantom limb pain may startle and frighten the patient. Knowing that others share his experience may lessen his fears.

3. Encourage weight bearing and ambulation if the patient has a temporary prosthesis. If he has no prosthesis, encourage independent activities of daily living (ADLs), ROM exercises, and a regular exercise program.

3. Activity reduces the severity of phantom pain. Phantom pain may be relieved by applying pressure to the stump.

4. Recommend that the patient use whirlpools, massage, and heat application after the incision has healed.

4. These measures are soothing, increase circulation to the stump, and help relieve pain experienced in between medication doses.

5. Teach the patient and family relaxation techniques.

5. Tense muscles exacerbate painful sensations. Such relaxation methods as diversion, backrubs, and guided imagery can bring pleasure and reduce the patient's awareness of painful stimuli.

6. If indicated, tactfully recommend that the patient undergo a psychological evaluation.

6. Such an evaluation may identify psychological factors contributing to phantom limb pain. The patient may experience social isolation, for example, indicating a need for acceptance by his family or society.

7. Discourage the use of analgesics for phantom limb pain.

7. Episodes of phantom limb pain may occur for years; long-term analgesic use can result in dependence or addiction.

8. If pain is intractable, refer the patient to a doctor for evaluation.

8. Intractable pain may require local anesthetics, nerve blocks, or surgical intervention.

Nursing diagnosis: *Impaired home maintenance management related to restricted mobility*

GOAL: To promote the patient's safety in the home

Interventions

1. Assess the patient's home for easy access to entrances and exits, bathrooms, kitchen, and bedroom.

Rationales

1. Some modifications, such as widening doors or providing a wheelchair ramp, may be required to facilitate the patient's access to essential or frequently used areas.

2. Assess the patient's need for durable medical equipment (DME), such as a hospital bed with trapeze bar and side rails, crutches, wheelchair, bedside commode, elevated toilet seat, bath stool, walker, sliding board, ramps, or grab bars. Arrange for provision of appropriate equipment.

2. Appropriate equipment promotes mobility and safety after discharge while the patient learns to use a prosthesis.

3. Assess the patient's need for occupational therapy.

3. An occupational therapist evaluates the patient's physical abilities, teaches self-care activities, assesses the home for safety, and assists in obtaining necessary equipment.

Nursing diagnosis: *Disturbance in self-concept: body image, related to the amputation*

GOAL 1: To help the patient examine feelings about the amputation and to promote acceptance

Interventions

1. Assess the patient's emotional response to changes in appearance and function.

2. Identify the patient's past coping mechanisms, which may involve interpersonal relationships, finances, illness, occupation, religion, and education, among others.

3. Encourage the patient and family to express their feelings and fears about the amputation.

4. Encourage the patient's involvement in choosing clothing to cover the amputation.

Rationales

1. The nurse must understand the patient's current attitudes and feelings to plan appropriate interventions.

2. Understanding past coping mechanisms helps in planning new coping strategies.

3. The patient and family will probably experience depression, anger, resentment, and hopelessness. Such feelings are normal, and discussing them openly may ultimately help the patient and family to accept the amputation.

4. Making decisions about self-care promotes the patient's self-confidence.

GOAL 2: To facilitate the patient's independence

Interventions

1. Assess the need for a home health aide to help the patient and relieve the family; arrange for the services of an aide only if necessary.

2. Discourage family members from helping the patient with tasks that he can perform independently.

Rationales

1. Although a home health aide can assist the patient and provide relief to the family, automatically assigning an aide can discourage independence in ADLs.

2. ADL accomplishments promote self-confidence and encourage further activity.

GOAL 3: To help the patient plan for the future

Interventions

1. Encourage the patient to pursue rehabilitation.

2. Assess the patient's need to change jobs.

3. If a job change is necessary, help the patient explore career interests and abilities.

Rationales

1. Rehabilitation promotes independence, improves self-image, and builds self-confidence, all of which help the patient look to the future with more optimism.

2. The patient's previous job may involve physical maneuvers beyond his ability, and he may need vocational retraining.

3. The patient is more likely to succeed in a new job if the job suits his interests and abilities.

Nursing diagnosis: *Altered bowel elimination: constipation, related to decreased mobility*

GOAL: To promote regular bowel movements of normal consistency

Interventions

1. Assess the patient's past and present bowel elimination patterns and identify causes of abnormal patterns.

Rationales

1. Such assessment and identification establish baseline data for developing the nursing care plan.

2. Instruct the patient to follow a high-fiber diet and, unless contraindicated, to drink at least 3 liters of fluid daily.

2. Inadequate fiber or fluid intake can cause constipation.

3. Advise the patient to use a stool softener, if necessary.

3. A soft stool is more easily evacuated.

4. Check the patient frequently for stool accumulation or impaction.

4. Improper bowel elimination can cause distention, anorexia, or cramping.

5. Avoid using enemas, and instruct the patient and caregiver not to use them.

5. Enemas remove electrolytes and disturb the body's pH balance.

6. Avoid overuse of laxatives to counter mild constipation.

6. Mild constipation poses no harm to the patient and may be preferable to the embarrassment and discomfort caused by having loose bowel movements at inappropriate times.

Nursing diagnosis: *Knowledge deficit related to exercise and positioning to prevent contracture and complications*

GOAL: To teach the patient proper positioning and preventive exercises

Interventions

1. Instruct the patient with a below-knee amputation to avoid sitting with knees flexed for long periods.

2. Instruct the patient with an above-knee amputation to avoid prolonged sitting, to lie in the prone position for 30 minutes four times each day, and to periodically extend the hip and knee.

3. Tell the patient not to elevate the stump on pillows.

4. Tell the patient to avoid abducted and externally rotated stump positions.

5. Teach the patient to adduct the stump frequently each day.

6. Tell the patient to avoid excessive use of the wheelchair. Encourage him to walk short distances, if possible, and to use other chairs in the home when relaxing or dining.

7. If the patient uses crutches without a prosthesis, warn against propping the stump in the V of the crutch.

8. Instruct the patient to change position often.

Rationales

1. Prolonged sitting can cause knee flexion contracture.

2. These actions prevent hip flexion contracture and strengthen the muscles needed to use a prosthesis.

3. Resting the stump on pillows can cause abduction-flexion contracture.

4. Abduction and external rotation can cause contracture. Externally rotated contracture adversely affects gait.

5. Adduction prevents abduction contracture.

6. Excessive wheelchair use can cause hip flexion contracture.

7. Propping the stump can cause flexion contracture.

8. Position changes prevent contracture and decubitus ulcer formation and help mobilize muscles and joints.

Nursing diagnosis: *Self-care deficit related to arm amputation*

GOAL 1: To improve the patient's self-care ability

Interventions

1. If the patient has unilateral arm amputation, determine whether the remaining arm is the dominant one.

2. Refer the patient to occupational therapy.

Rationales

1. This information helps in planning the patient's activities and restrictions. The patient with a unilateral amputation faces fewer self-care restrictions than does the patient with a bilateral amputation, and self-care activities are easier if the remaining arm is the dominant one.

2. An occupational therapist can help the patient achieve adequate mobility with the prosthesis to perform ADLs with greater independence and can assist in the patient's return to work, school, and community activities.

GOAL 2: To maintain current function and prevent complications

Interventions

1. Monitor for signs and symptoms of infection, such as redness, edema, foul odor, and exudate.

2. Encourage the patient to exercise the shoulder depressors, biceps, and triceps.

Rationales

1. Arm amputation typically is preceded by trauma, which increases the patient's risk of infection.

2. Exercise strengthens these muscles, preparing them for prosthesis use.

GOAL 3: To help the patient accept the amputation

Interventions

1. Assess the patient's progress in the grieving process.

2. Give the patient ample time to express feelings about the amputation, and discuss the grieving process with the caregiver, if possible. (See the "Grief and Grieving" care plan for more information.)

3. Urge the patient's family and friends to provide generous emotional support.

Rationales

1. Because arm amputation typically is preceded by trauma, the patient usually has no opportunity for preparation or anticipatory grief. Support and encouragement from the nurse can help the patient begin to accept the amputation.

2. The patient will probably experience severe body image disturbances because of the amputation; encouraging open expression of feelings may ease the grieving process. Explaining the grieving process to the caregiver helps prepare him for the patient's likely emotional responses.

3. Attention and encouragement from loved ones help the patient regain much-needed self-esteem.

ASSOCIATED CARE PLANS
• Diabetes
• Grief and Grieving
• Ineffective Coping
• Pain
• Sex and Sexuality
• Smoking Cessation

NETWORKING OF SERVICES
• Meals On Wheels
• DME supplier
• rehabilitation clinic
• vocational rehabilitation center
• local support group

CARE TEAM INVOLVED
• nurse
• doctor
• patient and family
• home health aide
• physical therapist
• occupational therapist
• medical social worker
• prosthetist

IMPLICATIONS FOR HOME CARE
• functional features of the home (wide doorways, wheelchair ramp)
• prevention of complications
• safety

PATIENT EDUCATION TOOLS
• written instructions on ROM exercises
• list of signs and symptoms of infection

DISCHARGE PLAN FROM HOME HEALTH CARE
Before discharge from home health care, the patient
should:
• post telephone numbers for the doctor, nurse, home
health agency, ambulance service, hospital emergency
department, and emergency medical team by the phone
• have a well-healed, well-shaped, mature stump
• use proper body alignment and positioning
• exercise regularly to promote muscle strength and
joint mobilization
• have a plan for keeping appointments with the doctor,
laboratory, and prosthetist
• participate in self-care and ADLs
• stop smoking (if patient smokes)
• have regular bowel movements
• institute necessary diet changes
• experience little or no phantom limb pain
• be adapting to the amputation and altered body image
• make changes necessary to facilitate mobility in the
home
• have a plan for vocational rehabilitation, if necessary.

SELECTED REFERENCES
Carpenito, L.J. *Handbook of Nursing Diagnosis.* Philadel-
phia: J.B. Lippincott Co., 1984.
Farrell, J. *Illustrated Guide to Orthopedic Nursing,* 3rd
ed. Philadelphia: J.B. Lippincott Co., 1986.
Gordon, M. *Manual of Nursing Diagnosis.* New York:
McGraw-Hill Book Co., 1987.
Mort, M. *Retraining for the Elderly Disabled.* Helm, N.H.:
Croom, 1985.
Price, S.A., and Wilson, L.M. *Pathophysiology: Clinical
Concepts of Disease Processes.* New York: McGraw-Hill
Book Co., 1986.
Schwartz, M.H. *Textbook of Physical Diagnosis, History
and Examination.* Philadelphia: W.B. Saunders Co.,
1989.

MUSCULOSKELETAL SYSTEM

Fractured Hip

DESCRIPTION AND TIME FOCUS

A fractured hip involves injury to the proximal third of the femur. Transcervical fracture is the most common type. Surgical repair involves an open reduction, internal fixation (ORIF) with a compression screw, pins, or rods, or hemiarthroplasty with a prosthesis, such as the Austin-Moore or bipolar implant. After surgery, the patient may be treated for osteoporosis and is at high risk for falls and fractures. Fracture can occur spontaneously.

This clinical plan focuses on the patient discharged home from an acute-care facility after surgery to repair a fractured hip. Postoperative care centers on rehabilitation to help the patient increase mobility while the bone and soft tissues are healing. The nurse monitors for complications and collaborates with the physical therapist to plan the patient's rehabilitation program. The home is an ideal setting for patient teaching, particularly for elderly patients, who are typically better oriented in a familiar environment.

- Typical home health care length of service for an uncomplicated hip fracture: 4 weeks
- Typical visit frequency: twice weekly

HEALTH HISTORY FINDINGS

In a health history interview, the patient may report many of these findings:
- osteoporosis
- thin, petite body frame
- history of falls
- history of vertebral or wrist fractures

PHYSICAL FINDINGS

In a physical examination, the nurse may detect many of these findings:

Musculoskeletal
- hip or posterior knee pain
- ecchymosis in groin
- limb rotation
- edema in thigh or groin
- pain and crepitation on movement
- impaired ability to move

Cardiovascular
- tachycardia
- hypertension or hypotension
- pallor and numbness in lower leg or foot
- diminished pedal pulse

Neurologic
- disorientation and confusion
- anxiety

DIAGNOSTIC STUDIES

The following studies may be performed to evaluate the patient's health status:
- hip X-ray—6 to 12 weeks after surgery, then every 3 to 6 months for first year, to evaluate bone healing, detect infection, and monitor alignment
- serum calcium studies—monthly until stable, then at least every 3 months, as ordered, to ensure continued stability; normal range 4.5 to 5.5 mEq/liter
- prothrombin time (if patient is on warfarin)—weekly until doctor discontinues medication or changes time span; normal range 9.6 to 11.8 seconds (males); 9.5 to 11.3 seconds (females)

Nursing diagnosis: *Potential for injury related to hip dislocation, avascular necrosis, thromboembolitic complications, fat embolism syndrome, neurovascular compromise, or wound infection*

GOAL 1: To prevent life-threatening complications and promote healing

Interventions

1. Assess neurovascular status of the legs by comparing the affected and unaffected legs. Assess color, temperature, movement, sensation, distal pulses, capillary refill, and degree of pain during passive and active motion.

2. Instruct the patient to avoid crossing his legs or ankles and to place a pillow between his legs when sleeping or lying on the nonoperative side. Tell him to do this for 6 to 12 weeks to prevent hip adduction.

Rationales

1. Neurovascular compromise can indicate hip dislocation or internal fixation failure. Prompt intervention is needed to ensure adequate tissue perfusion and prevent tissue necrosis.

2. Hip adduction can cause dislocation, particularly if a prosthetic device has been inserted.

3. Tell the patient he should prevent hip flexion beyond 90 degrees for 6 to 12 weeks by using an elevated toilet seat, avoiding leaning forward, and sitting in a high, firm chair.

4. Instruct the patient to wear thigh-high elastic stockings for 6 weeks or more.

5. Teach the patient to perform quadriceps-setting and ankle-pumping exercises every 1 to 2 hours during the day.

6. Encourage the patient to ambulate and use a walker, as ordered.

7. Monitor the patient for signs and symptoms of infection anywhere in the body. Assess wound status thoroughly, and record the patient's temperature.

3. Hip hyperflexion can cause hip dislocation until the fracture and soft tissues heal.

4. The risk of thigh thrombi, which readily become emboli, is greatest during the first 6 weeks after surgery.

5. Lower leg exercises increase venous circulation, which decreases the risk of deep vein thrombus formation.

6. Early and consistent ambulation decreases the risk of thromboembolitic complications.

7. Any infection (for example, of the urinary tract or upper respiratory tract) can migrate to the hip, cause a deep wound infection, and result in sepsis or the need to remove the hardware.

GOAL 2: To recognize and respond to signs of complication promptly

Interventions

1. Monitor for indications of hip dislocation, such as limb rotation and shortening or hip pain.

2. Assess the location and characteristics of the patient's pain.

3. Monitor the patient for subtle changes in neurovascular status.

4. Assess the legs for signs of deep vein thrombus formation, including Homans's sign.

Rationales

1. Dislocation is the most common complication of hip surgery, especially if a prothesis is used. Prompt treatment preserves tissue perfusion in the lower leg.

2. Sharp, intermittent hip pain can indicate loosening of the fixation or prosthetic device, avascular necrosis, or dislocation. Dull, continuous hip pain may indicate a deep wound infection. Sudden chest pain may indicate pulmonary embolus or fat embolism syndrome.

3. Early signs of acute neurovascular compromise include increased pain during passive motion of the foot and pain that is unrelieved by analgesics.

4. Deep vein thrombi can dislodge and migrate to the brain, heart, or lungs.

Nursing diagnosis: *Impaired physical mobility related to hip discomfort, surgical trauma, weight-bearing restrictions, and hip precautions*

GOAL 1: To facilitate mobility until the patient can ambulate independently

Interventions

1. Teach the patient weight-bearing restrictions, and stress their importance.

2. Reinforce proper use of a walker or other ambulatory aid and of such devices as reachers and dressing sticks.

3. Encourage the patient to perform daily exercises prescribed by the physical therapist, such as range-of-motion (ROM) and muscle-strengthening exercises.

Rationales

1. Weight-bearing restrictions are usually imposed until the fracture and soft tissues heal completely. Typically, a patient with ORIF or a cemented prosthesis can bear partial weight (or as much as is tolerable) during the first 6 to 12 weeks. A patient with a cementless prosthesis should not bear weight until bony ingrowth is confirmed by X-ray. Then the patient can progress from partial to full weight bearing.

2. Ambulatory aids help bear the patient's weight, placing less weight on the affected hip. Medical devices promote independence in self-care and increase mobility.

3. The patient must perform prescribed exercises daily to improve mobility and prevent contracture and muscle atrophy.

GOAL 2: To prevent complications associated with impaired mobility

Interventions	Rationales
1. Instruct the patient to change position frequently while in bed; help him change position if necessary. Also tell him to avoid sitting for prolonged periods.	1. Frequent position changes help prevent skin breakdown, flexion contracture, and respiratory complications.
2. Remind the patient to perform leg exercises and to wear elastic stockings.	2. Leg movement and elastic stockings promote venous circulation, which decreases the patient's risk of deep vein thrombosis.
3. Teach the patient the importance of drinking at least 1½ liters of fluid each day, unless contraindicated.	3. Adequate fluid intake helps prevent urinary tract infection and renal calculi formation.

Nursing diagnosis: *Altered comfort: pain related to surgical trauma and muscle spasm*

GOAL: To alleviate hip pain

Interventions	Rationales
1. Tell the patient to maintain proper leg alignment by avoiding extreme internal or external rotation.	1. Extreme leg rotation can increase hip pain.
2. Assess the intensity and duration of the patient's pain. (See the "Pain" care plan for more information on assessing pain tolerance.)	2. Increasing pain can indicate a surgical complication, such as infection.
3. Use pain management modalities other than medications when feasible (for example, distraction, guided imagery, or music).	3. Hip pain should be managed using alternative methods to prevent excessive use of analgesics, which can have potent adverse effects, especially in elderly patients.

Nursing diagnosis: *Impaired home maintenance management related to potential safety hazards*

GOAL: To help the patient prevent falls and other serious injuries

Interventions	Rationales
1. Assess the patient's home for potential safety hazards, such as stairs, scatter rugs, slippery floors, and cluttered rooms.	1. These hazards can cause a fall and subsequent injury. Climbing stairs is prohibited until the fracture heals.
2. Tell the patient to wear rubber-soled shoes that provide firm support.	2. Shoes with slippery soles and poor support can cause a fall.

Nursing diagnosis: *Knowledge deficit related to the prosthesis*

GOAL: To improve the patient's knowledge of his prosthesis

Interventions	Rationales
1. Briefly describe the hardware used in a prosthesis, and explain to the patient why he must report the prosthesis whenever he gives a health history interview in the future.	1. Certain medical procedures, such as diathermy and ultrasound, can heat metal parts used in the prosthesis.
2. Advise the patient who travels by airplane to report his prosthesis before walking through a metal detector.	2. Hardware in the prosthesis will activate the airport's metal detector alarm.

ASSOCIATED CARE PLANS
• Osteoarthritis
• Osteoporosis
• Pain
• Total Hip Replacement

NETWORKING OF SERVICES
• Lifeline
• Meals On Wheels
• physical therapy
• occupational therapy
• osteoporosis clinic
• durable medical equipment supplier

CARE TEAM INVOLVED
• nurse
• orthopedic surgeon
• patient and family
• physical therapist
• occupational therapist
• medical social worker

IMPLICATIONS FOR HOME CARE
• functional features of the home (raised toilet seat, access to bathroom and shower)
• telephone (communication)

PATIENT EDUCATION TOOLS
• list of permissible activities and precautions
• literature about osteoporosis
• literature about fall prevention
• literature about each medication prescribed
• instructions for prescribed exercises

DISCHARGE PLAN FROM HOME HEALTH CARE
Before discharge from home health care, the patient should:
• know permissible activities and precautions for hip positioning
• receive appropriate osteoporosis treatment
• ambulate independently with a walker
• know the signs and symptoms of potential complications
• require minimal medication for pain relief
• perform ADLs independently, using assistive devices
• perform prescribed exercises daily
• have a safe home environment
• know precautions for indwelling hardware, including medical procedures, such as diathermy and ultrasound (that can heat metal parts), and reporting prosthesis when passing through airport metal detector.

SELECTED REFERENCES
Doheny, M.O. "Porous-Coated Femoral Prosthesis: Concepts and Care Considerations," *Orthopedic Nursing* 1:43, January/February 1985.
Farrell, J. *Illustrated Guide to Orthopedic Nursing*, 3rd ed. Philadelphia: J.B. Lippincott Co., 1986.
Lackmann, J., and Sorensen, K.C. *Medical-Surgical Nursing: A Psychophysiologic Approach*, 3rd ed. Philadelphia: W.B. Saunders Co., 1987.
"Spotting a Dislocated Hip," *Emergency Medicine* 16:53, September 1984.

Spinal Compression Fracture

DESCRIPTION AND TIME FOCUS
Compression fracture resulting from intervertebral disc degeneration may be the primary cause of low back pain. The patient typically has a history of osteoarthritis with little or no history of injury, and reports sudden onset of pain usually localized to one area of the thoracolumbar spine.

This clinical plan focuses on the patient discharged home after hospitalization for a spinal compression fracture. Nursing care centers on controlling acute pain, teaching the patient about medications, and helping the patient follow a rehabilitation program.

■ Typical home health care length of service for a patient recovering from spinal compression fracture: 2 weeks

■ Typical visit frequency: Twice weekly for 2 weeks

HEALTH HISTORY FINDINGS
In a health history interview, the patient may report many of these findings:
• sudden onset of muscle spasm and pain in the thoracolumbar spine
• pain radiating to back of thigh, leg, and foot
• history of hyperflexion or excessive rotation of spine
• history of osteoarthritis
• history of calcium deficiency
• history of endocrine disorder, such as Cushing's syndrome, acromegaly, or hyperthyroidism

PHYSICAL FINDINGS
In a physical exaination, the nurse may detect many of these findings:

Musculoskeletal
• local tenderness on palpation of thoracolumbar spine
• stooped or otherwise deformed posture
• restricted lumbosacral flexion

Integumentary
• skin breakdown under brace at pressure points

DIAGNOSTIC STUDIES
None applicable to home care

Nursing diagnosis: *Altered comfort: pain, related to nerve impingement and muscle spasm*

GOAL: To control acute pain and promote healing

Interventions	Rationales
1. Instruct the patient to follow prescribed activity restrictions, which likely will include strict bedrest for at least 1 week.	1. Rest helps prevent the fracture from worsening and promotes healing.
2. Teach the patient proper positioning in bed. Instruct him to lie supine with knees and hips flexed, using pillows for support, or to lie on one side with knees and hips flexed. Tell the patient never to lie prone. Be sure the patient has a firm mattress and, if necessary, a bed board.	2. Proper positioning and firm support prevent excessive tension on the injured spinal column and relieve pain.
3. Instruct the patient to apply dry or moist heat to the lower back for 15 to 30 minutes, four to six times a day.	3. Heat relaxes muscles, provides local pain relief, and increases blood supply to the area, which promotes healing. (*Note:* Moist heat may be more effective than dry heat.)
4. Instruct the patient on the use of anti-inflammatory drugs or analgesics for pain control.	4. Anti-inflammatory drugs ease inflammation and swelling in the injured area, allowing it to heal. Analgesics provide pain relief and promote relaxation.

Nursing diagnosis: *Potential for impaired skin integrity related to prolonged immobility*

GOAL: To prevent skin breakdown

Interventions

1. Provide good skin care. Bathe the patient thoroughly, apply lotion as indicated, and massage bony areas. Teach these procedures to the family.

2. Inspect the skin for reddened areas, particularly the skin over bony prominences and under a brace or corset. Teach the family to do this and to report reddening promptly.

3. Encourage the patient to change position in bed at least every 2 hours. Assist with repositioning as necessary, using the logrolling technique and taking care to avoid damaging delicate skin. Teach the family these measures.

Rationales

1. Proper skin care prevents breakdown, a major complication of prolonged immobility.

2. Skin reddening is an early sign of breakdown and calls for prompt intervention to prevent further damage.

3. Periodic repositioning relieves pressure over bony prominences, which helps prevent skin breakdown. Logrolling prevents twisting and pressure on back muscles and the spinal column.

Nursing diagnosis: *Impaired physical mobility related to pain and limitations of the therapeutic regimen*

GOAL: To gradually increase mobility

Interventions

1. For a patient restricted to bed rest, teach exercises that he can do in bed, such as rolling from side to side and leg lifts. Caution against overactivity, however.

2. As the patient's condition improves, help him adhere to the prescribed physical rehabilitation program, which will include various leg- and back-strengthening exercises. Caution the patient not to bend, stoop, or lift until pain subsides.

3. Allow the patient to wear a corset or sacroiliac support at first, but tell him that he must gradually wean himself from this device.

4. Help the patient maintain adequate hydration and nutrition by encouraging him to drink plenty of fluids and to follow a well-balanced diet that includes foods high in calcium and fewer-than-usual calories.

5. Teach the patient back care measures, including good posture; proper body mechanics, such as bending at the knees and hips rather than the waist and carrying objects close to the body; getting adequate rest; sleeping in the supine or side-lying position on a firm mattress; and weight reduction (if necessary).

Rationales

1. These exercises can help maintain or improve mobility with a minimal risk of injury.

2. A good physical rehabilitation program helps strengthen muscles and promote improved mobility.

3. Such a device immobilizes the spinal column and maintains body alignment during activity, which minimizes pain, promotes healing, and prevents exacerbation. Extended use can lead to muscle weakness, which reduces the support needed to maintain spinal alignment.

4. Adequate fluid and calcium intake promotes healing and helps prevent complications. Restricted caloric intake helps prevent undesired weight gain linked to lowered metabolic needs during periods of prolonged immobility.

5. These measures help prevent injury recurrence.

ASSOCIATED CARE PLANS
• Osteoarthritis
• Osteoporosis
• Pain

NETWORKING OF SERVICES
• Meals On Wheels
• durable medical equipment supplier
• vocational rehabilitation center

CARE TEAM INVOLVED
• nurse
• doctor
• patient and family
• physical therapist
• home health aide

IMPLICATIONS FOR HOME CARE
• telephone at bedside
• functional features of the home (stairs, accessibility of bathroom and kitchen)
• safe home environment

PATIENT EDUCATION TOOLS
• information about proper body mechanics
• literature about each medication prescribed

DISCHARGE PLAN FROM HOME HEALTH CARE
Before discharge from home health care, the patient should:
• understand therapeutic activities and restrictions
• understand safety measures for the home
• understand and use proper body mechanics
• understand and implement measures to reduce discomfort
• know the name, action, dosage, and adverse effects of each medication prescribed
• understand the need for follow-up visits with the doctor, and know dates of scheduled visits
• have emergency phone numbers at bedside.

SELECTED REFERENCES
Farrell, J. *Illustrated Guide to Orthopedic Nursing*, 3rd ed. Philadelphia: J.B. Lippincott Co., 1986.
Jennings, M. (ed.) *Nursing Care Planning Guides for Home Health Care*. Baltimore: Williams & Wilkins Co., 1988.
Meinhart, N., and McCaffery, M. *Pain: A Nursing Approach to Assessment and Analysis*. East Norwalk, Conn.: Appleton-Century-Crofts, 1983.
Sutton, S. *Home Health Nursing Manual: Procedures and Documentation*. Baltimore: Williams & Wilkins Co., 1988.
Walsh, J., Persons, C., and Weick, L. *Manual of Home Health Care Nursing* Philadelphia: J.B. Lippincott Co., 1987.

MUSCULOSKELETAL SYSTEM
Osteomyelitis

DESCRIPTION AND TIME FOCUS
Osteomyelitis is a bone infection, usually caused by bacteria, that can result in bone destruction. *Staphylococcus aureus* is most often the cause, although *Escherichia coli, Pseudomonas, or Proteus* (including penicillin-resistant strains) can also be at fault. Osteomyelitis usually affects the long bones of children and vertebrae of adults, typically occurring within 2 years of bone surgery or trauma. Late onset (after 2 years) can result from hematogenous spread to a previously traumatized bone that has decreased resistance to infection. Osteomyelitis is classified as primary, secondary, or chronic.

In osteomyelitis, infected bone becomes avascular and scar tissue forms, creating a barrier against antibiotics. Unless controlled, the infection causes bone abscess and additional bone necrosis. Sequestra (separated, dead bone tissue) does not liquefy and drain; it may lead to chronic infection. Sequestrectomy (surgical debridement of dead and infected bone and cartilage) may be necessary.

Acute osteomyelitis usually occurs in children and can be caused by hematogenous spread of a bacterial infection from another source, such as boils, dental infections, or upper respiratory infection. An open fracture, bone surgery, or gunshot wounds also can cause acute bone infection. Chronic osteomyelitis is more common in adults and may develop when treatment for acute infection is delayed or ineffective.

This clinical plan focuses on the patient discharged home from a hospital after diagnosis and initial treatment of osteomyelitis. I.V. antibiotic therapy is usually anticipated.
■ Typical home health care length of service for a patient with osteomyelitis: 4 to 6 weeks
■ Typical visit frequency: twice weekly to assess the patient's wound healing and response to care. More frequent visits are needed to handle I.V. therapy. Frequency can range from once to five times daily, depending on treatment protocols and the patient's and caregiver's ability to learn I.V. skills.

HEALTH HISTORY FINDINGS
In a health history interview, the patient may report many of these findings:

• history of infection after open fracture, bone trauma, or systemic infection
• history of bone infection
• pain in affected part
• immobility
• malnourishment
• recent orthopedic surgery
• rheumatoid arthritis

PHYSICAL FINDINGS
In a physical examination, the nurse may detect many of these findings:

Musculoskeletal
• muscle spasm in affected part
• pseudoparalysis (inability to move joints near the affected area because of anticipatory pain)

Neurologic
• pain in affected area (long bones in children, vertebrae in adults)

Integumentary
• edema and erythema in affected area
• inflammation in affected area
• signs of systemic response (general weakness, fever, chills, diaphoresis)
• purulent drainage (indicates chronic osteomyelitis)
• chronically draining sinus tract (rare)

DIAGNOSTIC STUDIES
The following studies may be performed to evaluate the patient's health status:
• complete blood count (CBC)—weekly during antibiotic therapy and once after therapy ends to detect infection; increased white blood cell (WBC) count (leukocytosis) indicates infection
• drainage cultures—before antibiotic therapy begins and 1 week after it ends if drainage still present; positive for causative organisms
• X-ray—negative for 5 days to several weeks, then shows elevated periosteum or bone destruction
• bone scan—may be ordered during or after antibiotic therapy; may show bone changes before X-ray

---

Nursing diagnosis: *Altered comfort: pain, related to local inflammation and ischemia at the infection site*

GOAL: To promote comfort at the infection site

Interventions
1. Assess the patient's level of pain by having him rate

Rationales
1. Regular assessment helps in monitoring the patient's

it on a scale of 1 (minor) to 10 (severe). Evaluate the effectiveness of analgesics and comfort measures.

2. Immobilize the affected extremity, and have the patient remain in bed, as ordered.

3. Tell the patient to keep the affected extremity elevated at all times other than when using the bathroom.

4. Support the joints above and below the affected area when moving the patient.

5. Have a bed cradle installed if a lower extremity is affected.

progress and response to medications and treatment.

2. Immobilization and bed rest reduce stimulation to the affected area, thus reducing pain and episodes of muscle spasm. These interventions also minimize the patient's risk of further injury and promote healing.

3. Elevation reduces inflammatory edema and enhances venous return.

4. Support minimizes pain during movement and protects the bone from excessive stress.

5. The bed cradle protects injured parts from contact with bedclothes, reduces direct pressure, and minimizes discomfort.

Nursing diagnosis: *Potential for injury related to bone loss from infection or surgery*

GOAL: To prevent injury by minimizing complications

Interventions

1. Assess the neurovascular status of the affected extremity. Measure and record the circumference of the extremity.

2. Maintain proper positioning of the affected extremity. Apply splints if ordered, or use pillows and footboards.

3. Teach the patient the proper method of walking with crutches, with weight bearing as ordered.

4. Perform active or passive range-of-motion (ROM) exercises to uninvolved extremities and to the affected extremity if prescribed by the doctor.

5. Schedule rest periods and leisure activities the patient enjoys, such as puzzles, television, or painting. Be sure the activities conform to weight-bearing limitations.

6. Arrange support services, such as Meals On Wheels or home health aides, as needed.

Rationales

1. The patient's circulation may be compromised, and immobilization can cause muscle atrophy. Increased circumference may indicate increased inflammation.

2. Proper positioning prevents footdrop, outward rotation, and flexion contracture.

3. Proper technique minimizes the patient's risk for falls or further injury to the bone.

4. ROM exercises prevent muscle atrophy and bone resorption, minimize loss of muscle strength and endurance by maintaining adequate blood flow, and aid in bone remodeling.

5. Adequate rest is essential for healing. Leisure activities can divert the patient's attention away from pain and help him focus on pleasurable aspects of living.

6. Support services can provide help with many activities that the immobilized patient cannot complete independently.

Nursing diagnosis: *Potential for infection related to draining wound*

GOAL: To prevent the infection from spreading

Interventions

1. Teach the patient and caregiver how to administer antibiotics as ordered.

2. Monitor wound drainage and vital signs, especially temperature. Note any changes. Repeat drainage cultures as ordered. Teach the patient signs and symptoms of infection, such as purulent, copious drainage and foul odor.

Rationales

1. Antibiotic therapy is the primary treatment for the infection. The patient and caregiver must thoroughly understand the medication regimen, including method of administration, dosage, action, and adverse effects.

2. Increased pain, edema, or redness; purulent or copious drainage; and fever accompanied by malaise or weakness can indicate the infection is spreading. Careful monitoring and appropriate patient teaching help ensure prompt detection and treatment.

3. Instruct the patient and caregiver on all aspects of wound care. Review proper hand-washing technique, tell them to use gloves when handling infected materials, and show them how to properly dispose of contaminated dressings.

3. These interventions help prevent the spread of infection.

4. Caution the patient and family that immunosuppressed individuals must not come in contact with wound drainage.

4. Immunosuppression increases the risk of developing infection.

Nursing diagnosis: *Knowledge deficit related to the disease process and the treatment regimen*

GOAL: To help the patient adhere to the treatment regimen by increasing his knowledge of osteomyelitis

Interventions

1. Teach the patient about osteomyelitis, including the cause, risk factors, and need for prolonged treatments.

2. Explain the importance of drinking 3 liters of fluid daily and following a diet high in calories, protein, fiber, and vitamins C and D.

3. Tell the patient and caregiver to notify the doctor if the patient develops additional tender areas, increased temperature, increased joint stiffness, increased wound drainage or drainage having a foul odor, general malaise, boils, or a sore mouth.

4. Teach the patient and caregiver how to properly administer antibiotics. Tell the patient to take medication at appropriate intervals throughout the day and night, as indicated; to take oral antibiotics 1 hour before or 2 hours after meals; and to refer to the label instructions for mixing, storing, and administering antibiotics.

5. Tell the patient and caregiver to notify the doctor if the patient experiences any adverse reactions to the antibiotics. Respiratory distress, hives, vomiting, diarrhea, or edema can indicate hypersensitivity. Sore mouth, diarrhea, skin rash, itch, discharge, recurrence of fever, or malaise may indicate secondary infection or a superinfection.

Rationales

1. Understanding the long-term nature of the disease may reduce anxiety and promote compliance with treatment.

2. This diet provides a positive nitrogen balance and promotes healing. Extra calories spare proteins for tissue building. Fiber promotes normal peristalsis, which aids in bowel elimination resulting from immobility. Increased fluids promote bowel elimination and are especially important if the patient has a fever.

3. These signs and symptoms indicate that the infection is worsening or that a secondary infection is developing. Either condition requires prompt medical attention.

4. Periodic administration maintains therapeutic blood drug levels. Most oral antibiotics are absorbed better when taken on an empty stomach. Antibiotic effectiveness depends on strict adherence to instructions.

5. Hypersensitivity is most common with penicillin but can occur with any antibiotic. Superinfection, a common development, is serious because the causative organism may be drug-resistant and, therefore, hard to treat.

ASSOCIATED CARE PLANS
• Ineffective Coping
• Intermittent I.V. Therapy
• Pain

NETWORKING OF SERVICES
• Meals On Wheels
• in-home education for a school-age child
• vocational rehabilitation

CARE TEAM INVOLVED
• nurse
• doctor
• patient and family
• medical social worker
• I.V. therapist
• physical therapist
• spiritual advisor

IMPLICATIONS FOR HOME CARE
• ability of patient and caregiver to perform care and I.V. therapy
• suitability of home (uncrowded environment where aseptic technique for I.V. and drainage precaution can be managed)
• no immunosuppressed individuals in the home because of presence of infected materials

PATIENT EDUCATION TOOLS
• description of proper hand-washing technique
• information about signs and symptoms of new infection
• list of infectious disease precautions
• literature about home I.V. therapy

DISCHARGE PLAN FROM HOME HEALTH CARE
Before discharge from home health care, the patient should:
• understand proper wound care and precautions to take when handling and disposing of contaminated materials
• be using oral antibiotics
• demonstrate ambulation while bearing allowable weight
• know the method of storage and administration, dosage, action, and adverse effects of each prescribed medication
• know the signs and symptoms of recurrent infection
• demonstrate proper technique for walking with crutches
• understand the disease process and the need for prolonged treatment
• know the adverse effects that must be reported to the doctor
• demonstrate aseptic dressing change techniques
• comply with dietary requirements
• follow the prescribed exercise program
• know the date of follow-up appointments with the doctor
• post telephone numbers for the doctor, nurse, and home health agency in a prominent place.

SELECTED REFERENCES
Abrams, A.C. *Clinical Drug Therapy: Rationales for Nursing Practice*, 2nd ed. Philadelphia: J.B. Lippincott Co., 1987.

Brunner, L., and Suddarth, D. *Textbook of Medical-Surgical Nursing*, 6th ed. Philadelphia: J.B. Lippincott Co., 1988.

Carpenito, L.J. *Nursing Diagnosis: Application to Clinical Practice*, 2nd ed. Philadelphia: J.B. Lippincott Co., 1987.

Chrystal, C. "Making the NITA Standards Work for You," *NITA* 8(5):363-64, 1985.

Farrell, J. *Illustrated Guide to Orthopedic Nursing*, 3rd ed. Philadelphia: J.B. Lippincott Co., 1986.

Harris, L.F., et al. "Intravenous Antibiotics at Home," *Southern Medical Journal* 79(2):193-96, 1986.

Hoyt, N.J. "Infections Following Orthopaedic Injury," *Orthopaedic Nursing* 5(5):15-24, 1986.

Pagliaro, A.M., and Pagliaro, L.A. *Pharmacologic Aspects of Nursing.* St. Louis: C.V. Mosby Co., 1986.

Powell, M. *Orthopedic Nursing and Rehabilitation*, 9th ed. London: Churchill Livingstone, 1986.

Pozzi, M., and Peck, N. "An Option for the Patient with Chronic Osteomyelitis: Home Intravenous Therapy," *Orthopedic Nursing* 5(5):9-14, 1986.

MUSCULOSKELETAL SYSTEM

Osteoarthritis

DESCRIPTION AND TIME FOCUS

Osteoarthritis, also called hypertrophic arthritis or degenerative joint disease, is the most common form of arthritic disease. It can occur in any joint, but most commonly affects the hips, knees, and cervical and lumbar spine. The etiology is unknown, but aging, obesity, joint trauma, and family history may be predisposing factors. Most persons over age 60 suffer some degree of osteoarthritis.

Osteoarthritis occurs when joint hyaline cartilage is destroyed and adjacent bone ends hypertrophy, imposing into the joint space. Spurs, cysts, and nodes may form, and cartilage debris may occupy the joint. The arthritic joint weakens and becomes more susceptible to stress and further damage. In later, more severe stages, joint shape and mechanical structure may be destroyed, impairing joint function.

This clinical plan focuses on caring for a patient with a flare-up of osteoarthritis requiring medical and nursing intervention. Care after an acute flare-up centers on alleviating pain and fatigue, rehabilitating joint range of motion, and monitoring for such complications as muscle atrophy, contracture, persistent joint pain, joint immobility, skin breakdown, and psychosocial problems associated with prolonged immobility. Providing care in the patient's home helps minimize the patient's stress level and allows the nurse to plan home adaptations that will maximize the patient's ability to perform activities of daily living (ADLs) independently.

■ Typical home health care length of service for a patient with acute osteoarthritis: 2 weeks
■ Typical visit frequency: 2 visits weekly

HEALTH HISTORY FINDINGS

In a health history interview, the patient may report many of these findings:
• joint pain and stiffness
• limited mobility
• history of joint trauma or repeated joint stress
• family history of arthritic disease
• history of joint infection

PHYSICAL FINDINGS

In a physical examination, the nurse may detect many of these findings:

Musculoskeletal
• limited joint range of motion (ROM)
• joint structure deformity
• joint inflammation
• joint crepitation

DIAGNOSTIC STUDIES

The following studies may be performed to evaluate the patient's health status:
• X-rays—as ordered, to reveal increasing bony growths, decreasing joint spaces, and progressive joint deformity
• synovial fluid aspiration and analysis (less common)—as ordered, to monitor disease progression

---

Nursing diagnosis: *Impaired physical mobility related to pain, activity intolerance, and depression*

GOAL 1: To reduce joint pain and referred pain

Interventions

1. Administer prescribed antispasmodic, anti-inflammatory, or analgesic medications, as ordered. Teach the patient the route of administration, dosage, and adverse effects of each medication.

2. Massage the area surrounding the painful joint—not the joint itself. Provide traction, if ordered.

Rationales

1. These medications can reduce pain and inflammation. The patient's understanding of the medication regimen promotes compliance.

2. Massage promotes muscle relaxation and pain relief. Traction relieves joint stress and pain, especially in the cervical spine.

GOAL 2: To increase the patient's mobility and activity tolerance

Interventions

1. Work with a physical therapist to plan an exercise program in accordance with the doctor's orders. Such a program typically includes active and passive ROM exercises, isometric exercises, progressive resistance exercises, and aerobic exercise.

2. Teach the patient and family proper body alignment and joint support techniques.

3. Teach the patient the importance of slow, smooth movements, proper body mechanics, and safe transfer techniques. Instruct the patient to avoid heavy lifting.

4. Plan alternating periods of activity and rest each day. Scheduling is particularly important during peak stress times, such as late afternoon.

5. As necessary, help the patient obtain an assistive device, such as a cane or walker, and provide instructions on proper use.

6. Assess the patient's home for potential safety hazards, such as throw rugs that could slip, exposed electrical and telephone cords, and unsafe stairs. Intervene as necessary to eliminate or minimize any hazards.

7. Provide praise and positive reinforcement when the patient demonstrates improved activity tolerance. Encourage similar support and praise from family members.

Rationales

1. ROM exercises prevent muscle contracture and atrophy, maintain joint flexibility, and increase joint mobility. Isometric and progressive resistance exercises promote muscle tone and strength. Aerobic exercises promote endurance and a feeling of well-being.

2. Proper alignment promotes comfort and helps prevent muscle contracture and atrophy, both of which contribute to increased activity tolerance.

3. These techniques reduce joint stress and help slow joint degeneration, decrease pain, and reduce fatigue—all of which help increase activity tolerance and promote mobility.

4. A daily routine that includes adequate rest and exercise reduces the patient's fatigue and improves activity tolerance.

5. Assistive devices can increase the patient's mobility.

6. Elimination of hazards helps decrease the risk of falls and other accidents and encourages increased mobility.

7. Support and praise motivate the patient to continue working toward goals.

GOAL 3: To alleviate fatigue, frustration, and depression

Interventions

1. Teach the patient to recognize the early symptoms of stress and fatigue—such as joint pain, weakness, lethargy, numbness, tingling, tension, and anxiety.

2. Teach the patient relaxation techniques, and discuss the benefits of quiet reflection, self-reward, pet therapy, music therapy, and visualization.

3. Help the patient accept activity limitations. Focus his attention on remaining abilities, and suggest interesting alternative activities to replace former hobbies and interests he can no longer pursue.

Rationales

1. Early recognition of increased stress and fatigue enables the patient to take steps to decrease these problems.

2. These techniques help alleviate stress, which can exacerbate the patient's condition if unrelieved.

3. Productive and interesting activities help alleviate stress, loneliness, and depression.

Nursing diagnosis: *Self-care deficit: bathing/hygiene, dressing/grooming, feeding, toileting related to pain, decreased mobility, and activity intolerance*

GOAL: To improve the patient's self-care capabilities

Interventions

1. Schedule nursing visits at various times of day rather than at the same time each day.

Rationales

1. Visiting the patient at different times of the day facilitates comprehensive assessment of the patient's ability to perform ADLs and safety requirements.

2. Help the patient plan ADLs that promote health and self-esteem. Consider his privacy and dignity when discussing self-care deficits. Advise him to acquire necessary medical equipment and devices (for example, shower stalls for bathing transfers and padded utensils for feeding). Instruct him on their use, or reinforce the instructions provided by an occupational therapist.

2. Completing self-care activities increases the patient's sense of independence and self-esteem.

3. Advise the patient and family about the benefits of home modifications, such as grab bars and elevated toilet seats.

3. Such modifications promote safety and increased self-care ability.

Nursing diagnosis: *Impaired home maintenance management related to inadequate support system*

GOAL: To maximize the patient's support system

Interventions

1. Assess the household tasks that must be done and the availability of family, friends, or other support persons to complete these tasks if the patient cannot.

2. Teach the patient and family appropriate questions to ask when choosing an agency for in-home assistance. Provide information and guidance that will enable them to make an informed decision. Include a discussion of patients' rights.

3. If necessary, refer the patient and family to a social worker for counseling about available financial resources.

4. When appropriate, coordinate the activities of agencies involved in the patient's care (for example, Medicare, private homemaker care, physical therapy, Meals On Wheels).

Rationales

1. The patient's condition, life-style, and home environment determine whether tasks are few or many, simple or difficult. If family and friends are not available to help, a home health aide, housekeeper, or similar service may be needed.

2. Many states have no laws regulating home health agencies. The patient and family may require guidance in selecting a high-quality agency whose services meet their specific needs and economic resources.

3. Community resources can provide financial advice and assistance (such as sliding-scale government-subsidized programs).

4. Activities must be coordinated to prevent duplication of services and ensure goal-directed, regular care.

ASSOCIATED CARE PLANS
• Ineffective Coping
• Pain
• Sex and Sexuality

NETWORKING OF SERVICES
• durable medical equipment (DME) supplier
• Meals On Wheels
• home health aide service
• Arthritis Foundation
• Arthritis Information Clearinghouse, Box 9782, Arlington, Va. 22209

CARE TEAM INVOLVED
• nurse
• doctor

• patient and family
• physical therapist
• occupational therapist
• medical social worker

IMPLICATIONS FOR HOME CARE
• functional features of the home (stairs, ramps, accessibility of bathroom, kitchen, and bedroom)
• adequate support network of family and friends

PATIENT EDUCATION TOOLS
• Arthritis Foundation literature
• information about each prescribed medication
• literature about and a demonstration of DME
• written instructions for ambulation and ROM exercises

DISCHARGE PLAN FROM HOME HEALTH CARE

Before discharge from home health care, the patient should:
• understand the pathophysiology of osteoarthritis and the rationales for interventions
• recognize factors that may precede exacerbations, such as stress, weather changes, or eating certain foods
• know about potential surgical interventions, such as arthroplasty, arthrodesis, osteoplasty, and osteotomy
• be complying with a prescribed exercise regimen
• know techniques for managing stress and fatigue
• be performing ADLs adequately or have dependable, daily assistance as necessary
• know the dates of follow-up appointments with the doctor, laboratory, physical therapist, or occupational therapist
• understand the hazards of immobility and medically unreliable treatments, such as copper bracelets
• Have the names and telephone numbers or addresses of appropriate support services.

SELECTED REFERENCES

Eliopoulos, C. *A Guide to the Nursing of the Aged.* Baltimore: Williams & Wilkins Co., 1987.

Gioiella, E., and Bevil, C. *Nursing Care of the Aging Client: Promoting Healthy Adaptation.* Norwalk, Conn.: Appleton & Lange, 1985.

Humphrey, C. *Home Care Nursing Handbook.* Norwalk, Conn.: Appleton & Lange, 1986.

Hurley, M. *Classification of Nursing Diagnoses.* St. Louis: C.V. Mosby Co., 1986.

Taylor, C., and Cress, S. *Nursing Diagnosis Cards.* Springhouse, Pa.: Springhouse Corp., 1988.

Ulrich, S., et al. *Nursing Care Planning Guides.* Philadelphia: W.B. Saunders Co., 1986.

Walsh, J., Persons, C., and Wieck, L. *Manual of Home Health Care Nursing.* Philadelphia: J.B. Lippincott Co., 1987.

Osteoporosis

DESCRIPTION AND TIME FOCUS
Osteoporosis, a disease characterized by abnormal, progressive loss of bone tissue, occurs primarily in women between ages 45 and 70 and has been linked to more than 200,000 hip fractures suffered by women in the United States each year. The disease rarely affects men. Dowager's hump, a hallmark of osteoporosis, develops from repeated spinal vertebral fractures, causing gradual height loss and increased spinal curvature.

Women who have had their ovaries removed before menopause are at extremely high risk for developing osteoporosis. Most of the women affected are thin and of small stature. Incidence is highest among Caucasian and Oriental women. Other contributing factors include chronic calcium deficiency, smoking, lack of exercise, high alcohol intake, and a family history of the disease. Treatment usually consists of regular exercise, especially walking, and increased calcium and vitamin D intake.

This clinical plan focuses on the patient at home with osteoporosis. Nursing care centers on preventing further deterioration and teaching the patient about the disease's signs and symptoms. The patient's home is an excellent setting for patient teaching and monitoring for possible complications (for example, fractures or hazardous walk areas).

■ Typical home health care length of service: 3 weeks

■ Typical visit frequency: twice weekly

HEALTH HISTORY FINDINGS
In a health history interview, the patient may report many of these findings:
• menopause
• sedentary life-style
• kyphosis
• calcium-deficient diet
• prolonged immobility
• history of alcohol abuse
• tobacco use
• history of steroid use
• family history of osteoporosis
• excessive caffeine use
• history of excessive antacid or laxative use

PHYSICAL FINDINGS
In a physical examination, the nurse may detect many of these findings:

Musculoskeletal
• fracture
• lower back pain
• increased curvature of thoracic vertebrae
• height loss
• neck pain
• lost or reduced equilibrium

Respiratory
• dyspnea on exertion (rare)
• rapid, shallow respiration

Integumentary
• increased redness and warmth
• new pain sites
• increased tenderness in new sites

DIAGNOSTIC STUDIES
The following studies may be performed to evaluate the patient's health status:
• X-ray—on diagnosis of fracture and 4 to 6 weeks after fracture to assess loss of bone mass
• bone biopsy—at diagnosis to rule out bone malignancy
• serum calcium, phosphorus, and alkaline phosphatase studies—monthly (if levels are elevated) until normal range obtained

---

Nursing diagnosis: *Impaired physical mobility related to decreased activity or prolonged immobilization*

GOAL: To improve the patient's mobility

Interventions

1. Instruct the patient to perform active and passive range-of-motion (ROM) exercises, as ordered.

2. Advise the patient to use a walker or cane, if needed.

3. Apply a back brace or corset to the patient before ambulation.

Rationales

1. Exercise maintains bone density and muscle and joint strength and prevents further bone deterioration.

2. Ambulatory aids facilitate mobility and reduce damaging stress on bones.

3. A brace or corset can reduce pain and increase mobility.

4. Advise the patient to walk daily, and suggest she join an activity group or walking club.

4. Walking is of great benefit in treating osteoporosis. Scheduling daily walks promotes increased mobility and optimal health.

Nursing diagnosis: *Altered nutrition: less than body requirements, related to chronic calcium deficiency*

GOAL: To increase the patient's calcium intake

Interventions

1. Assess the patient's nutritional status, food preferences, and cultural restrictions.

2. Involve the patient in meal planning. Teach her the importance of a balanced diet that contains ample protein and increased amounts of calcium and vitamin D. Provide her with a list of foods high in calcium, such as milk, cottage cheese, peanuts, cheddar cheese, and green leafy vegetables.

3. Encourage the patient to use calcium and vitamin D supplements if needed.

Rationales

1. Knowing the patient's usual dietary intake facilitates planning areas for improvement.

2. A balanced diet with ample protein, calcium, and vitamin D helps prevent bone loss and aids bone formation.

3. The body needs calcium to build strong bone; without calcium, bones become porous and brittle. Vitamin D is necessary for calcium absorption. Adequate calcium and vitamin D promote normal bone mineralization.

Nursing diagnosis: *Potential for injury related to weak and brittle bones*

GOAL: To reduce the patient's risk of injury

Interventions

1. Teach the patient the proper body mechanics for bending or lifting.

2. Explain the importance of sleeping on a firm mattress or bed board.

3. Teach family members the proper way to move a bedridden patient.

4. Explain to the patient the importance of wearing sturdy shoes and using caution and common sense when walking.

Rationales

1. Using proper body mechanics helps prevent compression fractures of the vertebrae.

2. A firm surface supports the spine and may help reduce damaging stress to weak, brittle bones, minimizing risk of fracture.

3. The patient's bones are brittle; a slight bump or jar can cause fractures.

4. Bones weakened by osteoporosis are easily fractured. Icy sidewalks, loose rugs, wet or polished floors, and stairs without handrails should be avoided.

Nursing diagnosis: *Altered comfort: pain, related to pathological fractures or impaired mobility of joints*

GOAL: To alleviate the patient's pain

Interventions

1. Administer analgesics as ordered.

Rationales

1. Analgesics reduce the patient's pain and permit greater mobility.

2. Instruct the patient on the medication regimen, including method of administration, dosage, action, and adverse effects.

2. Knowing the medication regimen can promote compliance and alleviate anxiety.

3. Teach the patient to use a back brace or corset when walking.

3. A back brace or corset provides spinal support, thus reducing pain and promoting mobility.

Nursing diagnosis: *Impaired home maintenance management related to the disease process*

GOAL: To ensure adequate home maintenance within limitations of the patient's condition

Interventions

1. Assess the patient's home for safety hazards, such as loose rugs, protruding electrical wires, and wet or slippery floors. If the patient must use the stairs, note whether they have handrails.

2. Evaluate the patient's need for ambulatory aids, such as a walker or cane.

3. Evaluate the patient's need for community services, such as Lifeline or Meals On Wheels.

Rationales

1. This assessment helps determine whether the patient can function safely in the home.

2. Appropriate ambulatory aids provide support and help prevent falls.

3. Knowing that community services are available can allay the patient's fears of risks associated with the illness. Lifeline provides a link to immediate emergency care. Meals On Wheels can minimize the need for food preparation.

Nursing diagnosis: *Disturbance in self-esteem related to changes in physical condition and life-style*

GOAL: To enhance the patient's self-esteem

Interventions

1. Explain to the patient that osteoporosis is common in elderly people. Encourage her to join a support group and walking club.

2. Encourage the patient to wear clothing that disguises the effects of kyphosis.

Rationales

1. Interacting with others who share her condition can reduce anxiety and make the condition easier to live with on a daily basis.

2. Kyphosis occurs in advanced osteoporosis, increasing curvature of the thoracic spine. Because clothing does not fit as well, the patient's self-esteem may suffer.

ASSOCIATED CARE PLANS
• Diabetes Mellitus
• Fractured Hip
• Ineffective Coping
• Malnutrition
• Pain
• Spinal Compression Fracture

NETWORKING OF SERVICES
• durable medical equipment supplier
• Meals On Wheels
• community care services program

CARE TEAM INVOLVED
• nurse
• doctor
• patient and family
• medical social worker
• physical therapist

IMPLICATIONS FOR HOME CARE
• functional features of the home (raised toilet seat, access to kitchen, bedroom, and bathroom)
• environmental safety factors
• telephone (communication)

PATIENT EDUCATION TOOLS
• literature about each medication ordered
• literature on osteoporosis
• daily schedule of exercises
• dietary plan
• literature about proper body mechanics
• list of environmental safety precautions
• name, address, and phone number of nearest walking club

DISCHARGE PLAN FROM HOME HEALTH CARE
Before discharge from home health care, the patient should:
• know the method of administration, dosage, action, and adverse effects of each prescribed medication
• post telephone numbers for the doctor, home health agency, and ambulance service by the phone
• know the dates of follow-up appointments with the doctor and laboratory
• have Lifeline response in place, if needed
• understand the prescribed diet and the need for adequate protein, increased calcium, and vitamin D supplements
• have a daily exercise or walking program
• be sleeping on a firm mattress
• understand that keeping active strengthens muscles and prevents additional bone destruction
• know the signs and symptoms of new fractures
• know to report to the doctor any new pain sites, no matter how slight.

SELECTED REFERENCES
Carpenito, L. *Handbook of Nursing Diagnoses.* Philadelphia: J.B. Lippincott Co., 1984.

Farrell, J. *Illustrated Guide to Orthopedic Nursing,* 3rd ed. Philadelphia: J.B. Lippincott Co., 1986.

Kneisl, C., and Ames, S.A. *Adult Health Nursing: A Biopsychosocial Approach.* Menlo Park, Calif.: Addison-Wesley Publishing Co., 1986.

Professional Guide to Diseases, 3rd ed. Springhouse, Pa.: Springhouse Corp., 1989.

Thompson, J., et al. *Clinical Nursing.* St. Louis: C.V. Mosby Co., 1986.

ENDOCRINE SYSTEM
Diabetes Mellitus

DESCRIPTION AND TIME FOCUS
Diabetes mellitus is a chronic disease in which the pancreas fails to produce sufficient insulin to efficiently metabolize glucose. Etiology is multifaceted. Some forms of diabetes are genetically transmitted; viruses and obesity may be involved in other forms of its development. Diabetes may also occur after pancreatic disease, which affects insulin production. Ongoing treatment consists of diet therapy, weight control, and medications, including insulin or oral hypoglycemic agents. The patient must understand the disease and comply with disease management techniques. The doctor may order diagnostic testing to determine complications and their progress, such as retinopathy, renal vascular disease, peripheral vascular disease, accelerated atherosclerosis, and neurologic complications.

This clinical plan focuses on the patient at home with a diagnosis of insulin-dependent or non-insulin-dependent diabetes mellitus. The home is an ideal setting for the nurse to monitor the patient and provide patient teaching about the disease and its control.

■ Typical home health care length of service for a patient with newly diagnosed diabetes who is administering insulin or monitoring blood glucose daily: 7 weeks

■ Typical visit frequency: five visits during the first week, three visits during the second week, twice weekly for 2 weeks, then once weekly for 3 weeks

HEALTH HISTORY FINDINGS
In a health history interview, the patient may report many of these findings:
• family history of diabetes mellitus
• obesity
• history of hypoglycemia
• history of obstetric problems or delivering infant weighing more than 9 lb

PHYSICAL FINDINGS
In a physical examination, the nurse may detect many of these findings:

Cardiovascular
• signs and symptoms of coronary atherosclerosis
• intermittent claudication
• faint peripheral pulses
• cold extremities (peripheral vascular disease)
• capillary refill time more than 3 seconds

Neurologic
• reduced tactile sensation
• numbness or tingling in extremities
• fatigue and lethargy
• impotence

Gastrointestinal
• polydipsia
• polyphagia

Integumentary
• persistent skin ulcers on extremities
• thin, dry skin
• skin infections
• pruritus
• shin spots

Renal and urinary
• polyuria

Vision
• reduced visual acuity (may be intermittent)
• retinopathy

DIAGNOSTIC STUDIES
The following study may be performed to evaluate the patient's health status:
• blood glucose analysis—as necessary to determine effectiveness of treatment; normal range 80-120 mg/dl, depending on laboratory method; samples drawn over several days, with patient fasting for 12 hours before test; consistent levels over 120 mg/dl may indicate diabetes

---

Nursing diagnosis: *Potential for injury related to metabolic instability from inefficient glucose metabolism*

GOAL: To stabilize the patient's metabolism

Interventions

1. During each visit, assess for signs of hyperglycemia (polyuria, polydipsia, polyphagia, muscle cramps, altered level of consciousness, dehydration, and acetone breath) and hypoglycemia (tremors, nervousness, restlessness, and cold, clammy skin). If signs are present, obtain blood glucose levels.

Rationales

1. Blood glucose levels can vary widely in a newly diagnosed patient until diet, exercise, and medication are regulated. Changes in blood glucose affect each patient differently. Blood glucose measurements help determine the patient's symptomatic threshold. A patient with a blood glucose level of 70 mg/dl may have symp-

toms of hypoglycemia whereas another patient with a level of 50 mg/dl may be asymptomatic. Knowing the patient's symptomatic level can help the nurse, patient, and family to recognize and correct abnormalities.

2. Review the patient's hospital chart or medical records to determine the acceptable blood glucose range. Notify the doctor if the patient's blood glucose level falls outside this range.

2. Each patient has a different acceptable blood glucose level. The standard range is 80-120 mg/dl, but the doctor may feel the patient cannot be kept within this range and may determine that a level of up to 180 mg/dl is acceptable. If the level falls outside the acceptable range, the nurse should notify the doctor, who may alter the treatment.

3. Teach the patient and caregiver the signs of hyperglycemia and hypoglycemia and appropriate responses, such as giving the patient concentrated sugar in candy, glucose tablets, or sweetened orange juice. Tell them to notify the doctor immediately if the patient is unconscious or the condition does not improve in 30 minutes. Provide written instructions that the patient can post prominently in the home.

3. Metabolic instability can occur at any time. The patient must recognize and respond to hyperglycemic or hypoglycemic emergencies, which can occur suddenly and lead to death if untreated.

4. Tell the patient to record the time of day and types of activity that coincide with episodes of metabolic instability.

4. A newly diagnosed patient usually displays a reaction pattern. A written record of the pattern can facilitate diet and medication adjustments to control the instability.

5. Teach the patient measures to take during illness and conditions to report to the doctor. Encourage maintenance of diet and exercise habits if possible.

5. Illness disturbs the body's metabolic balance and may necessitate changes in the diabetic regimen. Nausea, vomiting, diarrhea, and increased metabolic rate from fever can cause sudden drops in the blood glucose level; alterations in diet during illness and certain medications can lead to increased blood glucose levels.

Nursing diagnosis: *Altered tissue perfusion: peripheral, related to the disease's effect on blood vessels*

GOAL: To achieve and maintain adequate peripheral tissue perfusion

Interventions

1. Assess the patient's pulse rate, temperature, and capillary refill time.

Rationales

1. Diabetes mellitus thickens the basement membrane in capillaries and arterioles, thereby reducing circulation, particularly in the lower extremities. An elevated pulse rate or temperature or an increased capillary refill time may indicate decreased peripheral circulation.

2. Tell the patient to wear loose, nonconstrictive clothing, to avoid crossing his legs, and to elevate his legs when sitting.

2. These measures promote circulation and help prevent vascular complications.

Nursing diagnosis: *Sensory-perceptual alteration: visual, related to diabetic retinopathy*

GOAL: To help the patient achieve and maintain optimal vision

Interventions

1. During the initial visit, ask the patient to evaluate his vision. Ask if he has had previous vision problems,

Rationales

1. Retinopathy is a common complication of diabetes. Because diabetes control depends, in part, on the pa-

such as cataract or glaucoma. Assess his vision by asking him to read newspaper print of different sizes or to identify objects held at varying distances.

tient's vision (for example, in monitoring blood glucose and preparing and administering insulin), the nurse must know his vision status to effectively plan self-care instruction. The patient with severe visual problems may need a caregiver or visual aid, such as a magnifier, to assist with these functions.

2. Reassess the patient's vision during each visit to detect changes.

2. Many patients with diabetes report daily changes in vision until the diabetes is brought under control. Changes in the patient's vision may require the nurse to alter her plan for a visit, such as postponing a demonstration of preparing insulin in a syringe until the patient can see well enough to learn and participate.

3. Encourage the patient to schedule regular appointments with an ophthalmologist and to keep the ophthalmologist informed of his progress in controlling diabetes.

3. Consistent eye care promotes vision maintenance. The ophthalmologist must know the patient's treatment regimen to provide appropriate eye care.

4. Help the patient obtain and learn to use vision aids, such as magnifiers and large-print reading material. Explain the importance of proper lighting, especially when he performs activities that require close scrutiny, such as reading.

4. Vision aids help the patient maintain independence and provide self-care. Proper lighting helps promote optimal vision.

Nursing diagnosis: *Sensory-perceptual alteration: tactile, related to diabetic neuropathy*

GOAL: To prevent injury to the extremities

Interventions

1. Using a cotton swab or ice cube, evaluate the degree of sensation in the patient's hands and feet.

Rationales

1. Diabetes inhibits the patient's ability to sense temperature and pain, particularly in the hands and feet. The nurse can evaluate the patient's degree of sensation by lightly touching him with a cotton swab or ice cube and noting his response.

2. Tell the patient to inspect his hands and feet daily for injury and to wear gloves and socks to protect against injury and temperature extremes.

2. Because of reduced sensation, the patient may sustain an injury without being aware of it. The nurse must emphasize the importance of protective measures.

Nursing diagnosis: *Potential for impaired skin integrity related to the disease process*

GOAL: To maintain skin integrity

Interventions

1. Teach the patient and caregiver the importance of meticulous skin care.

Rationales

1. Reduced circulation caused by diabetes slows healing. The patient and caregiver must understand that maintaining skin integrity minimizes the risk of infection and skin ulcers.

2. During each visit, assess the patient's skin for pressure areas, abrasions, and other threats to skin integrity. Teach the patient to inspect the skin and to prevent pressure areas.

2. Pressure areas develop quickly. Regular inspection can detect problems early. The patient should participate in the nurse's inspections to prepare for self-care.

3. Teach the patient about necessary foot care and the importance of regular appointments with a podiatrist for nail cutting and inspection.

3. Limited sensation and circulation in the patient's feet increase the risk of impaired skin integrity, which can lead to infection.

Nursing diagnosis: *Altered health maintenance related to lack of experience in diabetic care*

GOAL 1: To teach the patient and caregiver to monitor blood glucose levels

Interventions

1. Assess the patient's or caregiver's visual acuity, dexterity, and attitude toward learning.

2. Assemble the equipment and explain each item to the patient or caregiver. Have him handle each item.

3. Perform the procedure, explaining each step. Assure the patient or caregiver of your assistance until he can comfortably perform the procedure independently.

4. Transfer responsibility for the procedure to the patient or caregiver gradually. Observe his technique and assist when necessary.

5. Suggest that the patient or caregiver write the procedure down and then use these notes as instructions each time he performs the procedure.

6. Teach the patient and caregiver the importance of performing the procedure consistently, recording all results, and notifying the doctor of readings that fall outside the established range.

Rationales

1. The doctor may advise the patient to learn to monitor blood glucose levels using visual techniques or meters. Before teaching begins, the nurse must evaluate the patient's or caregiver's physical and emotional ability to perform the procedure.

2. Becoming familiar with each item facilitates learning and reduces anxiety about the procedure.

3. Watching the procedure facilitates learning.

4. Gradually involving the patient or caregiver in the procedure eases anxiety and permits mastery of one step at a time.

5. Writing the procedure down reinforces learning and enhances the patient's sense of control.

6. Compliance improves when the patient understands the significance of the procedure. Because a patient may lack the dexterity or visual acuity to perform the procedure, the nurse may need to work with the patient, caregiver, other family members, and the doctor to devise alternate methods of monitoring the patient's condition.

GOAL 2: To teach the patient and caregiver to administer insulin properly

Interventions

1. Assess the patient's capability for and attitude toward insulin self-administration.

2. Teach the patient and caregiver about the types of insulin, and verify that they know the action and duration of the insulin prescribed.

3. Encourage the patient and caregiver to handle the syringe, injector, or insulin pump and to practice the actions necessary to prepare an insulin dose.

4. Perform the procedure slowly, explaining each step. Gradually involve the patient or caregiver in the procedure.

5. Suggest that the patient or caregiver write the procedure down and then use these notes as instructions each time he performs the procedure.

6. Observe the patient or caregiver during the first few independent insulin administrations.

Rationales

1. Abilities and attitudes vary among patients. The nurse must consider the patient's specific abilities and attitudes when formulating teaching plans.

2. The patient and caregiver must understand that one type of insulin cannot be substituted for another.

3. The patient and caregiver may be unfamiliar with the equipment and procedures and require practice.

4. Watching the procedure facilitates learning. Gradually involving the patient or caregiver eases anxiety and permits mastery of one step at a time.

5. Writing the procedure down reinforces learning and enhances the patient's sense of control.

6. The nurse's presence reassures the patient or caregiver and allows the nurse to monitor the technique for accuracy and consistency.

GOAL 3: To teach the patient about dietary restrictions

Interventions

1 . Verify the doctor's orders for diet restrictions. Compile the patient's diet history, including food preferences, meal frequency, and his ability to prepare food. Determine if the home is equipped with kitchen appliances and cookware.

2. Explain the importance of eating regular meals and complying with caloric and food group restrictions. Tell the patient to measure foods and count calories accurately and to avoid high-sugar foods. Be sure he knows how to use exchange food lists.

3. Encourage diet variety by helping the patient identify foods and preparation methods that meet diabetic diet requirements. Include allowable fast foods and restaurant meals in the teaching plan.

4. Have the patient keep a food diary for several days after teaching is completed.

Rationales

1. Diabetic diets vary, and verification helps avoid confusion. The patient's dietary habits affect compliance with the necessary restrictions and should be considered before teaching begins.

2. Proper diet is a crucial element of diabetic treatment. Compliance improves when the patient understands the importance of dietary restrictions.

3. Diet variation—and knowledge that most foods can be included in a diabetic diet—promotes compliance.

4. Evaluating the patient's intake alerts the nurse to problems. A clinical dietitian can help resolve persistent problems, such as noncompliance or poor understanding of meal planning.

GOAL 4: To teach the patient and caregiver the importance of regular patient exercise

Interventions

1. Assess the patient's physical ability to perform exercise.

2. Explain to the patient the importance of exercise, and work with him to devise a reasonable exercise plan.

Rationales

1. Because diabetes is a metabolic disease, exercise is important to diabetes control. A baseline assessment helps the nurse develop an appropriate exercise program. The caregiver should be included in all instruction to reinforce the nurse's instruction between visits.

2. Exercise must be consistent in frequency and duration to be of value. Compliance with the exercise program improves if the patient helps develop the program.

Nursing diagnosis: *Disturbance in self-concept related to chronic illness and life-style changes*

GOAL: To help the patient achieve and maintain a healthy self-concept

Interventions

1. Encourage the patient to express his feelings (including anger) about the disease and required life-style alterations.

2. Help the patient place the disease and its management in proper perspective.

3. Maximize the patient's control of disease management.

Rationales

1. Diabetes management requires life-style changes and active patient participation. The patient may resent these impositions. Before he can actively learn and participate, he must resolve anger and denial.

2. The need for daily doses of insulin, regular blood glucose checks, and dietary restrictions can overwhelm the patient. Consequently, he may limit his attention to the disease and its management and ignore enjoyable aspects of life. The nurse must help him develop a balanced perspective.

3. A patient with a chronic illness may feel a loss of control. Restoring control whenever possible enhances the patient's self-esteem and promotes compliance.

ASSOCIATED CARE PLANS
• Angina Pectoris
• Cellulitis
• Chronic Renal Failure
• Functional hypoglycemia
• Hospice Care
• Hypertension
• Ineffective Coping
• Sex and Sexuality

NETWORKING OF SERVICES
• Lifeline
• outpatient diabetic program
• impaired vision program
• Meals On Wheels
• American Diabetic Association

CARE TEAM INVOLVED
• nurse
• doctor
• patient and family
• medical social worker
• clinical dietitian

IMPLICATIONS FOR HOME CARE
• functional features of the home
• telephone (communication)
• financial ability to obtain supplies needed for
ongoing care

PATIENT EDUCATION TOOLS
• literature about each medication ordered
• American Diabetic Association literature about
diet, skin care, foot care, exercise, and insulin
administration
• literature about blood glucose monitoring
• charts for recording blood glucose and insulin dosage

DISCHARGE PLAN FROM HOME HEALTH CARE
Before discharge from home health care, the patient
should:
• have a list of medications and an administration
schedule
• know the type of insulin prescribed, peak action time,
and effects
• be able to administer insulin properly without
assistance
• be able to monitor blood glucose without assistance
• know the acceptable range for blood glucose levels
• know the signs and symptoms of metabolic instability
and appropriate responses
• comply with diet restrictions
• comply with the treatment plan, especially exercise
and skin care programs
• post phone numbers for the ambulance service, doctor,
and home health agency in a prominent place
• know the dates of follow-up appointments
• know about available community resources
• know sources for equipment and supplies.

SELECTED REFERENCES
Birmingham, J.J. *Home Care Planning Based on DRGs.*
Philadelphia: J.B. Lippincott Co., 1986.
Brunner, L., and Suddarth, D. *Textbook of Medical-Sur-
gical Nursing,* 6th ed. Philadelphia: J.B. Lippincott
Co., 1988.
Eliopoulos, C. *A Guide to the Nursing of the Aged.* Balti-
more: Williams & Wilkins Co., 1987.
Iyer, P., et al. *Nursing Process and Nursing Diagnosis.*
Philadelphia: W.B. Saunders Co., 1986.
School, D.E. *Nutrition and Diet Therapy.* Oradell, N.J.:
Medical Economics Books, 1986.
Thompson, J., et al. *Clinical Nursing.* St. Louis: C.V.
Mosby Co., 1986.
Walsh, J., et al. *Manual of Home Health Care Nursing.*
Philadelphia: J.B. Lippincott Co., 1987.

Functional Hypoglycemia

DESCRIPTION AND TIME FOCUS
Hypoglycemia is an abnormally low blood glucose level. It occurs when excessive insulin enters the bloodstream, when glucose burns up too rapidly (from insufficient food intake), or when the glucose release rate falls behind tissue demands (from excessive physical activity).

Hypoglycemia can result from organic or inorganic problems. Functional hypoglycemia, of inorganic origin, may result from excessive insulin production after increased carbohydrate ingestion, leading to a rapid drop in blood glucose. Fasting hypoglycemia, an organic type not directly related to carbohydrate ingestion, usually is caused by excess insulin from such conditions as insulinomas, pancreatic hyperplasia, Addison's disease, and hypopituitarism.

This clinical plan focuses on the patient who has been discharged home from an acute care facility with functional hypoglycemia. The plan also can apply to the patient who requires follow-up teaching.

■ Typical home health care length of service for a patient with functional hypoglycemia: 7 weeks

■ Typical visit frequency: twice the first week, then once weekly for 3 weeks, then once every other week for 3 weeks

HEALTH HISTORY FINDINGS
In a health history interview, the patient may report these findings:
• steroid use
• history of hepatic disorder, such as Addison's disease or pancreatic disease

PHYSICAL FINDINGS
In a physical examination, the nurse may detect many of these findings:

Cardiovascular
• tachycardia
• increased blood pressure

Neurologic
• weakness
• shakiness
• headache
• restlessness
• blurred vision
• confusion
• incoherent speech
• bizarre behavior
• convulsions
• seizures
• coma

Gastrointestinal
• hunger

Integumentary
• sweating
• cold, clammy skin

DIAGNOSTIC STUDIES
The following studies may be performed to evaluate the patient's health status:
• 3-hour glucose tolerance test—to diagnose functional hypoglycemia; a blood glucose level of 40-60 mg/dl after 3 hours indicates functional hypoglycemia
• blood glucose—levels are measured at the time the patient is experiencing symptoms

---

Nursing diagnosis: *Altered nutrition: more than body requirements, related to excessive insulin secretion*

GOAL: To promote food intake that helps stabilize the patient's blood glucose level

Interventions

1. Assess the patient's dietary history; include food preferences and eating habits. Consider religious, ethnic, and budgetary constraints when planning the patient's menu.

2. Instruct the patient to avoid simple carbohydrates, to eat sufficient amounts of complex carbohydrates (grain products, raw vegetables, and legumes) and protein foods (milk, meat), and to consume adequate calories.

Rationales

1. A dietary history identifies problems and provides information necessary for planning dietary management.

2. A diet with sufficient amounts of complex carbohydrates, fiber, and protein helps stabilize blood glucose levels. The body needs adequate calories to meet energy requirements.

3. Instruct the patient to eat small, frequent meals at the same times each day.

3. Eating small, frequent meals on a regular schedule helps stabilize the blood glucose level because hypoglycemia usually occurs several hours after a meal.

4. Tell the patient to include a protein food source (such as meat, milk, or peanut butter) with each meal.

4. Protein foods help prevent hypoglycemia because protein breaks down slower than other energy-producing nutrients.

5. Tell the patient to eat snacks between meals and at bedtime. Encourage him to eat high-protein foods, such as cheese, nuts, or half a sandwich.

5. High-protein snacks, especially before bedtime, help prevent hypoglycemia during the night or in the early morning.

6. Identify factors that influence the patient's hypoglycemia, such as vigorous activity or exercise and inappropriate eating habits.

6. Contributing factors must be identified to plan preventive measures. For example, eating large amounts of carbohydrate foods at one time may result in excessive insulin secretion, which can lead to hypoglycemia.

7. Encourage the patient to establish regular schedules for eating and exercising. Explain the importance of eating a snack that contains carbohydrates and proteins before engaging in vigorous exercise.

7. Maintaining regular schedules for eating and exercising helps minimize the incidence of hypoglycemia. Vigorous exercise burns up available blood glucose, which results in excessive insulin in the blood.

Nursing diagnosis: *Knowledge deficit related to hypoglycemia management*

GOAL: To improve the patient's and family's knowledge of disease management and treatment alternatives

Interventions

1. Assess the patient's knowledge of hypoglycemia and his ability to learn.

2. Teach the patient and family the signs and symptoms of hypoglycemia. Review general signs and symptoms (weakness, hunger, shakiness, tachycardia, cold and clammy skin, and restlessness) and neurologic signs and symptoms (headache, blurred vision, confusion, incoherent speech, and convulsions).

3. Teach the patient and family to treat the signs and symptoms by eating complex carbohydrate and protein food sources, such as cheese with crackers or nuts.

4. Teach the family to administer a subcutaneous injection of glucagon, a necessary response if the patient loses consciousness during a hypoglycemic attack. Tell the patient to eat a complex carbohydrate food and a protein food when consciousness returns.

5. Teach the patient the importance of having a form of carbohydrate, such as cheese crackers, with him at all times.

6. Instruct the patient to wear a Medic Alert bracelet.

7. Teach the patient and family self–blood glucose monitoring.

8. Evaluate the patient's and family's progress in learning disease management and treatment alternatives.

Rationales

1. Assessing the patient's knowledge and learning ability helps in designing an appropriate teaching plan.

2. General signs and symptoms occur when blood glucose levels drop and the body releases epinephrine in an attempt to increase hepatic glycolysis. Neurologic signs and symptoms occur when glucose-deficient blood reaches the brain, impairing cerebral functions.

3. The body absorbs complex carbohydrates slowly, which slows insulin secretion, thereby minimizing the risk of a rebound hypoglycemic attack.

4. Glucagon accelerates hepatic glycogenolysis, which forms glucose from glycogen and thus increases the blood glucose level.

5. Readily available carbohydrates help the patient cope with an emergency.

6. The bracelet provides information about the patient's condition to health professionals in the event he is unconscious.

7. The patient and family must be able to monitor blood glucose levels during symptomatic episodes.

8. By evaluating what they have learned, the nurse can determine whether they need further teaching.

ASSOCIATED CARE PLANS
• Diabetes Mellitus

NETWORKING OF SERVICES
• hospital-based support groups
• Meals On Wheels

CARE TEAM INVOLVED
• nurse
• doctor
• patient and family
• dietitian
• medical social worker

IMPLICATIONS FOR HOME CARE
• diet regulation, diet teaching, exercise
• financial ability to purchase necessary food
and medical supplies
• food storage and preparation

PATIENT EDUCATION TOOLS
• American Dietetic Association literature
• activity guidelines

DISCHARGE PLAN FROM HOME HEALTH CARE
Before discharge from home health care, the patient
should:
• understand the disease process
• recognize the signs and symptoms of hypoglycemia
• know how to prevent or treat a hypoglycemic attack
• understand dietary management requirements
• know when to seek medical aid.

SELECTED REFERENCES
Birmingham, J.J. *Home Care Planning Based on DRGs.*
    Philadelphia: J.B. Lippincott Co., 1986.
Doenges, M.E., et al. *Nursing Care Plans.* Philadelphia:
    F.A. Davis Co., 1984.
Gordon, M. *Nursing Diagnosis: Process and Application.*
    New York: McGraw-Hill Book Co., 1982.
Morrissey, B.G. *Quick Reference to Therapeutic Nutrition.*
    Philadelphia: J.B. Lippincott Co., 1984.
Robinson, C.H., et al. *Normal and Therapeutic Nutrition.*
    New York: Macmillan Publishing Co., 1986.
Whitney, E.N., et al. *Understanding Normal and Clinical
    Nutrition,* 2nd ed. St. Paul, Minn.: West Publishing
    Co., 1987.
Williams, S.R. *Nutrition and Diet Therapy,* 6th ed. St.
    Louis: Times Mirror/Mosby College Publishing, 1989.

REPRODUCTIVE SYSTEM
Prostate Cancer

DESCRIPTION AND TIME FOCUS
Prostate cancer, typically a form of adenocarcinoma, is the second most common cancer among males, usually occurring in white males over age 50. Etiology is poorly understood, although androgens may promote cancer cell growth. The disease can spread via the lymphatic and hematologic systems or by direct extension of another cancer site. Signs and symptoms appear only in the disease's advanced stages; about 50% of all prostatic cancer patients exhibit locally advanced tumors or evidence of metastasis at the time of diagnosis.

Prostatic cancer is classified according to one of four disease stages. Treatment depends on the stage, the patient's physical condition, and the doctor's and patient's choice. A *Stage A* tumor, confined to the prostate gland, is too small to detect by physical examination or laboratory tests. The tumor usually is detected when a biopsy is performed during a transurethral prostatic resection for benign prostatic hypertrophy. Radical prostatectomy is the treatment of choice for localized lesions. External beam radiation therapy may be used for the patient who is a poor surgical candidate because of cardiac or respiratory compromise. A *Stage B* tumor, also confined to the prostate gland, is palpable on rectal examination. Treatment choices and restrictions are the same as those for Stage A tumors. A *Stage C* tumor extends through the prostatic capsule and may involve local lymph nodes. Treatment includes radical prostatectomy and radiation therapy to the pelvis and prostate. Chemotherapy may be used if other treatments fail. A *Stage D* tumor involves distant metastases. Treatment is limited to palliative measures, such as radiation therapy to the pelvis and metastatic bone regions to promote comfort and reduce tumor size, bilateral orchiectomy or estrogen treatment to decrease androgen production, transurethral resection to remove an obstructing tumor if radiation therapy proves ineffective, or chemotherapy if other treatments fail.

This clinical plan focuses on the patient discharged home from an acute-care hospital after diagnosis, management, and treatment of prostatic cancer. Nursing care centers on helping the patient accept necessary life-style changes after radical prostatectomy or other medical interventions. The nurse should encourage patients over age 40 to have annual rectal examinations to promptly detect tumor growth.

■ Typical home health care length of service for a patient with prostate cancer: varies according to disease stage and treatment

■ Typical visit frequency: for patients with Stages A to C, once weekly for 3 weeks; patients with Stage D are evaluated individually.

HEALTH HISTORY FINDINGS
In a health history interview, the patient may report many of these findings:

• diminution in caliber and force of urine stream
• hesitancy in voiding
• inability to terminate micturition
• dribbling
• urine retention

PHYSICAL FINDINGS
In a physical examination, the nurse may detect many of these findings:

Reproductive
• lymphedema in scrotum and inguinal region
• impotence (after surgery)
• sterility (after surgery or radiation therapy)

Cardiovascular
• anemia

Gastrointestinal
• unintentional weight loss
• cachexia
• liver enlargement

Musculoskeletal
• back pain with metastasis
• joint stiffness
• pathologic fractures
• costovertebral angle tenderness with bony metastasis

Renal and urinary
• decreased urine stream
• urinary frequency, urgency, or hesitancy
• nocturia
• dribbling
• difficulty starting urine stream
• urine retention (late stage)
• hematuria

DIAGNOSTIC STUDIES
The following studies may be performed to evaluate the patient's health status:
• serum alkaline phosphatase—elevated with bony metastases; normal range is 1.5 to 4 Bodansky units/dl
• hemoglobin and hematocrit—to detect anemia, which can indicate metastases; normal range: hemoglobin, 14 to 18 g/dl; hematocrit, 42% to 54%
• blood urea nitrogen (BUN) and creatinine—elevated with ureteral obstruction by tumor; normal range: BUN, 8 to 20 mg/dl; creatinine, 0.2 to 0.6 mg/dl
• bone scan—to detect metastases
• chest X-ray—to assess for lung metastases
• pelvic computed tomography (CT) scan—to determine local extension and lymph node involvement
• lymphangiography—to detect para-aortic and pelvic node involvement

Nursing diagnosis: *Altered urinary elimination patterns related to surgical intervention or tumor growth*

GOAL 1: To promote urinary control

Interventions

1. Explain to the patient that surgery diminishes bladder function and that he should anticipate temporary dribbling and incontinence.

2. Teach the patient to perform perineal muscle exercises (tighten buttocks and perineal muscles for 5 to 10 seconds, then relax; repeat 10 to 20 times hourly). Encourage him to void when he first feels the urge and to stop micturition in midstream for a few seconds before continuing. Explain why he should avoid caffeine and alcohol.

3. Teach the patient to recognize postoperative signs and symptoms of obstruction or decreased renal function, such as clot formation and hematuria. Explain why he should promptly report these to the doctor. Tell him that cloudy urine is normal after surgery and will clear with healing, usually in 10 to 14 days.

Rationales

1. Coping may improve if the patient understands why dribbling and urinary incontinence persist after surgery and if he knows the condition is temporary. Perineal muscle exercises (see next intervention) help restore bladder tone. Normal urinary function usually returns in 2 to 3 weeks.

2. Practicing perineal muscle exercises, voiding when the urge occurs, and stopping micturition in midstream can improve the patient's urinary control. Caffeine and alcohol may increase urine output.

3. Knowledge can alleviate the patient's fears and help promote compliance with treatment. Clot formation may result from dehydration, and hematuria can occur after strenuous activity or long automobile rides. Medical intervention is required if the urine stream is decreased or contains blood.

GOAL 2: To identify signs and symptoms of renal insufficiency or tumor growth

Interventions

1. Obtain laboratory data and diagnostic procedure results from the patient's hospital medical records.

2. At each visit, assess the patient's urinary elimination pattern. Document the findings.

Rationales

1. This information serves as a baseline to detect changes in the patient's status. Increased BUN and creatinine levels indicate ureteral obstruction. An excretory urogram can substantiate these data.

2. Assessment and documentation can measure improvement in the patient's elimination pattern or identify symptoms of renal insufficiency or tumor growth.

Nursing diagnosis: *Altered comfort: pain, related to surgery or disease metastasis*

GOAL: To alleviate the patient's pain

Interventions

1. Evaluate the cause, duration, intensity, and perceived location of the patient's pain, using a body diagram and asking the patient to rate his pain on a scale of 1 (minor) to 10 (severe).

2. Assess the patient for physiologic indications of pain, such as grimacing, bent posture, decreased mobility, elevated blood pressure, increased heart rate, rapid or irregular respirations, pupil dilation, and increased muscle tension.

Rationales

1. The nurse must evaluate these factors to provide effective pain relief. (See the "Pain" care plan for more information.)

2. Surgical manipulation or catheter placement can irritate bladder stretch receptors, causing painful bladder spasms. Indications of pain may last up to 3 weeks.

3. Work with the patient to implement an effective pain relief program. Include measures he has used successfully, and discuss additional measures, such as frequent position changes, heat application, exercises to reduce joint and muscle stiffness, adequate sleep, and relaxation techniques (soothing music, recreational therapy, guided imagery, and deep-breathing exercises). Consult with the doctor about using analgesics or antispasmodics.

3. An effective pain relief program typically includes measures that have worked in the past and new measures carefully selected and explained by the nurse.

4. Monitor vital signs before and after administering medications, and assess the patient's pain 30 minutes after he takes the medication. If pain persists, tell him to use several pain relief measures simultaneously, before pain becomes severe. Notify the doctor if all interventions fail to alleviate severe pain.

4. Monitoring vital signs and assessing pain aid in evaluating the effectiveness of the pain relief program and ensuring patient compliance. Using several pain relief measures at the onset of pain can prevent severe episodes. Unrelieved pain should be reported to the doctor, who may increase the dosage, change medications, or order radiation therapy, chemotherapy, or endocrine therapy.

Nursing diagnosis: *Disturbance in self-esteem related to incontinence, potential impotence, or sexual alterations*

GOAL: To enhance the patient's self-esteem

Interventions

1. Encourage the patient to express his feelings about body function changes resulting from medical and surgical interventions. Try to be empathetic and nonjudgmental. Provide positive reinforcement by noting his strengths and assets.

2. Advise the patient to use condom catheters or adult incontinence briefs.

3. Explain how surgical intervention, radiation therapy, and endocrine therapy can alter the patient's usual sexual responses.

4. Discuss alternative sexual methods and devices that can improve the patient's sexual satisfaction. Explain that sexual expression excluding intercourse can still be satisfying for both partners. Refer the patient and partner to a sex therapist, if needed, for counseling on sexual dysfunction.

Rationales

1. Expressing feelings about body function changes is the first step in developing healthy coping behaviors. Emotional support and positive reinforcement from the nurse can enhance the patient's self-esteem and may help him adjust more easily to changes in body function and life-style.

2. These devices help mask the effects of dribbling and urinary incontinence, preventing embarrassment and allowing the patient to remain socially active.

3. The patient must have accurate knowledge of the disease and treatment to make informed decisions. For example, he may decide to forgo a treatment option that adversely affects sexual function. Also, his self-esteem may improve more quickly if he understands that his sexual dysfunction is a physical—rather than psychological or emotional—problem.

4. Alternative sexual methods and devices provide the patient and partner with viable outlets of sexual expression. For example, a penile prosthesis may help the patient with impotence resulting from a surgical procedure. A sex therapist initiates open communication between partners to correct misinformation, decrease anxiety, and identify successful ways of coping with changes created by the illness. (See the "Sex and Sexuality" care plan for more information.)

Nursing diagnosis: *Impaired home maintenance management related to limitations imposed by prostate cancer*

GOAL: To promote the patient's independence and safety at home

Interventions

1. Interview the patient (and family members, if necessary) to assess his level of independence and responsibility before he was hospitalized.

2. Evaluate the patient's natural support system.

3. Assess the patient's ability to perform activities of daily living (ADLs) independently, such as shaving, bathing, dressing, shopping, and cooking. If the patient needs help, involve his natural support system, if possible, or refer him to appropriate support services, such as Meals On Wheels, homemaker services, or a home health aide.

4. Evaluate the patient's home for safety and convenience. Check for protruding electrical cords or other obstacles that can hinder walking. Advise the patient to place nonskid strips in the bathtub and to use an elevated toilet seat.

5. Refer the patient to appropriate community resources, such as social services, religious organizations, cancer support groups, or hospices, if necessary.

Rationales

1. Determining the patient's level of functioning before hospitalization helps the nurse evaluate his current needs and assess his potential to return to pre-illness functioning.

2. The patient's family and friends are significant resources for the home care plan. The nurse should involve family and friends before accessing formal support services, whenever possible.

3. Assessment helps the nurse establish the plan of care and aids in determining the patient's need for assistance with personal hygiene or household tasks.

4. Home modifications and special equipment can promote the patient's safety, convenience, and independence.

5. The home health nurse must adopt a holistic approach in caring for the patient, considering his physical, emotional, social, spiritual, and financial needs.

ASSOCIATED CARE PLANS
• Chronic Renal Failure
• Grief and Grieving
• Hospice Care
• Malnutrition
• Pain
• Sex and Sexuality

NETWORKING OF SERVICES
• hospice
• sex therapy
• durable medical equipment supplier
• Meals On Wheels
• transportation service
• cancer support group
• Lifeline (if patient is homebound)

CARE TEAM INVOLVED
• nurse
• doctor
• patient and family
• home health aide
• homemaker
• social worker
• radiologist

IMPLICATIONS FOR HOME CARE
• availability of competent caregiver (if patient cannot perform ADLs)
• functioning utilities (heat, electricity, plumbing, telephone)
• safety in the home (grab bars, shower chair, elevated toilet seat, adequate lighting)
• list of telephone numbers for appropriate community resources (hospice, sex therapist, cancer support group, transportation network)
• list of relaxation techniques

PATIENT EDUCATION TOOLS
• list of signs and symptoms the patient should report to the doctor
• list of side effects of radiation therapy, chemotherapy, or endocrine therapy, if applicable
• literature on each prescribed medication and instructions for their use

DISCHARGE PLAN FROM HOME HEALTH CARE
Before discharge from home health care, the patient should:
• know the signs and symptoms of urinary obstruction
• know which activities to avoid until healing occurs

• know how to administer medications properly and understand their side effects
• have a support system in place
• arrange to meet with a social worker to discuss financial assistance, if needed
• resume normal ADLs
• know the dates of follow-up appointments with the doctor and radiologist
• post emergency phone numbers for the doctor, ambulance service, and home health agency by the phone.

SELECTED REFERENCES

Ames, S., and Kneish, C. *Essentials of Adult Health Nursing.* Menlo Park, Calif.: Addison-Wesley Publishing Co., 1988.

Crawford, E.D., et al. *Genitourinary Cancer Surgery.* Philadelphia: Lea & Febiger, 1982.

Hood, G., and Dincher, J. *Total Patient Care: Foundations and Practice,* 6th ed. St. Louis: C.V. Mosby Co., 1984.

Lewis, S., and Collier, I. *Medical-Surgical Nursing Assessment: Management of Clinical Problems,* 2nd ed. New York: McGraw-Hill Book Co., 1987.

Peterson, R. *Urologic Pathology.* Philadelphia: J.B. Lippincott Co., 1986.

Thompson, F.D., and Woodhouse, C.R.J. *Disorders of the Kidney and Urinary Tract.* London: Edward Arnold Publisher, Ltd., 1987.

Thompson, J., et al. *Clinical Nursing.* St. Louis: C.V. Mosby Co., 1986.

Uterine Cancer

DESCRIPTION AND TIME FOCUS

Endometrial cancer is the most common uterine cancer, although other gynecologic cancers (cervical, vaginal, or vulvar) can spread to the uterus. The cause of endometrial cancer has not been identified, but its development has been linked with altered hormone production or metabolism that results in increased estrogen levels. Treatment for a patient with any gynecologic cancer usually begins with surgical intervention. For endometrial cancer, surgery consists of a total hysterectomy, frequently with a bilateral salpingo-oophorectomy. If the vagina or vulva is involved, additional resection is needed, with possible removal of pelvic lymph nodes. Other treatment may include hormone therapy, chemotherapy, or radiation therapy.

This clinical plan focuses on the patient discharged home from an acute-care hospital after diagnosis and initial surgical treatment of uterine cancer. Nursing care centers on teaching the patient about the disease, disease management, and possible complications.

■ Typical home health care length of service for a patient without complications or an open wound: 4 weeks

■ Typical visit frequency: twice the first week, then once weekly for 3 weeks

HEALTH HISTORY FINDINGS

In a health history interview, the patient may report many of these findings:
• history of breast cancer
• history of diabetes
• history of hypertension
• long-term estrogen therapy
• nulliparity
• late menopause or postmenopausal
• recent weight loss
• fatigue

PHYSICAL FINDINGS

In a physical examination, the nurse may detect many of these findings:

Reproductive
• irregular vaginal bleeding
• pelvic pain or pressure
• low back pain

Cardiovascular
• lymphedema
• anemia

Gastrointestinal
• anorexia
• obesity
• altered bowel function

Renal and urinary
• urinary frequency
• urgency
• pain on urination

DIAGNOSTIC STUDIES

The following studies may be performed to evaluate the patient's health status:
• endometrial biopsy—initially, to verify diagnosis
• cystoscopy—at any time to evaluate metastasis
• proctoscopy—at any time to evaluate metastasis
• computed tomography (CT) scan—at any time to evaluate metastasis
• complete blood count (CBC)—at any time to monitor anemia, white blood cell (WBC) count

---

Nursing diagnosis: *Activity intolerance related to the hypermetabolic disease process and postoperative restrictions*

GOAL: To improve the patient's activity tolerance

Interventions

1. Assess the patient's activity tolerance by having her perform a simple activity, such as walking across a room or washing her face and brushing her teeth. Monitor for signs of fatigue, such as dyspnea, tachycardia, or change in skin color.

2. Assess the patient's compliance with postoperative activity restrictions. Tell her not to lift or carry heavy objects for 4 to 6 weeks.

Rationales

1. A baseline assessment establishes the patient's initial activity tolerance, which aids care planning and progress evaluation.

2. A patient with endometrial cancer usually undergoes a hysterectomy, including removal of the ovaries and fallopian tubes. Complete healing takes 6 to 8 weeks. Too much activity can damage fragile new tissue; too little activity can contribute to complications of limited mobility, such as respiratory or circulatory problems.

3. Advise the patient to take short, frequent rests when performing daily activities.

3. Incorporating rest periods into the daily schedule can improve the patient's endurance.

4. Teach the patient to recognize signs of fatigue and to determine personal endurance limits. Tell her to stop any activity that causes increased heart rate, shortness of breath, or muscle trembling.

4. To increase independence in self-care, the patient must be able to recognize signs of fatigue and determine endurance limits without the nurse's intervention.

Nursing diagnosis: *Altered urinary elimination patterns related to proximity of affected organs to the urinary tract*

GOAL: To restore normal urinary elimination patterns

Interventions

1. Assess the patient's previous urinary elimination patterns. Ask her to recall how often she voided during the day and at night, and have her characterize the amount as small, moderate, or large.

2. Assess for urinary frequency or retention. Have the patient record when she voids and the amount of urine voided for 1 week. Notify the doctor if any urinary problems develop.

3. Monitor the patient for signs and symptoms of urinary tract infection (UTI), such as frequent voiding, burning on urination, voiding in small amounts, and bloody or foul-smelling urine. Teach the patient to recognize the signs and symptoms. Review hospital records for information about the patient's urinary function during hospitalization.

Rationales

1. The nurse must know the patient's previous elimination patterns, including any abnormalities, to assess current urinary function adequately.

2. Uterine cancer may spread to the bladder, causing decreased holding capacity and urinary frequency. The patient with a hysterectomy also may experience urinary frequency or retention because of postoperative inflammation of internal structures near the bladder. Urinary problems that develop in the first 4 weeks usually are related to surgery and resolve with little or no intervention, although the doctor should always be notified.

3. Most patients undergoing gynecologic surgery have an indwelling catheter during hospitalization. This invasion of the normally sterile urinary system may contribute to development of a UTI, which requires medical intervention.

Nursing diagnosis: *Altered bowel elimination: constipation, related to pelvic pressure from tumor growth or surgical intervention*

GOAL 1: To restore normal bowel function

Interventions

1. Ask the patient to describe previous and current bowel elimination patterns, noting frequency, color, and consistency of stools. Notify the doctor of any sudden changes in the patient's bowel function.

2. Instruct the patient on the bowel regimen. Tell her to drink six to eight 8-oz glasses of water daily, to include whole-grain cereals and fresh fruits and vegetables in her diet, and to use stool softeners, if needed. Warn against straining on elimination.

Rationales

1. Altered bowel elimination patterns can result from a tumor pressing on the bowel or metastasis to the bowel. In the patient with a hysterectomy, postoperative pain and decreased activity may contribute to altered bowel patterns. Knowledge of previous and current patterns helps in determining the patient's baseline status. A sudden change in bowel function may indicate the cancer is spreading.

2. Constipation or straining on elimination can cause pain and increase fatigue. Fluids, dietary fiber, and stool softeners can help alleviate constipation.

GOAL 2: To teach the patient to recognize bowel abnormalities and take appropriate action

Interventions

1. Teach the patient the signs and symptoms of constipation (straining on elimination, decreased frequency, and evacuation of small, hard stools) and appropriate treatment measures (increased fluid and fiber intake and, with the doctor's approval, use of stool softeners).

2. Assess for signs of bowel abnormalities, such as tarry stools or changes in stool shape. Teach the patient to recognize these signs, and tell her to notify the doctor promptly if any develop.

Rationales

1. Constipation must be recognized and treated promptly because enemas and harsh laxatives are usually contraindicated for a patient with uterine cancer.

2. Bowel abnormalities may indicate metastasis to the bowel, a potential complication of uterine cancer. The patient must be able to recognize abnormalities and report them to the doctor for prompt treatment.

Nursing diagnosis: *Altered tissue perfusion: peripheral, related to lymphatic drainage obstruction*

GOAL: To achieve and maintain adequate peripheral circulation

Interventions

1. During each visit, check the patient's legs for edema, and measure leg circumference. Document findings consistently.

2. Teach the patient ways to manage edema. Tell her to elevate her legs when sitting or lying down and to avoid tight clothing and shoes, which restrict circulation.

Rationales

1. Uterine cancer may metastasize through the pelvic lymphatic system, obstructing lymph flow and leading to pooling of fluid in the legs.

2. These measures help promote venous and lymphatic drainage and improve peripheral circulation.

Nursing diagnosis: *Altered nutrition: less than body requirements, related to hypermetabolic state and anorexia*

GOAL: To help the patient meet nutritional needs

Interventions

1. Assess the patient's eating habits and food preferences by having her keep a food diary for 3 days.

2. Tell the patient to add more protein (dairy products, legumes, meats) and calories (bread, macaroni) to her diet. Consult with a dietitian, if appropriate.

3. Tell the patient she can combat anorexia with small, frequent meals; nutritional supplements; attractively prepared foods; and high-protein snack foods, such as cheese cubes or peanut butter and crackers.

Rationales

1. Knowing the patient's eating habits and food preferences helps in setting realistic goals and planning effective teaching strategies to improve the patient's nutritional status.

2. Cancer and surgery can increase the patient's metabolism. Additional protein and calories help prevent malnutrition, maintain the patient's energy level, and promote tissue repair and maintenance.

3. Eating a large meal can increase fatigue and contribute to the patient's anorexia. Small portions and snacks are easier to manage and provide a sense of accomplishment for a patient who cannot finish a large meal.

Nursing diagnosis: *Disturbance in self-concept: body image, related to perceived loss of femininity*

GOAL: To improve the patient's self-concept

Interventions

1. Assess the patient's perception of herself as a woman.

2. Ask the patient to describe how she felt about herself and her relationships with family members before the diagnosis.

3. Encourage the patient to discuss concerns about sexual relationships and how they may affect—and be affected by—self-image.

4. Assess the patient's grooming and hygiene habits. Observe for clean skin, combed hair, use of makeup and perfume, and clean clothing. Teach her appropriate hygiene measures and energy-conserving grooming techniques, such as wearing clothing and hairstyles that are easy to care for. Determine if a home health aide is needed to assist with personal care.

Rationales

1. The patient may feel that her sexual identity as a woman has been diminished by removal of her uterus. To improve the patient's self-concept, the nurse must understand how the patient perceives herself.

2. Improving self-concept and body image can be particularly difficult for a patient who had a poor self-concept or strained family relationships before diagnosis.

3. After diagnosis of uterine cancer, the patient may have a lowered self-image resulting from psychosexual concerns. Discussing these concerns may help reduce the patient's anxiety and help in determining if the patient needs professional counseling.

4. Grooming and hygiene habits can be reliable indicators of self-concept. After gynecologic surgery, special hygiene measures, such as frequent changing of sanitary napkins and regular perineal cleansing, may be needed to control drainage and odor. Learning simple grooming techniques can increase the patient's pleasure in her appearance and improve her self-concept.

Nursing diagnosis: *Impaired home maintenance management related to limitations imposed by the disease*

GOAL: To ensure the patient's safety at home

Interventions

1. Assess the patient's home for safety and convenience, such as location of telephones, need for stair climbing, and bathroom and kitchen accessibility.

2. Evaluate the patient's support systems, financial status, and medical equipment needs. Refer the patient to a social worker or appropriate community resources, if necessary.

Rationales

1. A safe, convenient environment promotes independence. A patient just home from the hospital should not climb stairs and should have a telephone at the bedside. As the patient progresses, kitchen equipment within easy reach, grab bars in the bathroom, and a portable phone can further promote independence.

2. Adequate support systems, finances, and medical equipment can help the patient maintain a safe home. The patient may need assistance in obtaining the necessary services and equipment.

Nursing diagnosis: *Impaired skin integrity related to open surgical wound*

GOAL: To promote optimal wound healing, with the patient or caregiver gradually assuming responsibility for wound care

Interventions

1. Carefully assess the patient's wound size during each visit; measure its length, width, and depth in centimeters. Note the color, consistency, and odor of drainage. Document all findings precisely. For example, stating that the drainage "soaked two 4 x 4 gauze pads" provides more useful information than simply describing the drainage as "moderate" or "heavy."

Rationales

1. Accurate, consistent measurement and documentation of wound characteristics facilitate prompt recognition of significant changes in wound status.

2. Teach the patient and caregiver the signs and symptoms of wound complication or disruption (increased drainage, change in color of drainage, opening of the wound, fever, or chills). Tell them to notify the doctor immediately if any signs or symptoms develop.

2. Complications are common with perineal wounds. The patient and caregiver must understand the significance of the signs and symptoms and know how to react if problems occur.

3. Explain proper wound care to the patient and caregiver before starting the procedure. Help them select a well-lighted, private place to perform this care. Be sure the patient is as comfortable as possible before beginning.

3. A patient who has undergone extensive gynecologic surgery may have a large, disfiguring, draining wound. The nurse must be sensitive to the patient's feelings. Explaining wound care not only helps ensure proper care in the nurse's absence but also helps relieve the patient's anxiety about an unfamiliar procedure.

4. Ask the patient if she saw the wound at the hospital, and observe whether she looks at the wound during your visits. Note if she asks questions or appears interested in participating in wound care.

4. Eventually, the patient and caregiver must assume responsibility for wound care. Preparation should be gradual and should start as early as possible in the home care process.

5. Perform wound care exactly as ordered, using a consistent technique during each visit. Post written, detailed instructions for the procedure in the room where wound care is performed so the patient, caregiver, or relief nurse can refer to them.

5. Using a consistent technique reassures the patient that wound care is being performed correctly during each visit. Consistency also can enhance learning and may help the patient become comfortable with the procedure.

6. Store wound care supplies in one area, designated by the patient, rather than throughout the home. Dispose of soiled materials immediately in a trash container outside the home.

6. Storing supplies in one area chosen by the patient promotes efficiency of care and enhances the patient's participation. Proper disposal techniques can prevent infection.

Nursing diagnosis: *Potential for infection related to wound location and extent*

GOAL 1: To prevent wound infection

Interventions

1. Observe strict infection control techniques in all phases of wound care. Be sure the patient and caregiver wear sterile gloves and open sterile dressings properly.

2. Teach the patient and caregiver proper methods of perineal cleansing (depending on the doctor's orders, antiseptic wipes or an antiseptic in a squeeze bottle may be part of perineal care). Tell them to wash hands thoroughly before performing the procedure.

Rationales

1. The warm, moist perineal area is a good medium for organism growth, and the proximity of the rectum and urethra increases the risk of infection.

2. Properly cleansing the perineal area and thoroughly washing hands reduce the risk of infection. The nurse must check the patient's or caregiver's technique and compliance.

GOAL 2: To recognize and treat wound infection promptly

Interventions

1. Assess the patient for fever, tachycardia, or tachypnea during each visit. Check wound drainage for changes in color, consistency, or odor. Assess wound periphery for redness, edema, and fecal or urinary contamination. Report abnormalities to the doctor immediately.

2. Teach the patient and caregiver the signs of infection (see the signs in Intervention #1 above). Tell them to notify the doctor if the patient develops any of these signs.

Rationales

1. Perineal wounds are easily infected. Rectovaginal and vesicovaginal fistulas may also occur. The threat of infection must be addressed immediately.

2. Because the patient and caregiver are responsible for monitoring the wound between nursing visits, they must know the signs of infection and appropriate responses.

ASSOCIATED CARE PLANS
• Grief and Grieving
• Hospice Care
• Ineffective Coping
• Pain
• Sex and Sexuality

NETWORKING OF SERVICES
• Lifeline
• Meals On Wheels
• durable medical equipment supplier
• community support groups
• American Cancer Society (ACS)
• transportation service

CARE TEAM INVOLVED
• nurse
• gynecologist
• surgeon
• oncologist
• radiologist
• patient and family
• medical social worker
• home health aide
• dietitian

IMPLICATIONS FOR HOME CARE
• functional features of the home
• telephone (communication)

PATIENT EDUCATION TOOLS
• written instructions on wound care
• ACS literature on treatments
• literature on each prescribed medication
• list of signs and symptoms to report to doctor

DISCHARGE PLAN FROM HOME HEALTH CARE
Before discharge from home health care, the patient
should:
• understand uterine cancer etiology
• know the signs and symptoms of complications and
infection and appropriate responses
• know the method of administration, dosage, action,
and adverse effects of each prescribed medication
• comply with activity restrictions and other postoperative restrictions, if applicable
• demonstrate proper wound care
• know how to obtain supplies and equipment
• understand and plan to meet dietary needs
• have lists of high-protein and high-calorie foods
• post telephone numbers of the doctor, emergency medical service, home health agency, and local office of the
ACS by the phone
• know the dates and times of follow-up appointments
with the doctor or therapist
• arrange transportation for follow-up appointments.

SELECTED REFERENCES
Birmingham, J.J. *Home Care Planning Based on DRGs.*
    Philadelphia: J.B. Lippincott Co., 1986.
Eliopoulos, C. *A Guide to the Nursing of the Aged.* Balti-
    more: Williams & Wilkins Co., 1987.
Groenwald, S.L. *Cancer Nursing Principles and Practice.*
    Boston: Jones and Bartlett Publishers, 1987.
Iyer, P., et al. *Nursing Process and Nursing Diagnosis.*
    Philadelphia: W.B. Saunders Co., 1986.
Thompson, J., et al. *Clinical Nursing.* St. Louis: C.V.
    Mosby Co., 1986.

REPRODUCTIVE SYSTEM
Breast Cancer

DESCRIPTION AND TIME FOCUS
Treatment of breast cancer involves surgery, radiation therapy, cytotoxic chemotherapy, or hormonal therapy, alone or in combinations. Primary surgery removes diseased tissue. Options include total radical mastectomy, modified radical mastectomy, and simple mastectomy. Surgery is also used as an adjuvant treatment (for example, salpingo-oophorectomy) to create an environment hostile to tumor growth. Radiation therapy may take place before or after surgery to damage cancer cells and prevent their reproduction or to relieve metastatic pain. Cytotoxic chemotherapy, usually combined with surgery or radiation therapy, uses an alkylating agent to create an environment hostile to tumor growth. Hormonal therapy usually is combined with other therapies to inhibit tumor growth and disease advancement and occasionally is used to relieve pain or prevent recurrence.

This clinical plan focuses on the patient discharged home after diagnosis and initial treatment of breast cancer. Three clinical phases of care are addressed. In the curative phase, the goal is to preserve life and control the disease. In the remission phase, the goal is to prevent recurrence and prepare the patient for reconstructive surgery. In the decline and death phase, the goal is to promote comfort and preserve the patient's dignity. The relationship between the disease phase and the patient's emotional status is crucial to the development of an effective care plan. The nurse must assess the patient and intervene appropriately.

■ Typical home health care length of service for a patient with breast cancer: depends on the illness stage
■ Typical visit frequency: during the curative phase, once weekly unless complications exist, such as the need for dressing changes, when daily visits may be required until the wound heals; a patient in remission is rarely seen by the home health team unless treatment side effects necessitate care or blood work; during the death and decline phase, two to five times weekly

HEALTH HISTORY FINDINGS
In a health history interview, the patient may report many of these findings:
• early menses (before age 12)
• late pregnancy (first parity after age 30)
• late menopause (after age 50)
• family history of breast cancer
• history of ovarian, endometrial, or colon cancer

PHYSICAL FINDINGS
In a physical examination, the nurse may detect many of these findings:

Integumentary
• lump or mass on palpation
• change in breast size or shape
• altered skin appearance (dimpling, nipple retraction, edema, hardening, peau d'orange)
• increased skin temperature

DIAGNOSTIC STUDIES
The following studies may be performed to evaluate the patient's health status:
• breast self-examination—each month about the same time, for unaffected breast
• mammography—usually, once yearly for unaffected breast

Nursing diagnosis: *Powerlessness related to anger toward, fear of, and anxiety about the disease*

GOAL: To teach the patient about the disease and the importance of treatment

Interventions

1. Evaluate the patient's ability to understand the disease by encouraging her to express her emotions and fears.

2. Explain the importance of following the treatment program and its relationship to recovery.

3. Work with the patient to establish acceptable goals and a time frame for meeting the goals.

4. Praise the patient for her efforts in working with treatment protocols.

Rationales

1. The patient must be able to express emotions before she can absorb and process additional information. Fear, denial, or anger may prevent her from seeking medical treatment.

2. Showing the patient how her individual care plan relates to her recovery gives her hope, establishes her trust, and promotes compliance.

3. Establishing goals and time frames may help the patient regain control over life's events.

4. Positive reinforcement and reward systems are important methods of encouraging goal achievement.

Nursing diagnosis: *Impaired adjustment related to postoperative complications, radiation therapy, or chemotherapy*

GOAL: To facilitate adjustment by teaching the patient the signs and symptoms of complications and appropriate management techniques

Interventions

1. Assess the patient's knowledge about the disease and its management.

2. Assess the patient's previous and current nutrition and elimination patterns and ability to perform activities of daily living.

3. Develop a list of normal and abnormal treatment side effects experienced by the patient.

Rationales

1. The nurse must identify the patient's level of knowledge to determine necessary teaching and provide a baseline for evaluating the patient's learning progress.

2. A baseline assessment of functions and capabilities helps in monitoring physiologic and psychological changes that may occur.

3. This list and the baseline functional assessment help in verifying problems and explaining their significance to the patient.

Nursing diagnosis: *Potential for infection related to possibility of lymphedema*

GOAL: To minimize the patient's risk of lymphedema

Interventions

1. Have the patient elevate the affected arm above her head and exercise the arm and hand as often as tolerable, usually three to four times daily. Tell her that washing her face and combing her hair can be an effective exercise. Be sure the patient starts out slowly, gradually increasing frequency and duration without overexercising. Periodically assess the effects of the exercise program.

2. Teach the patient to care properly for the affected arm. Provide literature about arm care and restrictions. Tell her not to work near thorny plants or dig in the garden without heavy gloves nor to permit her affected arm to be used for injections, blood samples, or blood pressure monitoring.

Rationales

1. Elevation and exercise promote circulation and prevent blood pooling, which can cause infection. Exercise also strengthens muscles.

2. An arm with damaged or removed lymph nodes is more susceptible to infection.

Nursing diagnosis: *Knowledge deficit related to the disease process*

GOAL: To help the patient understand and adapt to remission

Interventions

1. Consult the doctor about the patient's prognosis; then interview the patient to determine her expectations about remission.

2. Explain the signs and symptoms that require medical attention. Teach the patient to monitor for these signs and symptoms and to schedule doctor visits as needed.

Rationales

1. A patient in remission may believe she has been cured. The patient may be disappointed with her performance as she tries to resume activities enjoyed before diagnosis and treatment. Although the nurse should not discourage hope, the patient must understand restrictions and develop achievable goals.

2. To live independently at home with few problems, the patient must be able to identify and report potential problems and be willing to schedule and keep follow-up medical appointments.

Nursing diagnosis: *Disturbance in self-concept: body image, related to feelings of mutilation*

GOAL: To help the patient improve her self-concept

Interventions	Rationales
1. Provide the patient with literature about prostheses and surgical options.	1. Most reconstructive surgery is performed during the remission phase. A prosthesis or surgical restoration can improve the patient's self-image and allow her to maintain a more natural life-style.
2. Discuss available support groups, and provide the patient with their telephone numbers and addresses.	2. Introducing the patient to others with similar problems can help prevent isolation and give her a sense of belonging.

Nursing diagnosis: *Altered sexuality patterns related to changes in body image resulting from the mastectomy*

GOAL: To help the patient and partner reestablish former sexual patterns and adapt to the mastectomy

Interventions	Rationales
1. Encourage the patient and partner to discuss their feelings about the mastectomy and to ask questions about its effect on their sex life.	1. The patient and partner may benefit from accurate information and reassurance that sex can be as enjoyable as it was before the surgery.
2. Discuss techniques they can use in resuming sex, such as assuming comfortable positions, having the partner caress the unaffected side, massaging the mastectomy site with lotion or cream, and choosing a time for sex that permits love, attention, and fun.	2. These techniques may help the patient and partner develop a more positive attitude toward resuming sex.
3. Suggest that the couple make love in the dark and that the patient wear a bra with a prosthesis.	3. These measures may decrease the patient's anxiety while giving her time to cope with the body image changes she is experiencing.

Nursing diagnosis: *Altered comfort: pain, related to the disease process*

GOAL: To maximize the patient's comfort

Interventions	Rationales
1. Assess the patient's skin for lesions, eruptions, abrasions, and chafing on bony prominences. Improve the patient's comfort by smoothing wrinkled sheets and applying lotions or powders. Monitor for infection.	1. Skin damage and rubbing or chafing on bony prominences usually cause pain or discomfort. Pain diminishes if nerve endings are damaged, but infection is still a possibility.
2. Assess the patient's respiratory status before administering pain-suppression medications. Adjust the dosage or change the medication as ordered.	2. Medications that depress the central nervous system also decrease organ function. The nurse must exercise caution to achieve maximum pain control without inhibiting functions such as respirations or heart rate.
3. Assess the patient's pain, its relationship to the disease, and appropriate pain control measures. Consider the patient's health status when treating the source of pain. Know the strength and effects of pain medication.	3. The nurse must avoid creating one problem while attempting to alleviate another. For example, providing pain medication for stomach discomfort can create another problem if the patient has a fecal impaction. The therapeutic effects of some medications fail at this time, and other medications may be needed to enhance the therapeutic effect.

4. Note the patient's environmental preferences; for example, light or dark environment, quiet or normal noise level. Help family members understand the patient's point of view and act accordingly. Encourage the use of night-lights, soft music, stuffed animals (if appropriate), and family contact to promote patient comfort.

4. Families frequently maintain a sickroom atmosphere in the home without realizing that it compounds the patient's depression and fear. Nighttime can be frightening for a dying patient who views silence and darkness, like death, as an unknown void.

Nursing diagnosis: *Spiritual distress related to inability to participate in religious practices and functions, anger at God*

GOAL: To help the patient resume practices associated with her religious beliefs

Interventions

1. Encourage the patient to discuss her spiritual needs, beliefs, and previous religious involvement.

2. If appropriate, explore the possibility of family participation in community spiritual activities, such as Bible reading, meditation, or clergy visits.

Rationales

1. Discussing the patient's spirituality helps the nurse identify unfulfilled spiritual needs.

2. When appropriate, encouraging the family to practice spiritual beliefs together can be beneficial to all family members. However, if the patient has practiced alone or has beliefs different from those of her family, the family's participation may be inappropriate.

ASSOCIATED CARE PLANS
• Grief and Grieving
• Hospice Care
• Ineffective Coping
• Osteoporosis
• Pain
• Sex and Sexuality

NETWORKING OF SERVICES
• durable medical equipment (DME) supplier for breast prosthesis
• hospice
• American Cancer Society's (ACS) Reach for Recovery program
• genetic counseling
• local religious group
• support groups

CARE TEAM INVOLVED
• nurse
• doctor
• patient and family
• medical social worker
• psychologist
• spiritual advisor
• home health aide
• hospice volunteers
• physical therapist
• occupational therapist
• sex therapist

IMPLICATIONS FOR HOME CARE
• telephone
• understanding of chemotherapy's side effects
• hospital bed and DME (final stage)
• wigs or turbans after chemotherapy or radiation treatment

PATIENT EDUCATION TOOLS
• literature about each medication ordered
• ACS literature
• information about prostheses
• literature about clothing for the postmastectomy patient
• exercise program
• pain control techniques, such as relaxation therapy or guided imagery (see "Pain" care plan)
• financial assistance and insurance information

DISCHARGE PLAN FROM HOME HEALTH CARE
Before discharge from home health care, the patient should:
• understand the disease process
• know the dosage, action, and side effects of each medication prescribed
• know when to communicate with the doctor
• be able to express her feelings to others
• understand the value and effect of therapeutic treatment
• have support systems
• know personal capabilities and limitations
• know about available community resources
• recognize potential risks
• establish an effective emergency care plan
• begin adapting to required life-style modifications
• have a sense of spiritual involvement, if applicable.

Before the patient is discharged from home health care, the family should:
• be able to cope with changes in their environment
• provide support for each other
• know about and schedule counseling, as needed
• reestablish pre-illness emotional bonds.

SELECTED REFERENCES

Archer, D.N., and Smith, A.C. "Sorrow Has Many Faces," *Nursing88* 43-45, May 1988.

Bernstein, L.H., et al. *Primary Care in the Home.* Philadelphia: J.B. Lippincott Co., 1987.

Billings, A.J. *Outpatient Management of Advanced Cancer.* Philadelphia: J.B. Lippincott Co., 1985.

Ferszt, G.G., and Taylor, P.B. "When Your Patient Needs Spiritual Comfort," *Nursing88* 48-49, April 1988.

U.S. Department of Health and Human Services. *When Cancer Recurs: Meeting the Challenge Again.* Bethesda, Md.: NIH Publication No. 87-2709, 1987.

RENAL AND URINARY SYSTEM
Indwelling Catheter Care

DESCRIPTION AND TIME FOCUS
Indwelling catheterization—which maintains urine drainage for weeks, months, or years—usually is required for a patient with neurogenic bladder, a spinal cord injury, or multiple sclerosis and may be required for a patient with urinary tract disease, cardiovascular disease, orthopedic problems, decubitus ulcers, chronic urinary incontinence, or urethral obstruction. Incidence of urinary incontinence and the probability of a neurologic cause for incontinence increase with age. Other age-related physiologic factors that increase the likelihood of indwelling catheterization include gradual failure of the bladder to concentrate urine, decreased muscle tone of the pelvic floor, and reduced ability to control urination.

Preventing urinary tract infection (UTI) is an important and difficult aspect of managing a patient with an indwelling catheter. Difficulties are common because any problem in urinary drainage—such as leaking, blocking, odor, irritation, encrustation, or bladder spasm—can cause a UTI. Studies indicate that most patients with indwelling catheters have bacteriuria within 30 days of catheterization.

This clinical plan focuses on the patient at home with an indwelling catheter. Routine patient care usually is provided by family members or other nonprofessional caregivers. The nurse performs the skilled procedure of catheterization and teaches the patient and family proper care techniques. Care centers on maintaining catheter patency and preventing UTI and other complications.

■ Typical home health care length of service for a patient with an indwelling catheter: varies from weeks to years, depending on the patient's condition

■ Typical visit frequency: once monthly, although the nurse should anticipate additional visits to address specific problems. The schedule for catheter change depends on the patient's condition and circumstances. Most patients need the catheter changed every 3 to 6 weeks.

HEALTH HISTORY FINDINGS
In a health history interview, the patient may report many of these findings:
• reduced mobility
• history of urine dribbling
• inability to start and stop the urine stream
• lack of urge to void
• history of surgery involving the bladder and urethra
• decreased level of consciousness
• confusion

PHYSICAL FINDINGS
In a physical examination, the nurse may detect many of these findings:

Renal and urinary
• residual urine (greater than 50 ml)
• reduced bladder capacity (less than 300 ml)
• reduced sensation in the perineal area
• palpable bladder
• enlarged prostate gland
• tumor in spinal cord resulting in neurogenic bladder
• congenital anomaly, such as hypospadias or epispadias
• loss of tissue and muscle tone

Neurologic
• cerebral atherosclerosis
• cerebrovascular accident
• brain tumor or trauma
• multiple sclerosis
• diabetic neuropathy
• alcoholic neuropathy
• inability to recognize bladder cues because of reduced attention span, depression, anxiety, or disorientation
• spinal cord disorder

Gastrointestinal
• fecal impaction

DIAGNOSTIC STUDIES
The following studies may be performed to evaluate the patient's health status:
• urine culture—to detect UTI if signs of infection occur; result greater than 100,000 organisms/ml indicates UTI
• urinalysis—specific gravity 1.001 to 1.003, cloudy or smoky color, unpleasant odor, pH greater than 7; may indicate proteinuria, hematuria, or abnormal red cell cast, white cells, white cell casts
• white blood cell count—greater than 10,000/mcl
• erythrocyte sedimentation rate—elevated

Nursing diagnosis: *Total incontinence related to motor impairment*

GOAL: To control urine flow

Interventions
1. Insert the smallest (14-18G) catheter possible for good drainage.

Rationales
1. The paraurethral glands, which bathe the urethra with a natural lubricant, are blocked if the catheter lumen is too large.

2. Use strict aseptic technique when inserting the catheter.

2. Proper technique prevents UTI.

3. Use a small catheter balloon (5-10 ml) when possible. If you must use a larger balloon, be sure to inflate it completely.

3. Smaller balloons minimize bladder irritation. Larger balloons may cause bladder neck necrosis. Incomplete inflation can cause the balloon to expand on one side only, causing irritation and pressure on the bladder mucosa.

4. Record the size of the catheter and balloon and the amount of water used to fill the balloon.

4. Proper documentation ensures continuity of care.

5. Change the catheter every 4 weeks or as needed.

5. The nurse should assess the patient to determine the change schedule required, although 4 weeks can be used as a guideline. Gritty deposits, frequent infection, or difficulty in removing the catheter may indicate the need for more frequent changes.

Nursing diagnosis: *Potential for impaired skin integrity related to catheter obstruction or leakage*

GOAL: To promote unobstructed urine flow

Interventions

1. Determine the cause of leakage or blockage. Assess for constipation, and establish a bowel retraining program, if indicated. Also assess for bladder spasticity, and consult with the doctor to determine if oxybutynin chloride is needed to treat bladder spasms.

2. Encourage the patient to drink 5 to 8 oz of cranberry juice three times daily. Consider implementing an acid-ash diet, including meat, eggs, whole-grain bread, prunes, and plums.

3. Encourage the patient to drink 2 to 3 liters of fluid daily, unless contraindicated.

4. Irrigate the catheter only when necessary, using a 0.25% acetic acid solution; avoid routine irrigation. Store irrigation fluids in a closed bottle in the refrigerator (never in an open bottle or at room temperature).

5. Milk the catheter as needed, gently squeezing the drainage bag's tubing proximally to distally (from the patient to the bag).

6. Use a silicone catheter instead of a latex catheter.

Rationales

1. Constipation or bladder spasticity can cause leakage.

2. Cranberry juice and an acid-ash diet lower the pH of the patient's urine, which helps prevent urinary calculi formation.

3. Fluids dilute urine and increase its flow.

4. Although irrigation can dislodge and dilute sediment that may be causing blockage, routine irrigation opens the system to bacteria and increases risk of infection. Storing irrigation fluids in a closed bottle in the refrigerator limits bacteria growth.

5. Milking minimizes the need for irrigation and maintains catheter patency.

6. A silicone catheter causes less irritation; can be left in place longer, thereby reducing urethral trauma; is less susceptible to encrustation; and has a larger lumen to which body salts do not easily adhere.

Nursing diagnosis: *Potential for infection related to catheterization and the drainage system*

GOAL: To prevent infection and related complications

Interventions

1. Cleanse the patient's urinary meatus daily. Wash around the catheter and remove any encrustations. Do not apply lotions or powders.

Rationales

1. Cleansing the urinary meatus daily helps prevent infection. Lotions and powders should not be used because they promote growth of microorganisms.

2. Assess for—and teach the patient and caregiver to recognize—signs and symptoms of infection (fever, abdominal pain, burning in the bladder or urinary meatus, chills, bladder or flank pain, tachycardia, cloudy or foul-smelling urine, disorientation, and nausea or vomiting) and abnormal changes in urine properties (increase in sediment, hematuria, or a change in color).

2. Signs and symptoms of infection warrant a urine culture. UTI must be diagnosed and treated promptly to prevent such complications as acute or chronic pyelonephritis; perinephric, vesical, or urethral abscesses; vesical and renal calculi; bacteremia; renal failure; and death. A urine culture can help the doctor identify the infection's cause and determine appropriate treatment.

3. Be aware that chronic bacteriuria is common in a patient with an indwelling catheter.

3. Urinalysis and a urine culture are warranted only if signs and symptoms of acute UTI appear.

4. Do not disconnect the catheter from the drainage bag.

4. Disconnecting the catheter from the bag opens the system to bacteria, increasing the risk of infection.

5. Wash your hands before emptying the drainage bag, or wear gloves to empty the bag if the urine contains blood. Do not allow the drainage or outlet tap to touch the floor. Consider rinsing the drainage tap with 3% hydrogen peroxide.

5. These measures prevent bacterial contamination of the drainage bag, which often precedes UTI, suggesting intraluminal spread of the organism.

6. Empty the drainage bag at least twice daily and more often if needed.

6. Organisms in the urine in the bag can lead to retrograde contamination of the urinary tract.

7. Carefully clean the patient after each bowel movement.

7. Organisms from the patient's bowel movement can cause UTI.

8. Clean the distal catheter or port with alcohol or povidone-iodine. Aspirate urine specimens, using a syringe and a 21G needle.

8. Using aseptic technique and aspirating specimens help prevent contamination of the system.

Nursing diagnosis: *Knowledge deficit related to indwelling catheter care*

GOAL: To teach the patient and caregiver about the condition, equipment, and self-care

Interventions

1. Assess the patient's equipment needs (leg bag, extra drainage bag, acetic acid, alcohol or povidone-iodine, syringes, catheters, catheter tray).

Rationales

1. Proper supplies enhance urinary drainage and help prevent contamination of the system.

2. Assess what the patient and caregiver know about catheters, and answer any questions they may have.

2. The patient and caregiver may not understand how the catheter works. Knowledge can allay fears of accidentally disconnecting or displacing the catheter when moving the patient or working with the catheter.

3. Teach the patient and caregiver how to maintain the catheter system. Instruct them to:

3. Instruction allows the patient and family members to participate in and assume responsibility for patient care.

• keep the drainage bag lower than the bladder at all times

• An unobstructed downhill flow must be maintained at all times to promote proper drainage.

• coil excess tubing on the bed so the tubing descends straight into the drainage bag

• Tubing that hangs over the side of the bed can impede urine flow.

• wash leg bags and drainage bags in soapy water, rinse them with clear water, and then soak them in a solution of 1 part sodium hypochlorite to 10 parts water for 30 minutes; empty and air dry the bags; close the bags with a cap soaked in alcohol; store the bags in a clean container and use within 3 days

• This cleaning procedure dissolves sediment and reduces odor.

• encourage frequent position changes

• Frequent position changes can increase urine flow.

• notify the doctor or nurse if the catheter becomes blocked; then deflate the balloon by cutting the balloon leg or by extracting air with a syringe.

• Deflating the balloon when the catheter is blocked prevents an emergency. The doctor or nurse must be notified to change the catheter.

4. Provide the patient and caregiver with the telephone number of an on-call agency nurse.

4. Many routine questions or problems, such as those relating to a change in amount or color of urine, can be handled over the phone.

Nursing diagnosis: *Impaired home maintenance management related to indwelling catheterization*

GOAL: To promote effective home maintenance management

Interventions

1. Assess the patient's home to ensure suitability for home catheter care. If the patient's bed is inappropriate, recommend a hospital bed. Be sure the home is sanitary and has running water.

2. Interview the patient to determine his ability to pay for necessary equipment and supplies. Refer him to a social worker, if necessary, for help in arranging delivery.

Rationales

1. A hospital bed is higher than a typical bed and has side rails, so positioning or moving the patient is easier. A sanitary home and running water are necessary for aseptic care of equipment and supplies.

2. Medicare will pay for equipment and supplies if the patient is elderly. Medicaid also covers equipment and supply expenses. Family, friends, or the nurse can pick up the items from a pharmacy or medical equipment supplier.

ASSOCIATED CARE PLANS
• Cerebrovascular Accident
• Multiple Sclerosis
• Neurogenic Bladder
• Prostate Cancer
• Sex and Sexuality
• Spinal Cord Injury

NETWORKING OF SERVICES
• durable medical equipment supplier
• support group

CARE TEAM INVOLVED
• nurse
• doctor
• patient and family
• urologist
• home health aide
• sex therapist

IMPLICATIONS FOR HOME CARE
• adequate bathroom facilities
• telephone (communication)
• extra catheter set for emergency

PATIENT EDUCATION TOOLS
• list of signs and symptoms of UTI
• literature about catheter care and use

DISCHARGE PLAN FROM HOME HEALTH CARE
Before discharge from home health care, the patient should:
• demonstrate proper use and care of indwelling catheter and supplies
• know that the drainage bag should never be higher than the bladder

• know to check for catheter obstruction and to notify the nurse if drainage stops
• know the complications of UTI
• know the signs and symptoms of UTI
• have the telephone number of the home health agency for follow-up care, if needed
• plan to have the catheter changed every 4 weeks, or more often if needed
• understand that sexual activity is allowed and know proper techniques (see "Sex and Sexuality" care plan).

SELECTED REFERENCES
Bradley, C., et al. "Taking Precautions: Urinary Tract Infection in Catheterized Patients Can Be Prevented," *Nursing Times* 82:70-73, 1986.
Carpenito, L.J. *Nursing Diagnosis: Applications to Clinical Practice,* 2nd ed. Philadelphia: J.B. Lippincott Co., 1987.
Conti, M.T., and Entropius, L. "Preventing UTIs: What Works?" *American Journal of Nursing* 87:307-09, 1987.
Doenges, M.E., et al. *Nursing Care Plans: Nursing Diagnoses in Planning Patient Care.* Philadelphia: F.A. Davis Co., 1984.
Fischbach, F. *A Manual of Laboratory Diagnostic Tests.* Philadelphia: J.B. Lippincott Co., 1984.
Potter, P.A., and Perry, A.G. *Fundamentals of Nursing: Concepts, Process, and Practice.* St. Louis: C.V. Mosby Co., 1985.
Steward, D.K., et al. "Failure of the Urinalyses and Quantitative Urine Culture in Diagnosing Symptomatic Urinary Tract Infection in Patients with Long-term Urinary Catheters," *American Journal of Infections Control* 134:154-60, 1985.
Wilden, M.H. "Living with a Foley," *American Journal of Nursing* 86(10):1121-23, 1986.

RENAL AND URINARY SYSTEM
Chronic Renal Failure

DESCRIPTION AND TIME FOCUS
In chronic renal failure, the kidneys fail to eliminate waste and maintain homeostasis, and normal function is not likely to return. Chronic renal failure can result from chronic glomerular disease, nephrotoxic agents, endocrine diseases, obstructive disorders, congenital anomalies, repeated infections, and vascular diseases. Disease progress is monitored by periodic urine and blood studies.

This clinical plan focuses on the patient at home with chronic renal failure. Nursing care centers on assessing the patient's condition, intervening to prevent complications, and teaching the patient self-care and dietary requirements. The patient may experience anxiety and fears about death or family issues, such as the financial burden of medical expenses. The nurse must help the patient and family cope with this chronic illness, which typically involves increasingly severe symptoms and eventually leads to death.

■ Typical home health care length of service for a patient with chronic renal failure: 4 to 6 weeks

■ Typical visit frequency: usually once or twice weekly. In the terminal stage, daily visits are needed, and hospice services should be arranged in accordance with the patient's and family's wishes. Rehabilitative services, Lifeline, Meals On Wheels, and other health team disciplines also may be needed.

HEALTH HISTORY FINDINGS
In a health history interview, the patient may report many of these findings:
• history of hypertension
• history of diabetes
• family history of renal disease
• recent gradual weight gain
• altered urinary patterns
• decreased appetite
• susceptibility to infection
• insomnia

PHYSICAL FINDINGS
In a physical examination, the nurse may detect many of these findings:

Renal and urinary
• polyuria
• oliguria
• nocturia
• chronic urinary tract infections

Cardiovascular
• hypertension
• dysrhythmias
• cardiomyopathy
• pericarditis
• congestive heart failure

Respiratory
• pulmonary edema
• pleurisy
• friction rub
• pleural effusion
• dyspnea
• Kussmaul's respirations

Neurologic
• pain, burning, or itching of legs and feet
• paresthesia
• muscle cramps or twitching
• short memory
• confusion
• coma
• convulsions

Gastrointestinal
• stomatitis
• gum ulceration
• parotitis
• esophagitis
• gastritis
• duodenal ulcers
• uremic colitis
• pancreatitis
• metallic taste in mouth
• anorexia
• uremic fetor
• vomiting
• constipation

Integumentary
• pallor
• yellow skin
• dry skin
• pruritus
• purpura
• uremic frost (rare)
• thin, brittle fingernails
• thin, brittle hair

Musculoskeletal
• calcium-phosphorus imbalance

Endocrine
- impotence
- decreased libido
- impaired carbohydrate metabolism
- amenorrhea

General
- anemia
- thrombocytopenia
- hyponatremia
- hyperkalemia

DIAGNOSTIC STUDIES
The following studies may be performed to evaluate the patient's health status:
- X-rays of kidney, ureter, bladder—to detect hydronephrosis
- intravenous pyelogram (IVP)—to detect obstruction
- nephrotomography—to detect congenital anomalies
- renal scan—to detect circulatory defects
- renal arteriography—to detect evidence of renal damage
- urinalysis—once weekly; may reveal proteinuria, glycosuria, erythrocytes, casts; specific gravity becomes fixed at 1.010
- biopsy—to identify pathology
- blood studies—once weekly; reveal increased blood urea nitrogen (BUN), creatinine, and potassium levels; decreased arterial pH and bicarbonate
- creatinine clearance test (24-hour sample)—once or twice monthly to detect gradual kidney dysfunction

---

Nursing diagnosis: *Fluid volume excess related to impaired kidney function*

GOAL 1: To reduce the work load of the damaged kidney

Interventions
1. Discuss the patient's case with the referring nurse or doctor. Review the discharge summary and pertinent medical records to obtain most recent diagnoses, laboratory values, and medication orders. Take the patient's health history, and perform a physical examination.

2. Encourage the patient to rest periodically throughout the day. Tell him to nap 1 hour for every 4 hours of activity.

3. Tell the patient to weigh himself unclothed at the same time each day, using the same scale. Explain that he must report a weight gain of more than 3 lb in a day or 5 lb in a week to the doctor or nurse.

4. Teach the patient to record intake and output daily, using standard fluid measurements. Give the patient a list of fluid values that includes measurements he uses at home, such as cups, pints, or quarts.

5. Teach the patient the importance of complying with fluid restrictions. Suggest ways to reduce thirst while maintaining compliance, such as brushing and flossing frequently, sucking on hard candy or cracked ice, eating frozen desserts, and avoiding foods that increase thirst.

Rationales
1. These sources provide information on the extent of disease, treatment plans (such as dialysis or a planned transplant), baseline laboratory values, and the patient's health status. The information helps in formulating a plan of care.

2. Napping increases circulation to the kidneys, conserves energy, and promotes endurance.

3. Weight gain may indicate fluid retention because of impaired kidney function. Daily weighings done consistently help detect problems quickly.

4. Accurately recording fluid intake and output helps monitor kidney function.

5. Limiting fluids reduces the kidneys' work load and helps maintain homeostasis by preventing extra fluid from circulating, which skews electrolyte values.

GOAL 2: To improve kidney function

Interventions
1. Monitor BUN, creatinine, electrolyte, hematocrit, and hemoglobin values and urinalysis results at least once weekly.

2. Teach the patient the signs and symptoms of metabolic imbalance, as evidenced by diabetes (polyuria, thirst, hunger, weight loss, anorexia, nausea, vomiting), anemia (weakness, vertigo, headache, tinnitus, drowsiness), and hyperkalemia (usually asymptomatic until cardiac toxicity occurs).

Rationales
1. Monitoring laboratory values alerts the nurse to changes in the patient's status.

2. Chronic renal failure inhibits other regulatory functions in the body. Prompt attention can alleviate life-threatening imbalances.

Nursing diagnosis: *Altered cardiac output: decreased, related to stroke volume reduction as kidney failure produces fluid overload*

GOAL 1: To maintain optimum cardiac output

Interventions

1. During each visit, monitor the patient's blood pressure while the patient stands, sits, and reclines. Monitor for pulse deficits and dysrhythmias. Listen for friction rub, and be alert to signs and symptoms of congestive heart failure (cough, shortness of breath, edema, orthopnea) and pericarditis (those of congestive heart failure plus pleuritic pain).

2. Teach the patient the signs of edema (swelling of legs, feet, and sacral area) and the importance of reporting these promptly. Review proper use of medications, especially diuretics and cardiac drugs.

3. Teach the patient to notify the doctor if he experiences paroxysmal nocturnal dyspnea, shortness of breath, orthopnea, or dyspnea on exertion.

Rationales

1. Renal disease usually affects the cardiovascular system. Assessing the patient's cardiac status at each visit can prevent complications or facilitate prompt intervention if complications occur.

2. Edema inhibits cardiac function, exacerbating the kidneys' inability to eliminate wastes. Knowledge of the medication regimen promotes compliance.

3. Changes in respiratory status can indicate more serious conditions, such as congestive heart failure, cor pulmonale, or decreased kidney function.

GOAL 2: To improve activity tolerance by conserving the patient's energy

Interventions

1. Assess the patient's sleep patterns at each visit, and, if necessary, teach him relaxation techniques, such as bathing in warm water, reading, listening to soft music, and taking a sleeping medication, if ordered.

2. At each visit, assess the patient's activity tolerance by watching him perform activities of daily living (ADLs). Note how many he can perform independently without tiring.

Rationales

1. Nocturia, insomnia, and metabolic imbalances can interfere with normal sleep patterns and result in fatigue.

2. If the patient has difficulty with self-care or basic activities, the nurse should arrange appropriate assistance to reduce stress and help him conserve energy.

Nursing diagnosis: *Potential for impaired skin integrity related to decreased kidney function and fluid imbalance*

GOAL: To maintain skin integrity

Interventions

1. Tell the patient to change positions frequently.

2. Teach the patient to inspect for skin breakdown daily (have the caregiver check areas the patient cannot see) and to perform meticulous skin care. Tell him to wash daily with warm water, to apply baby oil to dry skin, and to avoid harsh soaps or creams with alcohol.

Rationales

1. Lying or sitting in one position for a long time diminishes circulation, which can result in skin breakdown and infection.

2. A patient with renal failure usually has dry skin, anemia, and edema. Regular inspection can detect skin breakdown, facilitate prompt treatment, and minimize the risk of complications. Meticulous skin care promotes circulation to pressure areas and moisturizes the skin.

Nursing diagnosis: *Ineffective individual coping related to stress produced by chronic illness*

GOAL: To help the patient cope more effectively with his illness

Interventions	Rationales
1. Encourage the patient to talk about his illness and prognosis and to discuss coping behaviors used in the past. Promote coping by acknowledging his point of view and discussing topics at a comfortable pace.	1. Discussing the illness may help relieve some of the stress the patient is feeling. The discussion also may reveal that he does not fully understand his condition; if so, the nurse can provide additional, accurate information. The patient will probably cope better if he has no doubts about his illness or prognosis.
2. In your discussions with the patient, be alert to evidence that he is denying the illness (unrealistic plans for the future, refusal to discuss the illness).	2. Evidence of denial may indicate he has started the grieving process, which typically follows loss of body functions and alterations in body image. The patient may experience one or more of the five stages of grieving (denial, anger, bargaining, depression, and acceptance).
3. If appropriate, discuss the patient's wishes about advanced life support, intravenous feedings, antibiotic use, resuscitation, living wills, and durable power of attorney.	3. The patient should state his views on death-related issues while he is competent to do so. Specific measures can be taken to ensure that his wishes are carried out, especially in emergencies, and that family members are advised of these wishes.

ASSOCIATED CARE PLANS
- Chronic Congestive Heart Failure
- Diabetes Mellitus
- Grief and Grieving
- Hospice Care
- Hypertension
- Indwelling Catheter Care
- Kidney Transplant

NETWORKING OF SERVICES
- Lifeline
- Meals On Wheels
- durable medical equipment supplier
- hospice

CARE TEAM INVOLVED
- nurse
- doctor
- patient and family
- medical social worker
- professional homemaker or home health aide
- pharmacist
- clinical nurse specialist
- physical therapist
- occupational therapist

IMPLICATIONS FOR HOME CARE
- functional features of the home
- telephone or other access to help in an emergency
- reliable support system
- ability of the patient, caregiver, or other family members to provide necessary care

PATIENT EDUCATION TOOLS
- list of normal readings for pulse rate, blood pressure, and respiratory rate and instructions on how to monitor these
- literature on each medication ordered
- information on specialized diets and recipes
- American Kidney Association literature

DISCHARGE PLAN FROM HOME HEALTH CARE
Before discharge from home health care, the patient should:
- know that edema or signs and symptoms of congestive heart failure must be reported to the doctor immediately
- know the name, method of administration, dosage, action, and adverse effects of each prescribed medication
- carry a list of these medications, with the doctor's name and telephone number, and post a similar list by the phone for emergency use
- understand the need for daily weighings and notifying the doctor about abnormal weight gain
- perform ADLs with minimal help, using energy-conserving techniques
- understand why a special diet is needed, meet daily intake requirements, and follow other dietary restrictions
- undergo scheduled laboratory tests to evaluate his condition
- know the dates and times of follow-up appointments with the doctor and laboratory
- have Lifeline in place
- post telephone numbers of the doctor, ambulance service, hospital, and home health agency by the phone

• be able to express fears and concerns about chronic illness
• seek spiritual guidance, if desired
• wear a Medic Alert bracelet
• know about community-based support groups and rehabilitation services.

SELECTED REFERENCES

Lancaster, L.E., ed. *The Patient with End-Stage Renal Disease,* 2nd ed. New York: John Wiley & Sons, 1984.

Lerner, J., and Khan, Z. *Mosby's Manual of Urologic Nursing.* St. Louis: C.V. Mosby Co., 1982.

Nursing Diagnosis Cards. Springhouse, Pa.: Springhouse Corporation, 1989.

Oreopoulos, D. *Geriatric Nephrology.* Boston: Martin Nijhoff, 1986.

Tamplet-Ulrich, Beth, ed. *Nephrology Nursing: Concepts and Strategies.* Norwalk, Conn.: Appleton & Lange, 1989.

Neurogenic Bladder

DESCRIPTION AND TIME FOCUS
Neurogenic bladder is a dysfunction that occurs when a lesion in the central nervous system inhibits bladder innervation. The five types of bladder dysfunction, classified by the response or action of the bladder, are: uninhibited, reflex, autonomous, motor paralytic, and sensory paralytic. Complications of neurogenic bladder include lower urinary tract infection, renal disease secondary to lower urinary tract infection, autonomic dysreflexia, progressive hydronephrosis, urinary calculus disease, urethral strictures, bladder outlet dysfunction, vesicoureteral reflux, and prostatic hypertrophy.

This clinical plan focuses on the patient discharged home from an acute-care hospital after diagnosis, management, and initial treatment of a neurogenic bladder. Nursing care depends on the type of dysfunction and centers on implementing a bladder retraining program, preserving renal function, and preventing urologic complications. The home is a comfortable setting in which the nurse can teach the patient and family the bladder retraining program and monitor for complications, such as progressive renal deterioration.

■ Typical home health care length of service for a patient with neurogenic bladder: usually 3 to 4 weeks

■ Typical visit frequency: once daily

HEALTH HISTORY FINDINGS
In a health history interview, the patient may report many of these findings (or findings may be indicated in past medical records):
• cerebrovascular accident (CVA)
• multiple sclerosis
• syphilis
• brain trauma
• brain tumor
• Parkinson's disease
• delayed development during childhood
• cerebral atherosclerosis
• traumatic transection of the spinal cord
• lesion affecting sensory and motor tracts above the conus medullaris
• pernicious anemia
• spinal shock occurring after acute transection of the spinal cord
• spina bifida
• myelomeningocele
• trauma
• bacterial or viral infection
• neoplasm of the conus medullaris, cauda equina, or pelvic nerves
• spinal anesthesia
• recent radical pelvic surgery
• herniated intervertebral disc
• poliomyelitis
• Guillain-Barré syndrome
• neoplasms of sacral roots 2, 3, and 4 (parasympathetic fibers)
• diabetes mellitus
• tabes dorsalis

PHYSICAL FINDINGS
In a physical examination, the nurse may detect many of these findings:

Renal and urinary
• urinary incontinence
• urine retention
• uninhibited voiding
• chronic urine retention with overflow
• palpable distended bladder
• inability to void
• urinary urgency
• urinary frequency with minimal output
• poor bladder sensation
• infrequent voiding, with increased urine volume when detrusor muscle decompensates
• reduced urine output

Integumentary
• reddened skin in perineal area

DIAGNOSTIC STUDIES
The following studies may be performed to evaluate the patient's health status:
• urinalysis—monthly with intermittent catheterization, then four or more times each year after discharge from home health care; to assess for signs of infection (sediment, abnormal odor, cloudiness, mucus, hematuria) or calculus formation
• urine culture and sensitivity—monthly with intermittent catheterization, then four or more times each year after discharge from home health care; to assess for bacterial infection (*Escherichia coli, Proteus, Pseudomonas, Klebsiella, Staphylococcus*); 100,000 or more bacteria/ml indicates infection.
• serum creatinine—initially for baseline, then every 3 to 6 months, then annually after discharge from home health care; above normal levels indicate impaired renal function.
• blood urea nitrogen (BUN)—initially for baseline, then every 3 to 6 months, then annually after discharge from home health care; to assess renal glomerular function and urea production and excretion; above normal levels usually indicate impaired renal function.
• creatinine clearance—initially for baseline, then every

3 to 6 months, then annually after discharge from home health care; to assess glomerular filtration; below normal levels indicate impaired renal function.
• cystogram—after condition of patient with spinal cord injury has stabilized, when evidence of neurologic reflexes exists; to visually inspect bladder filling; differentiates between neurogenic and nonneurogenic bladder
• cystometrogram—after diagnosis of neurogenic bladder to determine the type; to assess neuromuscular function in the bladder by measuring the detrusor muscle reflex efficiency and intravesical pressure and capacity; uninhibited contractions with decreased bladder capacity indicate uninhibited or reflex bladder dysfunction; lack of uninhibited contractions with increased bladder capacity indicates autonomous, motor paralytic, or sensory paralytic bladder dysfunction.
• external electromyography (EMG)—usually performed with cystometrogram to assess electrical activity in external urinary sphincter voluntary muscles and pelvic floor muscles; external sphincter flaccidity indicates an autonomous bladder dysfunction.
• urethral pressure profile (UPP)—usually evaluated with electromyography to differentiate between striated and smooth muscle activity; low pressure indicates incontinence; high pressure indicates retention, strictures, or urethral narrowing.

• bulbocavernosus reflex—usually performed after cystometrogram and before removing indwelling catheter; reflex is positive (normal) when rectal sphincter contracts, indicating intact voiding reflex; uninhibited neurogenic bladder dysfunction has a normal reflex; hyperactive reflex indicates reflex bladder dysfunction; no reflex indicates autonomous or motor paralytic bladder dysfunction; variable reflex indicates sensory paralytic bladder dysfunction.
• catheterization for residual urine—immediately after each voluntary micturition during home care, then four or more times each year after discharge from home health care, to determine volume of urine remaining in bladder. No residual is normal; residual urine may indicate detrusor muscle dysfunction, obstructive uropathy, diverticula, or psychogenic inhibition.
• intravenous pyelogram (IVP)—performed during long-term home health care if laboratory studies indicate deterioration of renal function; visually inspecting kidney size and shape can detect hydronephrosis, renal calculi, chronic pyelonephritis, and vesicoureteral reflux.
• kidney ultrasonography—performed during long-term home health care if clinical obstructive symptoms indicate urinary tract infections or calculus formation; progressive hydronephrosis can indicate urinary tract infection or calculus formation.

Nursing diagnosis: *Altered patterns of urinary elimination related to weak detrusor muscle and lack of coordination between detrusor muscle contraction and external sphincter relaxation*

GOAL: To promote effective bladder emptying

Interventions

1. Administer drugs according to the doctor's orders.

2. Institute nonsurgical measures to promote effective bladder emptying, such as intermittent catheterization (using a clean technique) and anal stretch maneuver. Use Credés or Valsalva's maneuver, if necessary.

3. If surgery is required, help the patient prepare for such procedures as bilateral pudendal nerve block, neurectomy and transurethral resection of the external urinary sphincter, or ileal conduit urinary diversion.

Rationales

1. The doctor may order one or more drugs to promote effective bladder emptying. (For detailed information on their uses and mechanisms of action, see *Drugs that promote bladder emptying*, page 230.)

2. Nonsurgical measures promote bladder emptying when the patient has unacceptable levels of residual urine. Intermittent catheterization can empty the bladder without the complications associated with an indwelling catheter. Regular, frequent catheterization prevents bladder distention and ischemia. Anal stretch, Credés, and Valsalva's maneuvers overcome detrusor-sphincter dyssynergia, facilitating consistent bladder emptying and acceptable levels of residual urine.

3. Surgical intervention occasionally is required to reduce spasticity and resulting urethral resistance. Urinary diversion typically is used only after conservative management has been ineffective and persistent infection, obstruction, recurrent calculi formation, or bladder decompensation has resulted in renal function deterioration.

DRUGS THAT PROMOTE BLADDER EMPTYING

Drug	Major use	Action
bethanechol chloride *(Urecholine)*	To treat urine retention caused by detrusor muscle hypoactivity with no evidence of urinary outlet obstruction	Strengthens bladder muscle contraction to initiate voiding and to improve bladder emptying
diazepam *(Valium)*, dantrolene sodium *(Dantrium)*, baclofen *(Lioresal)*	To treat urine retention by improving bladder emptying	Decrease spasticity of the external urethra sphincter and relax the pelvic floor muscles
oxybutynin chloride *(Ditropan)*	To treat uninhibited and reflex bladders	Has a direct antispasmodic effect on smooth muscle, which inhibits the action of acetylcholine
propantheline bromide *(Pro-Banthine)*	To treat urinary frequency and incontinence caused by bladder muscle irritation and hyperactivity	Inhibits the action of acetylcholine on the nerve endings of parasympathetic fibers

Nursing diagnosis: *Reflex incontinence related to reflex neurogenic bladder*

GOAL 1: To alleviate reflex incontinence by emptying the bladder

Interventions

1. Assess the patient's health history for pernicious anemia or factors leading to a spinal cord lesion above T12, such as traumatic injury, infection, tumor, multiple sclerosis, or transverse myelitis.

2. Teach the patient techniques to stimulate reflex voiding, such as light, rapid or deep, sharp suprapubic tapping; gently tugging pubic hairs; massaging the abdomen; digital rectal stimulation; stroking the glans penis; lightly punching the abdomen above the inguinal ligaments; and stroking the inner thigh.

3. Tell the patient not to use Credé's maneuver.

Rationales

1. Pernicious anemia or a spinal cord lesion above T12 can result in reflex incontinence.

2. These techniques can stimulate spontaneous voiding.

3. Credé's maneuver can damage the urethra or cause vesicoureteral reflux if the external sphincter is contracted.

GOAL 2: To prevent or minimize episodes of autonomic dysreflexia and related complications

Interventions

1. Monitor the patient for—and teach him to recognize—signs and symptoms of autonomic dysreflexia, such as hypertension, anxiety, sweating, headache, bradycardia, chest pain, urine retention, pallor, piloerection, and diaphoresis.

2. Institute measures to lower the patient's blood pressure during an episode, such as elevating the head of the bed 90 degrees or having him sit down. Monitor his blood pressure every 3 to 5 minutes, and loosen tight-fitting clothing.

3. If the patient has an indwelling catheter, assess the urinary drainage system for possible obstruction from kinked or clamped tubing.

Rationales

1. Identifying signs and symptoms of autonomic dysreflexia facilitates prompt intervention.

2. Hypertension associated with autonomic dysreflexia can be life-threatening.

3. An obstruction can cause urine retention and lead to bladder distention, the most common cause of autonomic dysreflexia.

4. Insert an indwelling catheter if the bladder is distended and the patient is on intermittent catheter insertions.

4. An indwelling catheter can help alleviate urine retention.

5. If the patient's rectum is impacted, apply dibucaine hydrochloride (Nupercainal Ointment), and remove the impaction.

5. Dibucaine hydrochloride anesthetizes the rectum. Removing the impaction alleviates discomfort.

6. Institute bowel- and bladder-emptying programs, and encourage the patient to follow them.

6. Fecal impaction and bladder distention can lead to autonomic dysreflexia.

Nursing diagnosis: *Urge incontinence related to uninhibited neurogenic bladder*

GOAL: To minimize urge incontinence

Interventions

1. Assess for urge incontinence from uninhibited bladder contractions caused by or attributed to neurologic disorders, such as CVA, Parkinson's disease, or brain tumor, trauma, or infection.

2. Minimize or eliminate factors contributing to uninhibited bladder contractions. Establish a planned voiding program appropriate for the patient's bladder capacity and voiding patterns. Teach him to stimulate voiding by pouring water over the perineum or running water from the tap.

Rationales

1. A patient with uninhibited neurogenic bladder usually has cerebral cortex damage, which inhibits sensations of bladder fullness, resulting in urgency.

2. Brain damage may reduce the patient's ability to understand or comply with a bladder retraining program. Proper positioning relaxes the external sphincter and perineal muscles. Pouring water over the perineum or running water from the tap can relax the patient and stimulate voiding.

Nursing diagnosis: *Urine retention related to autonomic neurogenic bladder*

GOAL: To minimize urine retention and subsequent overflow incontinence

Interventions

1. Assess the patient's health history for CVA, demyelinating diseases, spinal cord injury, trauma, infection, or peripheral nerve damage.

2. Assess for signs of overflow incontinence, such as dribbling or urinary frequency.

3. Teach the patient methods that help empty the bladder, such as Valsalva's and Credés maneuvers. (See *Performing Valsalva's and Credé's maneuvers,* page 232.)

Rationales

1. These conditions can damage sensory and motor branches of the reflex arc, impairing afferent pathways and causing autonomic neurogenic bladder.

2. A patient with autonomic neurogenic bladder cannot sense a full bladder or control motor impulses to empty the bladder. Dribbling occurs when the bladder fills beyond its normal capacity.

3. Valsalva's and Credé's maneuvers are the most effective methods of emptying an autonomic neurogenic bladder.

Nursing diagnosis: *Sexual dysfunction related to physiologic limitations*

GOAL: To help the patient achieve sexual satisfaction

Interventions

1. Compile a history of the patient's sexual activity (including age, sex, partner, and usual activities and patterns), and assess his pre-illness sexual functioning.

Rationales

1. Compiling a history and assessing pre-illness functioning provide baseline information that facilitates planning.

2. Assess for medications that may affect sexual function.

2. Medications such as diazepam have adverse effects that can reduce the patient's libido or cause impotence.

3. Talk to the patient about alternatives for sexual intercourse, such as cuddling, massage, hugging, and kissing. Refer him to a sex counselor for further guidance, if necessary.

3. Alternatives can reduce stress and tension by helping the patient satisfy the need for sexual expression. Because of physical limitations, he may need a sex counselor to help him develop creative ways of expressing his sexuality.

Nursing diagnosis: *Knowledge deficit related to bladder retraining program*

GOAL: To implement a bladder retraining program

Interventions

1. Assess the patient's ability to participate in a bladder retraining program. Consider his cognitive skills, motivation to change behavior, and willingness to cooperate.

2. Assess the patient's voiding pattern. Monitor and record intake (time of day and type and amount of fluid) and output (time of day and amounts of void, incontinence, retention, residual, and triggered urine). Also identify behavior or activities that initiate or inhibit voiding, such as exercise or anxiety.

3. Encourage the patient to drink at least 2 liters of fluid daily, unless contraindicated. Advise him not to drink after 7 p.m. Initially, schedule voiding every 2 hours during waking hours and twice during the night. Gradually decrease daytime voiding to every 4 hours.

4. Assess the patient's residual urine levels.

5. If indicated, schedule an intermittent catheterization program.

• Have the patient drink at least 2 liters of fluid each day.
• Teach the patient to perform clean catheterization every 4 to 6 hours.

Rationales

1. This assessment helps in planning an appropriate bladder retraining program.

2. An assessment helps determine the patient's ability to void voluntarily.

3. These measures prevent dehydration.

4. Intermittent catheterization is indicated if residual urine is more than 100 ml.

5. An intermittent catheterization program maintains bladder muscle tone, prevents overdistention of the bladder, and empties the bladder completely.

• Adequate fluid intake maintains the patient's hydration status.

• Catheterization using clean technique is recommended for home care if done regularly by the same person and the bladder does not become distended.

PERFORMING VALSALVA'S AND CREDÉ'S MANEUVERS

Valsalva's and Credé's maneuvers are effective bladder-emptying measures, particularly for the patient with an autonomic neurogenic bladder. Review these steps with the patient to be sure he understands how to perform the maneuvers correctly.

Valsalva's maneuver
Tell the patient to:
• sit on the toilet and bend forward at the waist
• contract abdominal muscles and bear down as though defecating
• avoid breathing while bearing down until urine flow stops
• relax for 1 minute; then repeat the maneuver until urine flow stops.

Credé's maneuver
Tell the patient to:
• sit upright on the toilet
• place hands flat (one atop the other) on the abdomen just below the umbilicus
• press firmly down and toward the perineum six or seven times, until urine flow stops
• relax for 2 minutes; then repeat the maneuver until urine flow stops.

• Encourage the patient to attempt voiding before catheterization.

• This promotes voluntary micturition.

• Teach the patient to obtain urine residual levels every 6 hours.

• The patient should end intermittent catheterization when residual urine is 50 ml or less after each void.

6. Tell the patient to report urine that is cloudy or that contains blood, mucus, or sediment; elevated temperature; chills; shaking; lower front or middle abdominal pain; pain on voiding; urge to void; or small, frequent voids.

6. These are signs and symptoms of urinary tract infection (UTI), the most common complication of catheterization.

7. Teach the patient the importance of complying with the bladder retraining program, and provide positive reinforcement when he complies.

7. Compliance, which may improve with the nurse's encouragement, can minimize complications.

Nursing diagnosis: *Impaired home maintenance management related to limitations imposed by the disease*

GOAL: To promote the patient's health and safety at home

Interventions

1. Assess the patient's cognitive health status (such as brain damage from a CVA).

2. Evaluate the patient's need for support persons or services. Determine how much assistance and care the family members can provide, and advise the patient and family to contact community resources, such as Meals On Wheels, if necessary.

3. Determine the patient's need for equipment, such as a urinal, a commode, or catheterization and hygienic supplies.

4. Evaluate the patient's financial status. Refer the patient to a social worker for financial counseling, if necessary.

5. Give the patient a list of community services and organizations.

Rationales

1. Limited awareness and understanding may limit the patient's ability to maintain a healthful, safe home or participate in home care activities.

2. A support system of people and services can help the patient with home maintenance responsibilities.

3. The patient will need supplies for the bladder retraining program, and other medical equipment can enhance his independence.

4. Medical expenses can be substantial. Inadequate insurance or limited household income can create financial hardships. Social workers can help the patient locate financial resources.

5. Many local organizations provide education, services, and support for patients and their families.

ASSOCIATED CARE PLANS
• Brain Tumor
• Cerebrovascular Accident
• Chronic Renal Failure
• Hypertension
• Indwelling Catheter Care
• Ineffective Coping
• Multiple Sclerosis
• Parkinson's Disease
• Sex and Sexuality
• Spinal Cord Injury

NETWORKING OF SERVICES
• Meals On Wheels
• Head Injury Foundation
• Spinal Injury Learning Series Bladder Program
• durable medical equipment supplier

CARE TEAM INVOLVED
• nurse
• doctor
• patient and family
• urologist
• social worker
• sex therapist

IMPLICATIONS FOR HOME CARE
• functional features of the home
• telephone (communication)

PATIENT EDUCATION TOOLS
• list of signs and symptoms of autonomic dysreflexia and the patient's normal blood pressure reading
• list of normal urine residuals
• instructions for triggering techniques, Valsalva's

maneuver, Credé's maneuver, self-catheterization
• literature on each prescribed medication

DISCHARGE PLAN FROM HOME HEALTH CARE
Before discharge from home health care, the patient should:
• know the name, method of administration, dosage, and adverse effects of each prescribed medication
• know the latest residual urine volume
• know the date of latest kidney X-ray and relevant findings
• understand the signs and symptoms (no urination, distended bladder, high fever, bloody urine, severe headache) that must be reported immediately to the doctor, urologist, or urologic nurse specialist
• understand the importance of having at least four appointments with the doctor or urologist each year
• know the date of follow-up appointment with the doctor or urologist
• understand that laboratory studies are required four times each year and radiologic studies are performed annually
• have appointments scheduled for laboratory and radiology studies
• know behaviors and activities that inhibit or promote voiding
• know the signs and symptoms of autonomic dysreflexia and appropriate prevention measures
• understand and comply with the bladder retraining program
• practice thorough hygienic care
• know the signs and symptoms of UTI
• know the signs and symptoms of urinary calculus disease
• know the signs and symptoms of renal deterioration.

SELECTED REFERENCES
Carpenito, L.J. *Nursing Diagnosis: Application to Clinical Practice,* 2nd ed. Philadelphia: J.B. Lippincott Co., 1987.

DeRosa, S. "Urinary Incontinence" in *Signs and Symptoms in Nursing: Interpretation and Management,* edited by M.M. Jacobs and W. Geels. Philadelphia: J.B. Lippincott Co., 1985.

Diagnostics, 2nd ed. Nurse's Reference Library. Springhouse, Pa.: Springhouse Corporation, 1986.

Diagnostic Tests Handbook. Springhouse, Pa.: Springhouse Corporation, 1987.

Fischbach, F. *A Manual of Laboratory Diagnostic Tests,* 2nd ed. Philadelphia: J.B. Lippincott Co., 1984

Holland, N.J., et al. "Rehabilitation Research: Pathophysiology and Management of Neurogenic Bladder in Multiple Sclerosis," *Rehabilitation Nursing* 31-33, July/August 1985.

Long, M.L. "Incontinence," *Journal of Gerontological Nursing* 11(1):30-35, 41, 1985.

Niederpruem, M.S. "Autonomic Dysreflexia," *Rehabilitation Nursing* 29-31, January/February 1984.

Voith, A.M. "Conceptual Frameworks for Nursing Diagnoses: Alterations in Urinary Elimination," *Rehabilitation Nursing* 18-21, January/February 1986.

Voith, A.M., and Smith, D.A. "Validation of the Nursing Diagnosis of Urinary Retention," *Nursing Clinics of North America* 20(4):723-29, 1985.

Ziegler, S.M., et al. *Nursing Process, Nursing Diagnosis, Nursing Knowledge: Avenues to Autonomy.* Norwalk, Conn.: Appleton & Lange, 1986.

RENAL AND URINARY SYSTEM
Kidney Transplant

DESCRIPTION AND TIME FOCUS
Kidney transplant, or renal allograft, is the surgical transfer of a kidney from one person to another. Renal insufficiency or chronic renal failure are indications for renal transplant. Renal failure etiologies range from congenital diseases, such as polycystic kidney disease, to more common disorders, such as chronic glomerulonephritis or acute renal failure. Chronic renal failure can be a sequela of such conditions as diabetes mellitus, hypertension, sickle cell anemia, and autoimmune disease, such as systemic lupus erythematosus. Chronic diseases also affect the function of the graft (donated kidney).

This clinical plan focuses on the patient discharged home from an acute-care hospital after undergoing a kidney transplant. Potential complications include GI tract bleeding, hypertension, pneumonia, osteoporosis, and graft rejection. Graft rejection can be hyperacute, accelerated, acute, or chronic. Hyperacute and accelerated rejection typically occur during hospitalization and are not addressed here. Acute rejection can occur during the first 6 weeks after transplant, usually after 2 weeks. Chronic rejection, a slow, irreversible process occurring over months or years, characteristically resists therapy and results in the loss of the graft. Nursing intervention is similar for acute and chronic rejection with one exception; the nurse must help the patient with chronic rejection cope with the inevitable loss of the graft.

■ Typical home health care length of service for a patient with a kidney transplant: usually 8 weeks but may vary, depending on complications
■ Typical visit frequency: three times weekly

HEALTH HISTORY FINDINGS
In a health history interview, the patient may report many of these findings:
• fatigue
• diminished urine output
• history of hypertension
• paresthesias
• deep, rapid respirations

PHYSICAL FINDINGS
In a physical examination, the nurse may detect many of the findings below. Note that primary physical findings may be related to immunosuppressive drug therapy or graft rejection. Adverse effects are indicated as follows: of prednisone *; of cyclosporine **; of prednisone and cyclosporine ***.

Renal and urinary
• leakage from surgical anastomoses
• calculi
• fistula formation
• oliguria or anuria

Cardiovascular
• sodium and water retention **
• hypertension ***
• dependent edema
• congestive heart failure **
• anemia *
• hyperkalemia *
• thrombocytopenia *
• thromboembolism **
• hyperlipidemia
• uremia

Respiratory
• pneumonia ***
• pulmonary edema **
• pulmonary emboli **

Neurologic
• headache *
• hyperesthesia *
• tremors *
• euphoria **
• depression **
• convulsions *
• hearing loss *

Gastrointestinal
• peptic ulcer ***
• abdominal discomfort *
• nausea and vomiting *
• diarrhea *
• gastroenteritis *
• gum hyperplasia *

Integumentary
• acne ***
• hypertrichosis *
• moon face **
• graft site tenderness *
• brittle fingernails *
• buffalo hump **
• skin carcinomas ***

Endocrine
• hyperglycemia **

General
- fever ***
- sinusitis *
- tumors ***
- cataract **
- glaucoma **
- retinitis **
- infection ***
- leukopenia *
- hypocalcemia
- metabolic acidosis

DIAGNOSTIC STUDIES
The following studies may be performed to evaluate the patient's health status:
- glofil—at 1 week, 1 month, 3 months, and every 6 months to measure renal urine flow
- serum complete blood count (CBC)—at every outpatient checkup to monitor anemia, leukopenia, thrombocytopenia
- electrolytes—at every outpatient checkup to monitor fluid and electrolyte status, especially potassium levels
- creatinine—at every outpatient checkup to monitor glomerular function
- urea nitrogen—at every outpatient checkup to monitor for uremia and graft function
- glucose—at every outpatient checkup to monitor hyperglycemia from prednisone and cyclosporine
- urinalysis—at 1 week, 1 month, 3 months, and every 6 months to monitor specific gravity, urine glucose, and infection
- cyclosporine radioimmunoassay (RIA)—twice weekly for 2 months, then weekly for 4 months, then monthly for 6 months to monitor serum peak and trough levels for determining maximum therapeutic effect with minimum side effects. Trough should be greater than 100 ng/ml.

Nursing diagnosis: *Potential for injury related to graft rejection*

GOAL: To reverse acute rejection or slow chronic rejection

Interventions	Rationales
1. Administer immunosuppressive drugs, as ordered, and monitor for therapeutic and adverse effects.	1. Immunosuppressive drugs act generally or specifically on the immune system, depending on the prescribed drug.
2. Monitor for signs and symptoms of graft rejection, such as a swollen, tender kidney, weight gain, fever, increased blood pressure, decreased urine output, anorexia, drowsiness, or elevated serum creatinine.	2. Assessing and documenting early signs and symptoms of graft rejection help ensure prompt intervention to reverse the process.

Nursing diagnosis: *Potential for infection related to immunosuppressive drug therapy*

GOAL 1: To prevent viral or contagious infections

Interventions	Rationales
1. Arrange protective isolation for the patient, if necessary. Advise family or friends who are ill to stay away from the patient.	1. If the patient's white blood cell (WBC) count drops below normal, temporary isolation may be needed to minimize the risk of infection.
2. Tell the patient to wear a face mask when in a crowd or when visiting with family and friends who may have viral or bacterial infections.	2. Wearing a face mask reduces the patient's risk of infection.
3. Monitor the patient's vital signs at each visit, and assess for signs and symptoms of infection, such as fever, dyspnea, malaise, tachypnea, hypotension, or tachycardia.	3. Changes in vital signs are the first indicators of infection.

GOAL 2: To promote wound healing

Interventions	Rationales
1. Use strict aseptic technique when changing dressings, applying antibacterial ointments as necessary.	1. Immunosuppressive drug therapy reduces the patient's resistance to infection. Strict aseptic technique

2. Administer antibiotics, as ordered, during acute infection or prophylactically. Monitor for therapeutic and adverse effects.

3. Monitor for wound dehiscence, particularly 7 to 10 days after surgery.

GOAL 3: To prevent respiratory infection

Interventions

1. Monitor and document the patient's vital signs at each visit. Compare these findings to baseline values and previous findings. Refer the patient to the doctor, if necessary.

2. Monitor results of diagnostic studies, such as WBC count, WBC differential, and chest X-rays, for indications of respiratory infection.

3. Auscultate the patient's lungs to assess breath sounds at each visit. Document the findings.

GOAL 4: To prevent oral infection

Interventions

1. During each visit, assess the patient's mouth and oropharynx for signs and symptoms of infection, such as white, patchy areas; fever blisters; or a beefy, red tongue.

2. Explain the importance of brushing and flossing after each meal and scheduling regular dental checkups. Teach the patient how to use antifungal medications and antacid pastes, if necessary.

and antibacterial ointments help minimize the risk of infection.

2. Antibiotics are commonly prescribed for immunosuppressed patients because signs and symptoms of infection may not be evident.

3. Prednisone inhibits wound healing. Also, absorbable sutures dissolve at this time.

Rationales

1. Tachycardia is the first sign of respiratory infection, followed by fever and tachypnea. Recognizing early indicators of respiratory infection helps ensure prompt treatment.

2. Although laboratory results may be normal, comparisons to baseline values are useful. Chest X-rays can detect pneumonia, a common complication after surgery.

3. Crackles, rhonchi, or decreased breath sounds may indicate respiratory infection.

Rationales

1. A patient undergoing immunosuppressive drug therapy is at risk for fungal and viral infections.

2. Brushing and flossing after each meal and having regular dental checkups keep the mouth clean and can help prevent infection. Antifungal medications reduce oral fungi, and antacid pastes help soothe mouth ulcers and protect the oral mucosa.

Nursing diagnosis: *Knowledge deficit related to nutritional requirements after surgery*

GOAL: To help the patient meet his nutritional requirements

Interventions

1. Teach the patient and caregiver the importance of a diet low in sodium and simple carbohydrates and high in high-quality protein.

2. Tell the patient to avoid high-sodium foods, such as canned goods, condiments (sauces, ketchup), and snack foods (chips, pretzels). Caution the patient or food preparer not to use salt when preparing food and to check labels for sodium content when food shopping. Explain that many over-the-counter (OTC) medications (aspirin, cough medicines, laxatives) and toothpastes contain sodium.

Rationales

1. A low-sodium diet can help minimize adverse effects from steroids (such as sodium retention) and may also reduce hypertension. Limiting simple carbohydrates can reduce serum glucose levels. High-quality protein foods, such as chicken and fish, break down more easily and have fewer waste by-products.

2. A high sodium intake can lead to fluid retention, which increases blood pressure and aggravates adverse effects of steroids.

Nursing diagnosis: *Activity intolerance related to postoperative status*

GOAL: To improve the patient's activity tolerance while preventing complications from excessive activity or lifting

Interventions

1. Tell the patient not to lift anything weighing over 5 pounds for 3 months.

2. Tell the patient not to drive for at least 4 weeks after surgery.

Rationales

1. Lifting strains suture lines and anastomoses.

2. Sudden movements, such as sharp turns or hard braking while driving, can stress suture lines and anastomoses.

Nursing diagnosis: *Knowledge deficit related to immunosuppressive drug therapy*

GOAL 1: To promote proper understanding and use of cyclosporine

Interventions

1. Teach the patient and caregiver that cyclosporine is used to prevent graft rejection and that the patient must take the drug as ordered.

2. Tell the patient to avoid crowds and family members or friends who may have viral infections.

3. Teach the patient the importance of keeping laboratory appointments to monitor RIA levels.

4. Teach the patient and caregiver the adverse effects of cyclosporine and techniques to minimize them. Explain that:
• tremors usually resolve within a few weeks
• hyperesthesia may occur 2 to 4 hours after a dose and can be minimized by covering exposed body parts
• gum hyperplasia is aggravated by concurrent phenytoin therapy and can be prevented by proper oral hygiene, regular dental care, and breathing through the nose rather than the mouth
• hypertrichosis will disappear when therapy ceases; depilatories, shaving, and electrolysis can minimize its effects
• anemia and headaches may result from a lack of dietary iron and can be relieved by increasing dietary iron
• hypertension is a long-term adverse effect that can damage the graft and must be monitored and treated by the doctor
• nephrotoxicity often mimics graft rejection and requires close monitoring of RIA levels by the doctor.

5. Tell the patient and caregiver to use the supplied pipette when measuring each dose. Tell the patient to take the dose orally every 12 hours, 1 hour before a meal.

6. Teach the patient and caregiver to:

• use a glass container

Rationales

1. Understanding the purpose of the drug may improve compliance.

2. Cyclosporine suppresses killer T cells, thereby increasing the patient's susceptibility to viral infections.

3. Therapeutic cyclosporine levels must be maintained to prevent graft rejection and to minimize the drug's

4. Knowing how to minimize the adverse effects of cyclosporine can lessen the patient's discomfort and may alleviate his anxiety.

5. Accurate dosage is essential to prevent graft rejection and minimize the drug's adverse effects. I.V. administration is used only in acute care. I.M. administration causes inconsistent absorption and inferior trough levels.

6. Patient education promotes proper administration of cyclosporine.

• Cyclosporine is an oil-based medication that adheres to foam, paper, and plastic cups.

- mix the medication with a diluent, such as juice or chocolate milk
- stir well and then administer immediately
- refill the container with more diluent, stir, and administer.

7. Teach the patient and caregiver to store cyclosporine at room temperature, not in the refrigerator.

8. Tell the patient and caregiver to discard cyclosporine after 2 months.

- The drug is distasteful and may cause nausea and vomiting. Mixing the dose disguises the taste.
- Oil-based medications do not mix well with fluids.
- Cyclosporine is expensive, and the patient must receive a full dose.

7. Cold reduces the solubility of oil-based drugs.

8. The patient and caregiver should know the expiration date for each prescription.

GOAL 2: To promote proper understanding and use of prednisone

Interventions

1. Teach the patient and caregiver the therapeutic effects of prednisone, such as immune system suppression and graft rejection prevention.

2. Teach the patient and caregiver the adverse effects of prednisone, such as impaired response to infection, sodium and water retention, elevated serum glucose levels, and gastritis.

3. Teach the patient and caregiver how to monitor for signs and symptoms of graft rejection, such as fever and swelling and tenderness over the graft site.

4. Teach the patient and caregiver the importance of taking prednisone exactly as ordered and never abruptly discontinuing its use.

Rationales

1. Prednisone stabilizes cell walls, reduces migration of leukocytes into inflamed areas, and depresses T and B cell lymphocyte and phagocyte production. Knowing the purpose of the medication may promote compliance.

2. Many adverse effects of prednisone are dose related and can be alleviated by decreasing the dose. Sodium and water retention may lead to concurrent weight gain and increased blood pressure. A patient with diabetes may need to adjust hypoglycemic medications to compensate for increased serum glucose levels. Taking antacids with prednisone can help prevent gastric ulcer formation.

3. The patient and caregiver must recognize these signs and symptoms to facilitate prompt medical intervention.

4. Sudden cessation of prednisone therapy can cause adrenal crisis or graft rejection.

GOAL 3: To promote proper understanding and use of azathioprine

Interventions

1. Teach the patient and caregiver the therapeutic effects of azathioprine. Explain that it is a potent immunosuppressant that can prevent graft rejection.

2. Teach the patient and caregiver the adverse effects of azathioprine. Explain that:

- the azathioprine dose must be reduced to ¼ to ⅓ the normal dose if allopurinol is administered concurrently

- conception should be avoided during therapy and for 4 months after therapy
- signs and symptoms of liver toxicity (clay-colored stools, dark urine, itching, or yellowing of the skin or sclera) must be reported to the doctor
- hair loss is a common adverse effect

- any sign or symptom of infection (fever, localized pain or swelling, persistent tachycardia) must be reported to the doctor

Rationales

1. Knowledge of azathioprine's therapeutic effects helps the patient monitor for graft rejection and adverse effects of the drug.

2. The patient and caregiver must be familiar with azathioprine's adverse effects and necessary precautions to take.

- Allopurinol impairs inactivation of azathioprine; therefore, concurrent administration may require a decreased dose of azathioprine.
- Azathioprine may cause teratogenicity.

- Azathioprine may cause liver toxicity.

- The patient may want to use a wig or head covering to cope with alopecia. Hair will grow back when the drug is discontinued.
- Azathioprine is a potent immunosuppressant that increases the patient's susceptibility to infection.

• care must be taken to prevent bruising

• all scheduled laboratory work must be completed and monitored.

• Therapy may suppress the platelet count. The nurse should avoid giving I.M. injections to avoid I.M. hematoma formation.
• Hemoglobin level and WBC and platelet counts should be monitored each month. Therapy should cease if WBC count drops below 3,000/mm to prevent irreversible bone marrow depression.

ASSOCIATED CARE PLANS
• Chronic Congestive Heart Failure
• Chronic Renal Failure
• Diabetes Mellitus
• Grief and Grieving
• Hypertension
• Ineffective Coping
• Major Depression
• Pneumonia
• Sex and Sexuality

NETWORKING OF SERVICES
• American Council on Transplantation
• National Kidney Foundation

CARE TEAM INVOLVED
• nurse
• nephrologist
• surgeon
• patient and family
• medical social worker
• registered dietitian

IMPLICATIONS FOR HOME CARE
• hygienic environment
• control of patient exposure to individuals with infections
• patient's and family's ability to read and understand instructions
• vascular access patency for hemodialysis if the graft fails
• adequate supply of immunosuppressive drugs
• access to transportation

PATIENT EDUCATION TOOLS
• list of normal vital signs
• thermometer, sphygmomanometer, and stethoscope and instructions for their use
• list of signs and symptoms of graft rejection
• National Kidney Foundation literature on transplantation
• outpatient clinic literature

DISCHARGE PLAN FROM HOME HEALTH CARE
Before discharge from home health care, the patient should:
• know the method of administration, dosage, therapeutic effects, and adverse effects of all prescribed medications
• know the adverse effects that must be reported to the doctor
• know the signs and symptoms of acute and chronic graft rejection, and be free of such signs and symptoms
• know the signs and symptoms of infection and methods to prevent it
• understand dietary restrictions and supplements
• demonstrate adjustment to a new body image and to life-style changes
• understand the importance of maintaining vascular access patency
• know the date, time, and place of the next follow-up outpatient or laboratory appointment.

SELECTED REFERENCES
Ames, S.W., and Kneisl, C.R. *Essentials of Adult Health Nursing.* Reading, Mass.: Addison-Wesley Publishing Co., 1988.
ANNA Clinical Practice Committee. "Outcome Criteria and Nursing Diagnosis in ESRD Patient Care Planning," *American Nephrology Nurses' Association Journal* 14(3):197-212, 1987.
Fairman, J.A. "Sexual Concerns of the Renal Transplant Patient in the Ambulatory Care Setting: A Format for Nursing Intervention," *American Association of Nephrology Nurses and Technicians Journal* 9(12):45-48, 1982.
Harwood, C.H., and Cook, C.V. "Cyclosporine in Transplantation," *Heart & Lung* 4(6):529-40, 1985.
Kinney, M.R., et al. *AACN's Clinical Reference for Critical-Care Nursing.* New York: McGraw-Hill Book Co., 1988.
Lancaster, L.E. *The Patient with Renal Disease.* New York: John Wiley & Sons, 1984.
Levitz, B.A., and Parker, T.F. *Patient Information Manual for Kidney Transplantation.* Dallas: Dallas Transplant Institute, 1987.
Nursing89 Drug Handbook. Springhouse Pa.: Springhouse Corporation, 1989.
Rivers, R. "Nursing the Kidney Transplant Patient," *RN* 46-58, August 1987.
Waley, L.F., and Wong, D.L. *Nursing Care of Infants and Children.* St. Louis: C.V. Mosby Co., 1987.

Major Depression

DESCRIPTION AND TIME FOCUS
Major depression is a syndrome of persistent sad, dysphoric mood with accompanying psychological and somatic symptoms. One of the most common psychological disturbances, major depression affects people of all ages, races, and socioeconomic groups, but is especially prevalent in women and elderly persons.

Depression often is associated with dysfunctional grieving over a loss, such as of a spouse or other close person from death or breakup of a relationship, of a job or other significant role, or of physical function or ability. This form of depression, known as *situational* or *reactive* depression, is typically treated by psychotherapy that focuses on identifying the loss and facilitating the patient's completion of the grieving process. *Endogenous depression* is linked to an intrinsic biological process—for example, dysregulation of cholinergic and catecholamine neurotransmission—and represents a more complex problem. Treatment for endogenous depression goes beyond psychotherapy and typically involves drug therapy with tricyclic antidepressants and monoamine oxidase inhibitors and possibly electroconvulsive therapy.

This clinical plan focuses on a patient discharged home from an acute-care hospital after diagnosis and treatment of major depression. Care focuses on assessing the scope of the problem and its contributing factors, enhancing the patient's sense of self-esteem, maintaining adequate nutrition and personal hygiene, encouraging self-care and physical activity, and identifying potential suicidal behavior and taking steps to prevent it.

■ Typical home health care length of service for a patient recovering from major depression: 6 weeks

■ Typical visit frequency: three times the first week, then twice each week for 3 weeks, then once each week for weeks

HEALTH HISTORY FINDINGS
In a health history interview, the patient (or the patient's family) may report many of these findings:
• recent loss (a loved one, a way of life, a work role, or a change in physical health, such as reduced independent functioning)
• recent diagnosis of life-threatening illness
• lack of adequate social support
• feelings of sadness, despair, guilt, worthlessness, powerlessness, hopelessness
• thoughts of or attempts at suicide
• problems caring for family or holding a job
• withdrawal, social isolation
• anxiety
• fatigue and lethargy
• inability to concentrate
• memory loss
• preoccupation with physical ailments
• low libido; impotence or amenorrhea
• irritability
• emotional lability
• insomnia, sometimes hypersomnia
• anorexia or, less commonly, increased appetite
• bowel function changes, usually constipation
• noncompliance with medical regimen

PHYSICAL FINDINGS
In a physical examination, the nurse may detect many of these findings:

Neurologic
• psychomotor retardation (slowed speech and movement, lethargy) or psychomotor agitation (inability to sit still, pacing, hand-wringing, hair-tugging)
• poor concentration
• poor short-term memory
• confusion
• disorientation

Musculoskeletal
• "sagging" posture
• muscle weakness and wasting

General
• sad facial expression
• poor personal hygiene
• inappropriate dress
• weight loss or, less often, weight gain

DIAGNOSTIC STUDIES
None applicable to home care

Nursing diagnosis: *Potential for self-directed violence related to altered thought processes and feelings of despair, hopelessness, and worthlessness*

GOAL: To prevent the patient from acting on suicidal impulses and to provide a safe environment during treatment

Interventions

1. Assess for suicidal ideation. Ask the patient direct questions: "Since you've been feeling depressed, have you wanted to hurt yourself?" or "Do you ever just want to go to sleep and not wake up?"

2. Assess for evidence of passive self-destructive behavior.

3. Assess the home environment for weapons or dangerous medications, and be sure the patient is complying with the medication regimen rather than stockpiling medications with the intent of taking an overdose.

4. Assess the patient for characteristics associated with a higher potential for suicide: male; divorced or widowed; living alone; feelings of isolation, helplessness, and uselessness; chronically ill; history of substance abuse and previous suicide attempts; a definite plan, violent means, and sufficient energy; inattentiveness to self-care; and no referrals to future plans or events.

5. If the patient expresses suicidal feelings, establish a contract with him stipulating that he must contact the doctor, nurse, or a community support group, such as a suicide prevention center, before acting on impulse. Renew the contract at each home visit.

6. Enlist family support, if available.

7. If the patient cannot or will not make a contract, arrange for immediate psychiatric hospitalization. Always refer a suicidal patient to a mental health professional, such as a psychiatric clinical nurse specialist, psychiatrist, psychologist, or social worker.

Rationales

1. Most patients will answer a direct question honestly. The depressed patient's safety depends on the nurse's ability to identify a patient considering suicide.

2. A patient can commit suicide slowly through self-destructive behavior, such as not complying with the medical regimen, reducing his intake of food or fluids, or abusing alcohol or drugs.

3. A depressed patient can become suicidal at any time during treatment, particularly as antidepressants begin to increase his activity level. Maintaining a safe environment reduces the likelihood of the patient acting on impulse.

4. Evaluating these risk factors helps the nurse evaluate the patient's potential for acting on suicidal impulses.

5. Entering into a contract makes the patient an active participant in the treatment plan and helps restore feelings of control and responsibility.

6. Increasing the number of social contacts may be an effective crisis intervention method for a suicidal patient.

7. The patient may be asking for rescue and a safe, protected environment but is unable to express these feelings. Safety in the home is doubtful if the patient is unable to make this contract.

Nursing diagnosis: *Altered thought processes related to temporary cognitive impairment*

GOAL: To provide a safe environment, reduce the patient's anxiety level, and preserve the patient's self-esteem during episodes of cognitive impairment

Interventions

1. Assess for cognitive impairment by checking for disorientation and short-term memory loss.

2. If memory loss is significant, reorient the patient to time, person, place, and current situation.

3. Encourage caregivers to use practical reorientation devices, such as calendars and newspapers. Stress the importance of maintaining an organized and predictable environment.

Rationales

1. The patient may try to hide the impairment out of shame, guilt, or fear. Evaluating orientation level and short-term memory provides an objective assessment of cognitive ability.

2. Reorientation helps reduce the patient's fears and anxieties.

3. Involving the family or caregiver in the treatment plan helps them become supportive. Reorientation devices help maintain the patient's self-esteem. An organized, predictable environment promotes patient safety.

4. Communicate in a way that enhances the patient's comprehension; for example, maintain eye contact and provide clear, brief messages.

4. Anxiety about the cognitive impairment can interfere with the patient's comprehension. These measures can help improve comprehension.

5. Encourage the patient to engage in activities that generate self-satisfaction, such as hobbies or exercise.

5. Successful performance of activities helps build self-confidence in a patient who may otherwise be easily frustrated.

6. Explain to the patient that the cognitive impairment is temporary and reversible.

6. This reassurance can help reduce the patient's anxiety level and accelerate resolution of the condition.

Nursing diagnosis: *Self-care deficit related to low energy level and psychomotor retardation*

GOAL: To have the patient resume baseline activities of daily living (ADLs) with balanced activity and rest

Interventions

1. Assess the patient's ability to provide self-care during episodes of depression. If the patient cannot manage self-care and if a family member cannot provide sufficient assistance, arrange for the services of a home health aide.

2. Explain to the patient the importance of getting dressed and attending to personal hygiene and other ADLs each day. Work with the patient and family to develop a schedule for ADLs.

3. Encourage the patient to balance periods of activity with periods of rest.

4. If the patient's self-care deficit is linked to somatic complaints, such as fatigue, lethargy, muscle aches, and weakness, encourage the patient to focus on ADLs and other forms of physical activity.

Rationales

1. Depression typically impairs a patient's self-care abilities.

2. A depressed patient may feel that wearing night-clothes during the day and staying in bed are appropriate behaviors for a "sick" person. Having the patient attend to ADLs reduces the risk of complications associated with poor self-care and inactivity and provides much-needed structure in the patient's daily life.

3. A proper balance between rest and activity helps reduce fatigue and enhances the patient's self-care abilities.

4. Physical activity can help distract the patient's attention from somatic complaints and may improve his self-care abilities.

Nursing diagnosis: *Knowledge deficit related to antidepressant medication regimen*

GOAL: To improve the patient's and family's understanding of antidepressant drug therapy and thus help ensure compliance with the medication regimen

Interventions

1. Explain the purpose and action of prescribed antidepressants; emphasize that antidepressants carry no risk of addiction.

2. If the patient complains that the antidepressants don't seem to be working, determine the duration of drug therapy. If appropriate, reassure him that beneficial effects will eventually occur.

3. Teach the patient and family to watch for and report adverse effects of antidepressants, such as decreased intestinal motility and constipation, dry mouth, blurred vision, hypotension, and urine retention.

Rationales

1. Many patients think that antidepressants are potentially addictive stimulants or tranquilizers.

2. Most antidepressants must be taken for 4 weeks or more before therapeutic response occurs. Explaining this to the patient may allay any doubts he has about the efficacy of treatment.

3. Early recognition and reporting of adverse effects facilitates prompt intervention to manage them. Understanding potential adverse effects may improve the patient's sense of control over the illness and its treatment and may enhance compliance with the medication regimen.

4. Reassure the patient and family that many adverse effects will subside as the patient's tolerance to the medication increases.

4. A patient may be tempted to discontinue taking prescribed antidepressants if adverse effects occur. The patient's understanding that many of these effects are transient may help improve compliance.

5. Encourage the patient and family to discuss the medication regimen with a psychiatrist or internist regularly to determine whether the dosage should be lowered or discontinued.

5. In antidepressant therapy, periodic dosage adjustments may be necessary to maintain the therapeutic effect. Antidepressant therapy often is prescribed for a limited time and then discontinued as the patient's condition improves.

Nursing diagnosis: *Sleep pattern disturbance related to depression and anxiety*

GOAL: To promote adequate sleep

Interventions

1. Identify the patient's present and pre-illness sleep patterns.

2. Determine whether the patient is now or has been using sleep medications.

3. Encourage the patient to minimize the use of sleep medications.

4. Teach the patient and family about relaxation techniques to use before bedtime, such as drinking warm milk; eating a high-protein snack, such as crackers and peanut butter; performing conscious relaxation techniques; listening to soothing music; reading; and receiving a massage.

5. If appropriate, suggest that the patient perform sleep rituals that previously proved successful.

6. Discourage the patient from retiring too early at night.

7. Ensure that the patient receives adequate mental stimulation and exercise during the day.

Rationales

1. Such determination helps the nurse differentiate between acute and chronic sleep disturbances and identify any bedtime rituals the patient may have.

2. The patient may experience rebound insomnia if he has recently stopped taking a sleep medication.

3. Sleep medications interfere with the normal sleep cycle.

4. Relaxation before bedtime helps promote restful sleep.

5. Depression may interfere with the patient's ability or desire to perform usual sleep rituals.

6. Retiring too early may impair the patient's ability to fall asleep, or may cause the patient to awaken too early the next morning—both of which may increase his anxiety and lead to further sleep pattern disturbance.

7. Boredom and lack of exercise may lead to increased napping during the day, which can interfere with the patient's normal sleep cycle.

Nursing diagnosis: *Disturbance in self-esteem related to feelings of worthlessness and impaired role performance*

GOAL: To enhance the patient's self-esteem and reestablish an appropriate social role

Interventions

1. Spend time talking with the patient, encouraging him to identify and express his feelings and concerns. Use therapeutic communication skills such as active listening.

Rationales

1. Open, honest communication helps establish a good nurse-patient relationship and builds a sense of rapport and mutual trust. It also helps increase the patient's self-awareness.

2. Assess for contributing factors to the patient's low self-esteem. Consider such factors as forced isolation, changes in interpersonal relationships, feelings of non-productivity, reduced physical abilities, and fear of falling or other concerns for personal safety.

2. Identifying contributing factors helps the nurse define the scope of the problem and establish appropriate interventions to build the patient's self-esteem.

3. Evaluate the patient's ability to alter such contributing factors. Explore the patient's mental and physical abilities, coping mechanisms, and available support systems.

3. Mental or physical impairment, ineffective coping mechanisms, and lack of support or poor support may interfere with efforts to increase the patient's self-esteem. Identification of such impediments helps the nurse develop realistic goals and interventions.

4. Help the patient set attainable functional goals and to progress at his own pace.

4. Attainable goals help instill a sense of mastery and control, which improves self-esteem.

5. Provide positive reinforcement and encouragement by focusing on the patient's strengths rather than weaknesses, praising accomplishments, encouraging positive statements about self and discouraging negative comments, and discouraging comparison with others.

5. Positive reinforcement helps build the patient's self-esteem; encouraging the patient to focus on his strengths can help him develop effective coping mechanisms and thereby regain a sense of control.

6. Encourage the patient's family or other support persons to reinforce the patient's self-esteem. If necessary, refer the patient to support groups.

6. Support and encouragement from others can help decrease the patient's feelings of social isolation and worthlessness and promote increased self-esteem.

ASSOCIATED CARE PLANS
• Chronic Mental Illness
• Grief and Grieving
• Ineffective Coping
• Malnutrition
• Pain
• Substance Abuse

NETWORKING OF SERVICES
• Lifeline
• Meals On Wheels
• geriatric outreach program
• senior centers
• adult day treatment program
• support group

CARE TEAM INVOLVED
• nurse
• doctor
• patient and family
• psychiatrist
• physical therapist
• occupational therapist
• medical social worker
• home health aide
• psychiatric nurse consultant or psychiatric clinical nurse specialist

IMPLICATIONS FOR HOME CARE
• safe, structured environment
• adequate social support systems

PATIENT EDUCATION TOOLS
• literature on prescribed medications, including dosage schedule, potential interactions, and adverse effects
• suicide prevention literature, if necessary

DISCHARGE PLAN FROM HOME HEALTH CARE
Before discharge from home health care, the patient should:
• be free of suicide ideation and know actions to take if suicide ideation returns
• understand the early signs and symptoms of emotional decompensation
• know the name, dosage schedule, potential interactions, and adverse effects of all prescribed medications and know which adverse effects to report
• resume ADLs, including personal hygiene, and balance activity with rest
• express a willingness to contact the doctor or other support person at the first sign of relapse.

SELECTED REFERENCES
Baily, D., et al. *Therapeutic Approaches to Care of the Mentally Ill*, 2nd ed. Philadephia: F.A. Davis Co., 1984.

Baldwin, B.A. "Gerontological Psychiatric Nursing," in *Principles and Practice of Psychiatric Nursing*. Edited by Stuart, S., and Sundeen, S. St. Louis: C.V. Mosby Co., 1987.

Beck, C., et al. *Mental Health and Psychiatric Nursing*, 2nd ed. St. Louis: C.V. Mosby Co., 1988.

Ebersole, P., and Hess, P., eds. *Toward Healthy Aging: Human Needs and Nursing Response*. St. Louis: C.V. Mosby Co., 1985.

Gurland, B.J., and Cross, P.S. "Epidemiology of Psychopathology in Old Age: Some Implications for Clinical Services," in *Essentials of Clinical Geriatrics*. Edited by Kane, R., et al. New York: McGraw-Hill Book Co., 1984.

Haber, J., et al. *Comprehensive Psychiatric Nursing*, 3rd ed. New York: McGraw-Hill Book Co., 1987.

PSYCHOLOGICAL PROBLEMS
Manic-Depressive Illness

DESCRIPTION AND TIME FOCUS
Manic-depressive illness, also called bipolar affective disorder, is marked by severe pathologic mood swings from euphoria to sadness, by spontaneous recoveries, and by a tendency to recur. The disorder consists of separate episodes of mania (elation) and depression, either of which can predominate. The patient usually expresses regret about his behavior immediately before or during hospitalization. He may experience an emotional letdown after feeling euphoric during the manic episode or may still be more talkative or irritable than usual at time of discharge.

The cause of manic-depressive illness is not clearly understood, but hereditary, biological, and psychological factors may play a part. Incidence is 20% to 25% in siblings, and the illness is nearly twice as common among women as men. Onset usually occurs between ages 20 and 35, with an 80% recurrence rate. As the patient ages, episodes recur more frequently and last longer.

Treatment typically includes lithium therapy, which can dramatically relieve symptoms of mania and hypomania and may prevent recurrence of depression. Because lithium tends to flatten all moods and because therapeutic doses commonly produce adverse effects, the patient may resist taking the medication. Therapy usually is required indefinitely.

This clinical plan focuses on the patient discharged home from the hospital after treatment for a manic or hypomanic episode. Nursing care centers on improving the patient's self-esteem, teaching the patient and family about the condition and treatment, and providing generous emotional support.
- Typical home health care length of service for a

patient recovering from a manic or hypomanic episode: 4 weeks
- Typical visit frequency: once weekly

HEALTH HISTORY FINDINGS
In a health history interview, the patient may report many of these findings:
- family history of mental disturbance
- emotional lability
- history of hospitalization for or treatment of a manic-depressive illness

PHYSICAL FINDINGS
In a physical examination, the nurse may detect many of these findings:
- euphoria
- expansiveness
- irritability
- aggressiveness
- quick movements
- sadness
- chagrin over behavior during manic phase
- reticence
- inability to concentrate
- anger
- anxiety

DIAGNOSTIC STUDIES
The following study may be performed to evaluate the patient's health status:
- lithium serum level—as needed until satisfactory blood levels have been established, then every 4 to 6 weeks

---

Nursing diagnosis: *Disturbance in self-concept: personal identity, related to altered patterns of emotion and behavior*

GOAL: To help the patient adapt successfully to euphoria-free moods, including sadness

Interventions

1. Assess the patient's emotional balance, as indicated by appropriate food intake, sleep, and attention to physical appearance; nonhostile social interaction; and an ability to establish and carry out realistic plans.

2. Assess the family's ability to detect and respond to the patient's mood swings toward depression.

Rationales

1. After a manic episode, the patient probably will be unhappy to find his confidence and grandiosity diminished. In short, he may not like his "new" self and may express this dislike through self-neglect, hostility toward others, or irrational conversation or behavior.

2. Depressive episodes sometimes follow episodes of elation. The family should contact the therapist or doctor if the patient's demeanor changes markedly or he alludes to self-harm, death, or departing.

3. Assess the family's knowledge of the need for medical intervention if the patient exhibits such characteristics as hyperactivity, insomnia, excessive and impulsive spending, unrealistic planning, or physical aggression.

3. When the family knows the signs of decompensation, they can seek appropriate medical intervention to avert a full-blown episode of the illness.

Nursing diagnosis: *Knowledge deficit related to the medication regimen*

GOAL: To improve the patient's and family's knowledge of the medication regimen

Interventions

1. Teach the patient about necessary precautions while taking lithium, such as drinking 2 to 3 liters of fluid daily, maintaining usual sodium intake, regularly monitoring lithium serum level by testing 12 hours after a prescribed dose, avoiding excessive perspiration, and consulting the doctor before taking any over-the-counter (OTC) medications.

2. Review lithium's common adverse effects (such as GI irritation and dry mouth), and teach the patient and family measures to counter these effects. Advise the patient to take the medication with meals, and explain the benefits of good oral hygiene, frequent sips of water, sugarless gum, and saliva substitutes.

3. Teach the patient and family to recognize the effects of lithium toxicity (blurred vision, diarrhea, vomiting, increased urination, impaired coordination, slurred speech, or drowsiness), and tell them to notify the doctor immediately if the patient experiences any.

Rationales

1. Reduced fluid and sodium intake and excessive perspiration can lead to dehydration, which increases the patient's lithium serum level and, therefore, his risk of lithium toxicity. OTC medications that contain nonsteroidal anti-inflammatory agents also can increase the lithium serum level. Regularly monitoring the level can help detect potential problems.

2. Lithium can effectively prevent manic-depressive episodes, but the patient may stop taking it to avoid unpleasant adverse effects. Taking the medication with meals can minimize GI irritation. Proper oral hygiene, frequent sips of water, sugarless gum, and saliva substitutes can alleviate dry mouth.

3. Lithium toxicity may require emergency admission.

ASSOCIATED CARE PLANS
• Major Depression
• Schizophrenia

NETWORKING OF SERVICES
• day hospital
• outpatient group therapy
• self-help group
• social club
• religious group

CARE TEAM INVOLVED
• nurse
• doctor
• patient and family
• therapist
• medical social worker

IMPLICATIONS FOR HOME CARE
• family members who can be sympathetic and helpful without becoming overly involved with or burdened by caring for the patient
• family members who are knowledgeable about and sensitive to hints of suicide
• plan for replenishing food and other necessities during acute exacerbations

• adequate support for the family

PATIENT EDUCATION TOOLS
• Mental Health Association literature about manic-depressive illness
• written information on each prescribed medication, including administration, dosage, action, and adverse effects

DISCHARGE PLAN FROM HOME HEALTH CARE
Before discharge from home health care, the patient (or family members, if appropriate) should:
• be able to state the dosage, common adverse effects, and toxic effects of all prescribed medications
• understand the importance of maintaining proper lithium serum levels (if taking lithium)
• have names of local support groups
• know dates and times of scheduled appointments with the therapist, doctor, and laboratory
• have returned to work or to a sheltered workshop, as appropriate
• recognize mood and behavior changes that typically precede manic or depressive episodes
• have the telephone number of the home health agency for counsel.

SELECTED REFERENCES

Doenges, M., and Moorhouse, M. *Nursing Diagnoses with Interventions,* 2nd ed. Philadelphia: F.A. Davis Co., 1988.

Haber, J., et al. *Comprehensive Psychiatric Nursing,* 3rd ed. New York: McGraw-Hill Book Co., 1987.

Murray, R., and Huelskoetter, M. *Psychiatric/Mental Health Nursing,* 2nd ed. Norwalk, Conn.: Appleton & Lange, 1987.

Shives, L. *Basic Concepts of Psychiatric-Mental Health Nursing.* Philadelphia: J.B. Lippincott Co., 1986.

Townsend, M. *Nursing Diagnosis in Psychiatric Nursing.* Philadelphia: F.A. Davis Co., 1988.

Schizophrenia

DESCRIPTION AND TIME FOCUS

Schizophrenia is characterized by withdrawal into self and failure to distinguish reality from fantasy. Genetic vulnerability, brain chemistry imbalance, and internal and external stress are involved in the disease's development. The disorder is equally prevalent among men and women, with onset usually occurring before age 45.

The community health nurse occasionally works with a patient with a history of schizophrenia. In some communities, an agency may be charged with the responsibility of providing health supervision to patients with chronic psychiatric conditions as primary diagnoses.

This clinical plan focuses on the patient with a history of schizophrenia. Nursing care centers on meeting the patient's physical needs, providing emotional support, and helping the family understand his symptoms and cope with his behavior. Support from professionals and self-help groups may enable the family to care for the patient in the home.

■ Typical home health care length of service for a patient with schizophrenia: 6 months

■ Typical visit frequency: once every 2 weeks for 8 weeks, then once monthly for 4 months (after this time, the patient should phone the agency every 3 months to report on progress)

HEALTH HISTORY FINDINGS

In a health history interview, the patient may report (or the nurse may detect) many of these findings:

• history of hospitalization for treatment of schizophrenia
• reputation as the "troublemaker" for family, friends, and social service agencies
• impaired thinking, such as difficulty grasping ideas or focusing on important aspects of a situation
• conversation that is difficult to follow
• hallucinations
• delusions (somatic, grandiose, religious); feelings of being controlled by something or someone
• impaired decision-making ability
• lack of facial and vocal expression
• disturbed emotions, such as lack of emotion, occasional episodes of rage, inability to enjoy formerly enjoyable activities
• physical and emotional withdrawal

PHYSICAL FINDINGS
None

DIAGNOSTIC STUDIES
The following studies may be performed to evaluate the patient's health status:
• liver function studies—performed annually (antipsychotics rarely impair liver function)
• complete blood count (CBC)—performed annually or if patient develops sore throat, fever, or malaise (agranulocytosis is rarely associated with antipsychotics)

Nursing diagnosis: *Knowledge deficit related to the disorder*

GOAL: To improve the patient's and family's understanding of schizophrenia and prescribed treatments

Interventions

1. Assess the patient's and family's understanding of the patient's illness and fill in knowledge gaps. Explain that conditions within the patient's brain cause disturbances in normal thoughts and feelings. These disturbances include:
• distraction (difficulty separating personal thoughts from stimuli in the environment)
• a need to concentrate on tasks usually requiring little thought
• equal response to important stimuli (such as conversation) and unimportant stimuli (such as the hum of an air conditioner)
• a feeling that the mind is "playing tricks"
• altered perceptions (colors may seem brighter, images may appear more detailed and vivid, familiar objects may appear different or ominous)
• internal perceptions so vivid that the patient "hears" hallucinations
• withdrawal as the patient tries to block out intense external stimuli and avoids school or work, where stimulation is high; the patient shows little expression.

Rationales

1. Psychosocial support is vital to maintaining the patient at home and in the community. Understanding salient aspects of the disease helps the family develop a sense of control in an otherwise chaotic and unmanageable process.

2. Assess the patient's and family's understanding of prescribed medications.

3. Teach the patient and family about antipsychotics; explain common adverse effects and how to control them. For example, explain that drowsiness and lethargy are common and precautions should be taken to prevent injury; dry mouth and lips can be controlled using sugarless gum and a lip moisturizer; nasal dryness is alleviated by applying a moisturizer; constipation can be controlled with a mild laxative.

4. Monitor the patient for less common adverse effects, such as tremors, muscle weakness, restlessness, drooling, and (rarely) acute muscle spasms of the tongue, neck, face, and eyes. Report these to the doctor immediately.

5. Tell the patient to avoid or minimize alcohol use and to consult with the doctor before altering the medication dosage or adding medications.

2. An assessment of current knowledge establishes a baseline for teaching and planning. Compliance with the antipsychotic regimen is vital to prevent recurrent exacerbations of schizophrenia.

3. Antipsychotics control the activity of dopamine, a chemical that regulates brain function. Lifetime compliance with the medication regimen is essential to prevent exacerbations. Teaching the patient and family to control common adverse effects may improve compliance.

4. The doctor may prescribe an antiparkinsonian agent to counteract these symptoms. If the symptoms are left unchecked, the patient may stop taking the antipsychotics.

5. Alcohol potentiates the action of antipsychotics. Altering the dosage or adding medications can adversely affect the patient's response to the prescribed medication.

Nursing diagnosis: *Ineffective individual coping related to stress or an inadequate support system*

GOAL: To help the patient and family understand the relationship between stress and disease symptoms

Interventions

1. Explain to the patient and family that the patient's environment should be low-key. Tell them to avoid scheduling too many activities, too much change, or too many visitors at one time. Gauge the patient's response to these stressors over time.

2. Let the patient learn to know you as a concerned professional. Avoid appearing either cold or too friendly. Tell him how long you expect to be working with him and his family, and remind him of the time frame periodically.

3. Teach the patient and family the importance of clear communication through example and direct instruction. Advise them to specify house rules for such activities as sleeping, eating, cleaning, and dressing so the patient knows what is expected.

4. Encourage family members to maintain satisfactory relationships outside the family and to make time for leisure and personal enrichment.

5. Help the patient and family adopt a long-term perspective about the patient's illness. Tell them not to expect the patient to fit into a normal age-related role. Explain that setbacks are not failures, simply indications that a longer adjustment period is necessary. Refer the family to a therapist for a discussion of the patient's prognosis, if necessary.

Rationales

1. A stressful environment increases the patient's risk of relapse.

2. Because all relationships are stressful to the patient, he may approach them cautiously and with some misgivings. He may interpret coldness as disapproval; excessive friendliness as a sexual advance. Reminding him of the relationship's time frame is important because terminating an established relationship can be traumatic for an unprepared patient.

3. A clearly defined routine lets the patient know what is expected of him, which helps minimize stress and strengthen his sense of security.

4. Family members must meet their own needs if they hope to help the patient over time.

5. Schizophrenia is a chronic illness with lasting effects. The patient and family should avoid unrealistic expectations, such as complete recovery. Talking with a therapist may help them adjust their expectations.

6. Suggest that the family join a support group through a local psychiatric hospital or branch of the Mental Health Association.

6. Support groups offer emotional support and can provide ideas about adjusting to the patient's condition.

Nursing diagnosis: *Social isolation related to an inability to engage in personal relationships*

GOAL: To improve the patient's work and social relationships

Interventions

1. Explain that the patient should prepare to resume work responsibilities gradually.

2. Explore the possibility of the patient attending a day hospital or sheltered workshop.

Rationales

1. The patient's vulnerability to stress mandates that this process be gradual. Too much pressure to resume full-time work too soon may result in a relapse.

2. A day hospital or sheltered workshop can help the patient develop social and work skills and provide respite for the family.

Nursing diagnosis: *Potential for violence directed at others related to rage reactions*

GOAL: To help the patient and family recognize escalating episodes of anger as a symptom requiring medical intervention

Interventions

1. Tell the patient and family that physical separation is required when violence is threatened. Suggest that one or both persons leave the room and go for a walk.

2. Advise the family to consult a therapist if angry exchanges seem to be increasing.

3. If the patient makes threatening remarks or displays verbal or physical violence in your presence, leave the home and notify police and the patient's therapist.

Rationales

1. Separating angry family members helps them regain control. Walking helps dissipate anger.

2. An increase in episodes of anger may indicate that the patient is not complying with the medication regimen, that the dosage needs to be altered, or that the family and patient need respite from each other.

3. Police intervention to ensure the safety of the nurse, family, and patient may be necessary if the patient resists treatment.

ASSOCIATED CARE PLANS
• Major Depression
• Manic-Depressive Illness

NETWORKING OF SERVICES
• group home
• sheltered workshop
• day hospital
• halfway house
• state bureau of vocational rehabilitation
• support group such as the local chapter of Families of the Mentally Ill (affiliated with the National Alliance for the Mentally Ill, 1901 N. Fort Myer Dr., Suite 500, Arlington, Va. 22209)
• local Mental Health Association

CARE TEAM INVOLVED
• nurse
• doctor
• therapist
• patient and family
• medical social worker

IMPLICATIONS FOR HOME CARE
• family members who are interested in providing a home for the patient and who are not exhausted by other problems
• family members who are not highly critical or hostile
• patient who is motivated to follow the medication regimen

PATIENT EDUCATION TOOLS
• Mental Health Association literature
• written information about each prescribed medication, including administration, dosage, and adverse effects

DISCHARGE PLAN FROM HOME HEALTH CARE
Before discharge from home health care, the patient

(or family members, if appropriate) should:
• be able to state the dosage and adverse effects of each prescribed medication
• post telephone numbers of the home health agency, therapist, and doctor by the phone
• have a schedule for daily activities
• engage in various activities, including a program of regular exercise, such as walking
• contact support groups, such as a sheltered workshop, day hospital, social group, or religious group.

SELECTED REFERENCES

Anderson, C., Reiss, D, and Hogarty, G. *Schizophrenia and the Family*. New York: The Guilford Press, 1986.

Barofsky, I., and Budson, R., eds. *The Chronic Mental Patient in the Community*. New York: S.P. Medical and Scientific Books, 1983.

Govani, L.E., and Hayes, J.E., eds. *Drugs and Nursing Implications*. Norwalk, Conn.: Appleton & Lange, 1988.

Kerr, A., and Snaith, P. *Contemporary Issues in Schizophrenia*. London: The Bath Press, 1986.

McFarland, G.K., and Wasli, E.L. *Nursing Diagnoses and Process in Psychiatric Mental Health Nursing*. Philadelphia: J.B. Lippincott Co., 1986.

Menuck, M., and Seeman, M. *New Perspectives in Schizophrenia*. New York: Macmillan Publishing Co., 1985.

Murray, R., and Huelskoetter, M. *Psychiatric/Mental Health Nursing*, 2nd ed. Norwalk, Conn.: Appleton & Lange, 1987.

Neal, M.C., et al. *Nursing Care Planning Guides for Psychiatric and Mental Health Care*, 2nd ed. Pacific Palisades, Calif.: Nurseco, 1985.

Reighley, J.W., ed. *Nursing Care Planning Guides for Mental Health*. Baltimore: Williams & Wilkins Co., 1988.

Shives, L. *Basic Concepts of Psychiatric-Mental Health Nursing*. Philadelphia: J.B. Lippincott Co., 1986.

Stuart, G.W., and Sundeen, S.J., eds. *Principles and Practice of Psychiatric Nursing*, 3rd ed. St. Louis: C.V. Mosby Co., 1987.

Townsend, M. *Nursing Diagnosis in Psychiatric Nursing*. Philadelphia: F.A. Davis Co., 1988.

Section III

General Care Plans

Pain

DESCRIPTION AND TIME FOCUS

Pain is the most prevalent—and least understood—symptom treated by nurses. No two patients respond to a common pain stimulus in the same way. Each patient's attitude toward pain and his levels of anxiety, fear, depression, stress, and fatigue during pain help shape his response to it. Some experts even suggest that environmental and psychosocial factors can influence this response. Although health professionals classify pain as acute, chronic, or terminal, the nurse cannot precisely and objectively measure a patient's pain nor compare it to that of another patient. Perhaps for this reason, nothing is more frustrating than being unable to alleviate a patient's pain, and nothing is more satisfying than relieving it.

In home health care, the nurse encounters many different causes of pain, such as surgery, disease, trauma, or pregnancy and delivery. This clinical plan addresses invasive and noninvasive pain-control measures, including medications, transcutaneous electrical nerve stimulation (TENS), hypnosis, biofeedback, and guided imagery.

■ Typical home health care length of service for a patient with pain: varies according to the cause of pain

■ Typical visit frequency: *acute pain*—three times weekly for 3 weeks; *chronic pain*—twice weekly for 6 weeks; *terminal pain*—daily visits or until the pain is relieved

HEALTH HISTORY FINDINGS

In a health history interview, the patient may report many of these findings:
• history of hypertension
• anxiety
• emotional stress
• decreased mobility
• irritability
• anorexia
• depression
• diaphoresis
• insomnia
• fatigue
• inability to perform activities of daily living (ADLs)
• decreased ambulation

PHYSICAL FINDINGS

In a physical examination, the nurse may detect many of these findings:

Cardiovascular
• hypertension
• restlessness
• tachycardia

Respiratory
• shallow, rapid respirations
• shortness of breath
• gasping

Neurologic
• inability to concentrate
• depression
• low self-esteem
• tension
• disorientation
• crying
• moaning
• isolation

Gastrointestinal
• indigestion
• heartburn
• anorexia
• nausea
• vomiting
• pain on defecation

Integumentary
• pallor
• diaphoresis
• flushed skin
• grimacing

Musculoskeletal
• pacing
• writhing
• stiffness
• guarding
• spasms
• tremors

DIAGNOSTIC STUDIES

Radiologic and laboratory studies vary according to the disease. For detailed information, see "Diagnostic Studies" in the applicable care plan.

Nursing diagnosis: *Altered comfort: acute pain, related to trauma pressure, ischemia, spasm, or other disease*

GOAL: To alleviate acute pain

Interventions

1. In the health history interview, ask the patient to describe the character, intensity, location, duration, and frequency of pain. Rank findings in each category on a scale of 1 (mild) to 10 (severe). Determine whether acute pain is related to trauma, pressure, ischemia, spasm, or other disease entity.

2. Assess the patient for nonverbal indications of pain, such as restlessness, writhing, or grimacing.

3. Anticipate the patient's need for pain relief (for example, before such potentially painful experiences as walking, a dressing change, or a bowel movement); do not wait for him to ask for medication.

4. Reassure the patient that medication will be available when he needs it.

5. Promote a calm, restful environment. For example, encourage the patient and family to minimize noise from the television or radio and to limit the number of visitors the patient can see at one time or in one day.

6. Position the patient for the highest possible level of comfort. Encourage him to change position each hour to minimize stress on individual muscle groups.

7. Help the patient explore noninvasive pain-relief techniques. Ask him about techniques that have worked in the past, and teach him other pain-relief measures, such as relaxation techniques and deep-breathing exercises.

Rationales

1. Health history findings help in identifying the patient's pain pattern and developing a specific pain-control program.

2. The patient may not want to admit he has pain because he may fear becoming addicted to pain medications.

3. Analgesics—the primary tool for combatting acute pain, such as postoperative pain—are more effective when administered before the pain becomes severe.

4. The patient may worry that his complaints of pain will be ignored or that analgesics will not be available. Reassurance allays these fears.

5. A calm, restful environment is conducive to pain relief.

6. Position changes reduce muscle discomfort by promoting circulation and may prevent complications of decreased mobility, such as thrombophlebitis and atelectasis.

7. Noninvasive pain-relief techniques enhance medicinal measures. Relaxation techniques and deep-breathing exercises promote the brain's release of endorphins, opiatelike hormones that reduce stress and tension, provide pain relief, and potentiate narcotic analgesics.

Nursing diagnosis: *Altered comfort: chronic pain, related to an incurable disease accompanied by depression*

GOAL: To alleviate chronic pain

Interventions

1. In the health history interview, ask the patient to describe the character, intensity, location, duration, and frequency of pain and pain-relief methods he has tried.

2. Teach the patient the importance of mobility and regular exercise.

3. Assess the patient's pain at each nursing visit to determine the current pain pattern. Show him a body diagram so he can visualize the pain site.

Rationales

1. The nurse uses baseline data to plan an individualized pain-control program.

2. Mobility and regular exercise promote increased circulation to painful areas. Many patients in pain tend to avoid movements, unknowingly exacerbating pain.

3. Assessing the patient at each visit helps the nurse monitor the healing process and evaluate pain treatment effectiveness. A body diagram can help the patient explain the location and severity of his pain.

4. Have the patient keep a pain diary. Tell him to use a 1-10 line bar, ranking the pain on a scale of 1 (no pain) to 10 (severe pain).

4. Keeping a pain diary may help the patient anticipate when pain is most likely to occur so he can schedule important tasks and ADLs during pain-free periods.

5. Teach the patient to apply heat or cold to affected areas, as indicated, and to apply ice contralaterally if it cannot be placed directly on the painful area.

5. Heat relaxes painful muscle spasms by increasing blood flow to the area. Cold helps reduce swelling and its associated pain. Applying ice contralaterally to the pain triggers release of endorphins.

6. Teach the caregiver how to massage the patient.

6. Massage increases blood flow to painful areas and limits pain impulses by blocking ascending pain pathways and increasing release of endorphins.

7. Suggest that the patient drink one or two glasses of wine to relieve pain, unless contraindicated.

7. Alcohol releases serotonin in the brain; this stimulates release of enkephalins, which inhibit transmission of pain impulses.

8. Encourage the patient to maintain his sense of humor and to pursue enjoyable activities, such as listening to music, painting a portrait, or playing with the family pet.

8. These measures help refocus the patient's attention away from pain and toward more pleasurable aspects of life.

9. Discuss with the patient and doctor the use of TENS as a pain-relief method.

9. TENS effectively relieves many forms of chronic pain by stimulating the release of endogenous opiates from the brain.

10. Determine the patient's degree of referred pain.

10. After prolonged use of narcotic analgesics and sedative hypnotics, the patient will feel less energetic and motivated and more depressed and dependent; this can inhibit the drugs' effectiveness, as the patient's pain coincides with signs and symptoms of withdrawal.

11. Identify factors that may reinforce illness (such as increased attention from family members or disability payments), and discuss these with the patient.

11. Emotional or monetary reinforcements may interfere with the patient's recovery.

Nursing diagnosis: *Altered comfort: terminal pain, related to an incurable disease and impaired body systems*

GOAL: To alleviate terminal pain

Interventions

1. In the health history interview, ask the patient to describe his pain, including time of onset and pain patterns, and pain-relief measures he has tried. Use a 1-10 line bar to assess his pain.

2. Teach the patient to use a patient-controlled analgesic (PCA) pump. Set the dosage and timing controls as ordered.

3. Evaluate the patient's response to pain-relief measures, and notify the doctor of unrelieved pain.

4. Tell the caregiver to change the patient's position every 2 hours unless the patient is sleeping.

5. Teach the caregiver to massage the patient several times daily.

Rationales

1. The nurse uses baseline data to plan an individualized pain-control program.

2. A PCA pump allows the patient to control pain relief by releasing analgesic doses within preset limits.

3. Unrelieved pain may indicate the need for a medication change.

4. Rest and sleep are top priorities for a dying patient. Frequent position changes during waking hours help relieve discomfort.

5. Massage increases blood flow to painful areas and limits pain impulses by blocking ascending pain pathways and increasing release of endorphins.

6. When possible, use positive suggestion as a pain-relief measure. For example, after administering an analgesic, tell the patient, "You should be feeling some relief shortly."

6. Positive suggestion can enhance the effectiveness of other pain-relief measures and assures the patient and family that some degree of relief is possible.

Nursing diagnosis: *Altered comfort: pain, related to adverse effects of analgesics*

GOAL: To alleviate the patient's discomfort

Interventions

1. Advise the patient to increase his fiber intake, to drink at least 2 liters of fluid daily, to exercise if possible, to use stool softeners if needed, and to defecate when he feels the urge.

2. If the patient has nausea, try to minimize offensive odors, such as paint fumes, cooking odors, and tobacco smoke.

3. Administer antiemetics, as ordered. Teach the patient deep-breathing exercises, and tell him to avoid sudden movements.

4. Encourage the patient to drink a small glass of juice or soda water every hour, to brush his teeth every 2 hours, to breathe through his nose rather than his mouth, and to avoid alcohol.

5. Tell the patient to drink at least 2 liters of fluid daily and to suck on ice chips periodically.

Rationales

1. These measures help prevent or eliminate constipation.

2. Offensive odors may exacerbate nausea.

3. Antiemetics inhibit vomiting. Deep breathing reduces the strength of the vomiting reflex. Sudden movements may trigger the vomiting center in the medulla.

4. These measures help alleviate a dry mouth.

5. These measures help alleviate stomatitis by maintaining a clear, moist oral cavity.

ASSOCIATED CARE PLANS
• Grief and Grieving
• Hospice Care
• Ineffective Coping
(see also the applicable disease care plan)

NETWORKING OF SERVICES
• Lifeline
• durable medical equipment supplier
• organization relevant to the patient's condition, such as the American Cancer Society
• local pain clinic or pain center
• hospice

CARE TEAM INVOLVED
• nurse
• doctor
• patient and family
• medical social worker
• physical therapist
• pharmacist
• hospice staff

IMPLICATIONS FOR HOME CARE
• telephone (communication)

• adaptive equipment
• pillows for comfort

PATIENT EDUCATION TOOLS
• literature on each prescribed medication
• list of noninvasive pain-control techniques
• literature on the pathophysiology of the disease

DISCHARGE PLAN FROM HOME HEALTH CARE
Before discharge from home health care, the patient should:
• be free of signs and symptoms of pain
• know the signs and symptoms of pain that warrant medical attention
• understand the pathophysiology of his disease
• know the method of administration, dosage, action, and adverse effects of each prescribed medication
• be familiar with noninvasive pain-relief techniques
• understand his personal pain patterns and psychosocial and environmental factors that may influence his response to pain
• perform as many ADLs as possible
• post telephone numbers for the doctor and home health agency by the phone.

SELECTED REFERENCES

Holloway, N., and Gregory, C. "Pain," in *Nursing the Critically Ill Adult,* 3rd ed., edited by N. Holloway. Menlo Park, Calif.: Addison-Wesley Publishing Co., 1988.

McCaffrey, M. "Understanding Your Patient's Pain," *Nursing80* 10:26-31, September 1980.

Meyer, T.M. "Relieving Pain Through Electricity," *Nursing82* 12:57-59, September 1982.

Perry, A.G., and Potter, P.A. *Clinical Nursing Skills and Techniques.* St. Louis: C.V. Mosby Co., 1986.

Sandroff, N. "When You Must Inflict Pain on a Patient," *RN* 47:35-39, January 1984.

Tucker, S. *Patient Care Standards,* 4th ed. St. Louis: C.V. Mosby Co., 1988.

West, B.A. "Understanding Endorphins: Our Natural Pain Relief System," *Nursing81* 11:50-53, February 1981.

Ineffective Coping

DESCRIPTION AND TIME FOCUS

Ineffective coping is an impairment of adaptive behaviors and problem-solving abilities to meet life's demands and roles. A serious illness or injury, such as cerebrovascular accident or amputation, usually forces the patient and family to make difficult adjustments in life-style and role performance. This clinical plan focuses on the patient who is having difficulty coping with these adjustments. The nurse may determine that the patient's environment is conducive to effective coping only to discover that he exhibits poor coping techniques. Nursing care centers on helping the patient identify factors that impede effective coping, take positive steps to make his life as comfortable as possible, establish reliable support systems, and adapt successfully to life-style changes effected by his illness.

■ Typical home health care length of service for a patient with impaired coping skills: depends on the underlying disease

■ Typical visit frequency: depends on the underlying disease

HEALTH HISTORY FINDINGS

In a health history interview, the patient may report many of these findings:
• severe anxiety
• erratic or unstable attitudes and emotional responses
• illness in the family
• role changes in the family
• loss of self-control
• insomnia

PHYSICAL FINDINGS

In a physical examination, the nurse may detect many of these findings:

Cardiovascular
• high blood pressure
• tachycardia
• dysrhythmia

Respiratory
• hyperventilation

Neurologic
• restlessness
• lethargy
• insomnia

Gastrointestinal
• vomiting
• diarrhea
• stress ulcer
• GI bleeding
• constipation

Integumentary
• diaphoresis
• rash

Musculoskeletal
• muscle tension
• pain

DIAGNOSTIC STUDIES

Studies vary according to the disease. For detailed information, see "Diagnostic Studies" in the applicable care plan.

Nursing diagnosis: *Ineffective individual coping related to role change*

GOAL: To improve the patient's coping ability

Interventions

1. Perform a brief physical examination, and assess the patient's emotional response to the role change.

2. Evaluate the patient's sleeping patterns, dietary habits, and bowel patterns.

3. Use focused communication to help the patient identify factors causing anxiety. For example, if his illness forced him to find a new job, ask him several questions about his tasks, responsibilities, supervisor, co-workers, and working conditions. Ask him how anxious he feels

Rationales

1. A baseline assessment helps the nurse establish a plan of care.

2. Uninterrupted sleep, sound nutrition, and adequate bowel elimination are important to the patient's health. Deficiencies in these areas may reduce his ability to cope with role changes brought on by illness.

3. Focused communication, sometimes called targeted exchange, can be an effective technique in which the nurse thoroughly explores one topic with the patient to help him better organize his thought processes.

about the job change, and have him rate his anxiety on a scale from 1 (mild) to 10 (severe).

4. During discussions, observe the patient for memory loss or poor concentration. Pace the conversation accordingly, and restate questions or comments to be sure he understands.

5. Assess the patient for mood swings, and document his mood at each visit (for example, "depressed and uncooperative" or "happy and responsive"). Teach coping techniques when he is in a receptive mood.

6. Establish a relationship with the patient that is based on mutual trust. Speak candidly to him about his condition, arrive on time for scheduled visits, and provide accurate information (such as photocopies of recent articles on his condition) in response to his questions.

7. Help the patient identify positive aspects of his personality by asking him questions like these: "What do you like about yourself? What do others like about you? What do you wish others would admire you for, and how can you become that type of person? Who can help you do this? How can others help you?"

8. Encourage the patient to discuss fears or concerns he may have about his sexual identity. Provide educational information (books, pamphlets, or other current literature) relevant to his condition.

9. Help the patient identify stress-producing situations that hinder progress in coping more effectively.

10. Teach the patient appropriate ways to express hostility and anger, such as pounding pillows, doodling, or keeping a diary of his moods and feelings.

11. Provide generous emotional support to the patient, and encourage him to remain hopeful about the future. If possible, point out potential benefits of his new role, such as having more time to spend with family members or developing new skills to accomplish household tasks normally handled by others.

4. Memory loss and poor concentration may indicate regression of coping skills.

5. Assessing mood swings helps the nurse schedule visits during times when the patient is most receptive to learning.

6. Trust provides emotional support for the patient as he undergoes changes in personal identity associated with the role change.

7. An honest self-assessment gives the patient new insights about his personality and may suggest new goals to accomplish.

8. A patient facing a sexual identity crisis needs opportunities to express his fears and concerns openly. Discussing these issues usually helps decrease fears about impaired sexual performance and can positively influence the relationship between the patient and partner.

9. A patient who is mindful of potential stressors can take steps to avoid them when possible and, with the nurse's guidance, can develop effective methods of coping with unavoidable stressors.

10. Venting hostility and anger prevents personality deterioration and helps the patient develop effective coping skills.

11. The patient may adjust to his new role more readily—and feel more secure about his identity—if he realizes his life can still be rewarding and meaningful.

Nursing diagnosis: *Ineffective family coping: compromised, related to inadequate resources*

GOAL: To promote effective family coping by coordinating available resources

Interventions

1. Assess the patient's relationship with each family member. Identify those on whom the patient relies most often for support and guidance, particularly the primary caregiver.

2. Assess the family's financial ability to meet the patient's medical needs. Refer them to a social worker for

Rationales

1. Assessing family relationships helps the nurse employ members effectively in caring for the patient. Usually, one member emerges as the primary caregiver, and the nurse must work closely with this person to enhance the patient's health.

2. The family's financial status may influence decisions they must make about health care. A social worker can

financial counseling, if necessary, and give them a comprehensive list of community resources that can assist with other needs.

help them explore private- and community-funding options. Other community resources—such as support groups, mental health clinics, religious organizations, libraries, and Meals On Wheels—can provide emotional support, information on the patient's disease, and assistance with transportation, medical equipment, or homemaking needs.

ASSOCIATED CARE PLANS
• Developmental Disabilities
• Grief and Grieving
• Hospice Care
• Pain
• Sex and Sexuality

NETWORKING OF SERVICES
• Meals On Wheels
• mental health organizations
• religious organizations
• libraries

CARE TEAM INVOLVED
• nurse
• doctor
• patient and family
• social worker
• recreational therapist

IMPLICATIONS FOR HOME CARE
• functional features of the home
• telephone (communication)

PATIENT EDUCATION TOOLS
• list of necessary medical equipment
• literature on each prescribed medication, particularly mood-altering medications
• audiocassettes or videocassettes on relaxation techniques, self-improvement, and (if permitted) moderate exercises

DISCHARGE PLAN FROM HOME HEALTH CARE
Before discharge from home health care, the patient should:
• know the method of administration, dosage, action, and adverse effects of each prescribed medication, especially mood-altering medications
• understand dietary requirements
• know personal stressors and methods to minimize or eliminate them
• know how to reach care team members or community resources if necessary
• post telephone numbers for the doctor and home health agency by the phone for follow-up care, if necessary
• understand the problems that may occur in sexual functioning
• develop effective coping skills
• feel that he has control over many aspects of his life.

SELECTED REFERENCES
Carpenito, L. *Handbook of Nursing Diagnosis.* Philadelphia: J.B. Lippincott Co., 1989.
Shives, L.R. *Basic Concepts of Psychiatric Health Nursing.* Philadelphia: J.B. Lippincott Co., 1986.
Stuart, G., and Sundeen, S.J. *Principles and Practices of Psychiatric Nursing.* St. Louis: C.V. Mosby Co., 1987.
Townsend, M.C. *Nursing Diagnoses in Psychiatric Nursing.* Philadelphia: F.A. Davis Co., 1988.
Wilson, H.S.K., and Kneisel, C.R. *Psychiatric Nursing,* 3rd ed. Menlo Park, Calif.: Addison-Wesley Publishing Co., 1988.

GENERAL CARE PLANS
Grief and Grieving

DESCRIPTION AND TIME FOCUS
Grieving is the psychological process by which the patient and family gradually learn to cope with a loss, such as death, amputation, or loss of body function. Adjusting to a significant loss can be overwhelming, particularly when the loss is sudden and unexpected. Signs and symptoms of grief may include a choking sensation or tightness in the throat, shortness of breath, muscle weakness, intense distress, GI complaints, emotional distancing, guilt, anger, and irritability.

The normal grieving process usually consists of anticipatory grief (beginning as soon as the condition is known), acute grief (usually lasting 2 to 4 months but sometimes persisting for up to 1 year), and resolution (the mourner accepts the reality of the loss and establishes a new identity). In abnormal grieving, which usually lasts longer than 4 months, the mourner shows no signs of grieving but displays excessive denial; manic escape, evidenced by inappropriate cheerfulness and frenzied activity; dysfunctional hostility; and clinical depression.

This clinical plan focuses on the patient and family who must cope with a significant loss. Nursing care centers on helping them accept the loss and prepare for life-style changes that probably will result. The nurse should refer the patient and family for psychological or spiritual counseling, if appropriate.

■ Typical home health care length of service: varies according to the primary diagnosis

■ Typical visit frequency: varies according to stage of grief; usually, once or twice monthly (with weekly phone contact, if appropriate)

HEALTH HISTORY FINDINGS
In a health history interview, the patient or family may report many of these findings:
• altered life-style because of health status and activity restrictions
• loss of body function(s)
• death of a loved one
• altered body image after surgery
• amputation
• stress

• anxiety
• vertigo
• palpitations
• tightness in chest or throat
• preoccupation with the loss
• guilt
• headache
• inability to maintain organized daily patterns
• persistent sense of worthlessness and self-blame
• prolonged social isolation
• irresponsible or self-destructive behavior
• prolonged insomnia
• use of alcohol and over-the-counter drugs
• exhaustion
• nausea
• anorexia

PHYSICAL FINDINGS
In a physical examination, the nurse may detect many of these findings:

Neurologic
• increased emotional distance
• poor relationships
• restlessness
• limited concentration
• excessive sighing
• inability to relax
• lethargy
• prolonged denial (may take several forms, such as undertaking constant activity to avoid recognizing the loss or projecting a new object or person into the role of the lost object or person)
• psychosomatic illness
• prolonged, unreasonable blame and hostility toward care team members

Gastrointestinal
• vomiting
• diarrhea

DIAGNOSTIC STUDIES
None

Nursing diagnosis: *Anticipatory grieving related to death, amputation, or loss of body function*

GOAL: To help the patient and family participate in constructive grieving and, if possible, accept the loss

Interventions

1. Explain the stages of grieving to the patient and family. Identify which stage(s) they are currently experiencing.

Rationales

1. Knowledge of normal behavior during grieving may lessen their anxiety. Nursing interventions must be appropriate for their stage(s) in the grieving process.

2. Assess the patient and family for physical problems.

3. Help the patient and family begin to accept the loss. Encourage them to express their feelings, and let them know you are willing to listen. Reassure them that crying is a normal and beneficial response. If the patient is dying, urge him to complete unfinished personal business, and offer your assistance, if appropriate.

4. Help the patient and family members prepare for the life-style changes that will accompany the loss.

5. After the patient and family have begun to accept the inevitability of the prognosis, avoid reinforcing hopes that the prognosis will change.

6. Encourage the patient and family to participate in activities they enjoy.

7. Promote the patient's participation in activities of daily living (ADLs).

8. Encourage the patient to participate in decision making, especially about issues affecting his health.

9. Assess the patient's natural support network, and offer help as needed.

10. Refer the patient and family for psychological or spiritual counseling, if appropriate.

2. Grieving can inhibit proper nutrition, sleep, activity, and sexual desire.

3. Open discussion can alleviate feelings of isolation and denial and may help the patient adjust more easily to his loss. Crying aids in decreasing tension and may provide some measure of comfort. Resolving unfinished personal business further advances the dying patient's acceptance of his condition and may bring him peace of mind.

4. Adequate preparation may reduce stress by encouraging them to recognize and address potential problems.

5. At this point, offering hope is inappropriate and provides no consolation.

6. Engaging in enjoyable activities can help reduce stress by temporarily allowing the patient and family to focus their attention on pleasant situations.

7. Performing ADLs enhances self-control, independence, and self-esteem.

8. Active involvement in decision making allows the patient to maintain a measure of control over his situation.

9. The patient will probably need much emotional support during the grieving process. Friends within community and religious groups can help him adjust to the loss.

10. A therapist or religious advisor can provide the patient and family with additional guidance and support.

Nursing diagnosis: *Dysfunctional grieving related to death, amputation, or loss of body function*

GOAL: To identify the pathologic grieving process and provide treatment

Interventions

1. Assess the patient and family for unresolved feelings of guilt, anger, sorrow, and sadness.

2. Be alert for increased use of or dependence on drugs or alcohol, and document your observations.

3. Assess and document the patient's ability to resume his former role.

4. Observe the patient for signs and symptoms of suicide ideation, such as agitation, anxiety, insomnia, hopelessness, and helplessness.

5. Assess the patient's suicide potential, and consult with his doctor if appropriate.

6. Refer the patient to a social worker if necessary.

Rationales

1. Unresolved guilt, anger, sorrow, and sadness are common symptoms of pathologic grief. Untreated, they can lead to major depression.

2. Substance abuse contributes to dysfunctional resolution of the loss. (See the "Substance Abuse" care plan for more information.)

3. Chronic grieving often is accompanied by withdrawal and social isolation.

4. Chronic grieving often leads to suicide attempts.

5. Discussion of suicide potential can help identify patients at risk.

6. A social worker can help coordinate community resources and introduce the patient to an appropriate support group for further assistance in successfully working through the grieving process.

ASSOCIATED CARE PLANS
• Acquired Immunodeficiency Syndrome
• Amputation
• Hospice Care
• Ineffective Coping
• Sex and Sexuality
• Sleep Disorders

NETWORKING OF SERVICES
• hospice
• religious organizations
• support groups

CARE TEAM INVOLVED
• nurse
• doctor
• patient and family
• therapist
• religious advisor

IMPLICATIONS FOR HOME CARE
• safe environment
• telephone (communication)
• support network (friends, groups, hotlines)

PATIENT EDUCATION TOOLS
• literature on effectively resolving grief and grieving
• information on support group meetings and activities

DISCHARGE PLAN FROM HOME HEALTH CARE
Before discharge from home health care, the patient
and family should:
• be able to discuss the patient's condition openly
• be able to sleep, eat, and (if possible) work
• experience reduced anxiety
• know appropriate coping mechanisms
• know the steps to take if unable to cope.

SELECTED REFERENCES
Amenta, M., and Bohnet, N. *Nursing Care of the Termi-
    nally Ill.* Boston: Little, Brown & Co., 1986.
Doenges, M., and Moorhouse, M. *Nurse's Pocket Guide:
    Nursing Diagnoses with Interventions,* 2nd ed. Phila-
    delphia: F.A. Davis Co., 1988.
Doenges, M., et al. *Nursing Care Plans: Nursing Diag-
    noses in Planning Patient Care.* Philadelphia: F.A.
    Davis Co., 1984.
Gonda, T., and Ruark, J. *Dying Dignified: The Health
    Professional's Guide to Care.* Menlo Park, Calif.: Addi-
    son-Wesley Publishing Co., 1984.
Interdisciplinary Care Plans (unpublished document).
    Tampa, Fla.: Hospice of Hillsborough, 1987.
Ulrich, S., et al. *Nursing Care Planning Guide: A Nursing
    Diagnosis Approach.* Philadelphia: W.B.Saunders Co.,
    1986.

GENERAL CARE PLANS
Sleep Disorders

DESCRIPTION AND TIME FOCUS
This clinical plan focuses on the patient whose recovery or rehabilitation is affected by a sleep pattern disturbance. Although a home health nurse rarely sees a patient primarily to treat a sleep disorder, many patients experience sleep disorders during their home care. The home provides an excellent setting for the nurse to evaluate and treat sleep disorders because the patient feels comfortable and secure there.
■ Typical home health care length of service and visit frequency depend on the underlying illness.

HEALTH HISTORY FINDINGS
In a health history interview, the patient may report many of these findings:
• irritability
• excessive sleeping during the day
• loss of concentration
• anxiety
• chronic fatigue

PHYSICAL FINDINGS
Physical findings specific to a sleep disorder are rarely apparent during a nursing assessment.

DIAGNOSTIC STUDIES
The following studies may be performed to evaluate the patient's health status:
• complete blood count (CBC)—once to rule out infection and anemia
• Multiple Sleep Latency Test—once for diagnosis; abnormal results signify narcolepsy

---

Nursing diagnosis: *Sleep pattern disturbance related to external stimuli or poor understanding of normal sleep habits*

GOAL: To help the patient get adequate sleep

Interventions

1. Ask the patient how much sleep he feels he needs and why he is concerned about current sleep habits.

2. Teach the patient the relationship between daytime activity and nighttime rest. Explain that inactivity and napping during the day can result in sleeplessness at night.

3. Have the patient keep a written record of his sleep habits for 24 hours.

4. Assess the patient's medical regimen, life-style, and home for disruptive stimuli, and help him make changes conducive to sleep.

Rationales

1. Sleep patterns vary from person to person and change with age. The patient may believe that everyone needs 8 hours of sleep or that his sleep patterns should never change, even though 6 hours may satisfy his current physiologic needs.

2. Determining the patient's need for sleep and adjusting daytime activities may be the only interventions required to alleviate a sleep disorder.

3. Written evidence of excessive sleep during the day may convince the patient that his daytime sleep habits are interfering with his sleep at night.

4. Slight alterations in medication and treatment schedules may promote uninterrupted sleep. The patient's bedroom may require modifications to create a dark, quiet, and comfortable environment.

Nursing diagnosis: *Altered nutrition, less than body requirements, related to inappropriate use of stimulants and inadequate caloric intake*

GOAL: To promote adequate nutrition as a means to improve the patient's sleep

Interventions

1. Teach the patient why he should avoid stimulants, such as caffeine, nicotine, and alcohol. Provide him with a list of foods that contain stimulants, and tell him to avoid any food that he suspects may be causing insomnia.

Rationales

1. Caffeine, nicotine, alcohol, and certain foods stimulate the central nervous system, thereby inhibiting sleep. Compliance with dietary restrictions may alleviate sleep disturbances.

2. Teach the patient the importance of eating well-balanced meals and spacing them appropriately.

2. Inadequate food intake during the day may cause the patient to wake at night feeling hungry.

Nursing diagnosis: *Diversional activity deficit related to illness, isolation, or chronic fatigue*

GOAL: To help the patient cultivate stimulating daytime activities

Interventions

1. Assess the patient's life-style and current activity level.

2. Talk to the patient about activities that would provide mental and physical stimulation. Assess his level of interest and ability to participate in various activities. Refer him to a social worker if necessary.

Rationales

1. Insufficient mental and physical stimulation can cause fatigue and interfere with normal rest. A baseline assessment helps the nurse plan necessary changes.

2. Activities must interest the patient and be within his physical and financial abilities to participate. A social worker can acquaint him with community programs and resources.

Nursing diagnosis: *Ineffective individual coping related to anxiety caused by sleep disturbance*

GOAL: To promote effective coping behaviors

Interventions

1. Help the patient identify emotional concerns and sources of stress that may interfere with normal sleep.

2. Teach the patient effective techniques for coping with anxiety, such as biofeedback, guided imagery, and music or pet therapy.

Rationales

1. The sleep disorder may stem from anxiety about financial, emotional, or health problems. Identifying problems may help ease his anxiety.

2. Nighttime sleeplessness and daytime fatigue may be the patient's method of coping with existing problems. Improving the patient's coping techniques can reduce stress and may alleviate the sleep disorder.

ASSOCIATED CARE PLANS
• Grief and Grieving
• Ineffective Coping
(See also the care plan applicable to the patient's condition.)

NETWORKING OF SERVICES
• support groups
• Meals On Wheels
• mental health clinic

CARE TEAM INVOLVED
• nurse
• doctor
• patient and family
• medical social worker

IMPLICATIONS FOR HOME CARE
• functional features of the home
• telephone (communication)
• support system of family and friends

PATIENT EDUCATION TOOLS
• list of items to ensure a restful sleep, such as dark curtains and relaxation tapes
• list of stimulants that may interfere with sleep
• information on well-balanced, properly spaced meals

DISCHARGE PLAN FROM HOME HEALTH CARE
Before discharge from home health care, the patient should:
• participate in daytime activities that provide adequate stimulation
• know coping mechanisms to reduce anxiety
• eliminate stimulants from his diet
• understand personal sleep requirements and know that normal sleep time varies from person to person.

SELECTED REFERENCES

American Medical Association. *Straight Talk, No-Non-sense Guide to Better Sleep.* New York: Random House, 1984.

Guilleminault, C., ed. *Sleep and Its Disorders in Children.* New York: Raven Press, 1987.

Moore-Ede, M.C., et al. *The Clocks That Time Us: Physiology of the Circadian Timing System.* Cambridge, Mass.: Harvard University Press, 1982.

Parkes, J.D. *Sleep and Its Disorders.* London: W.B. Saunders Co., 1985.

Saunders, N.A., and Sullivan, C.E., eds. *Sleep and Breathing* (Lung Biology in Health and Disease, vol. 21). New York: Marcel Dekker, Inc., 1984.

GENERAL CARE PLANS
Sex and Sexuality

DESCRIPTION AND TIME FOCUS
Illness often requires that a patient alter customary sexual activities. The need to modify or change customary activities should not be confused with sexual dysfunctions. Activity changes may be temporary or permanent, depending on the patient's clinical problem. Temporary changes may resolve quickly if related to relatively minor illnesses, such as infections, or require more time if related to chronic illness or disorders requiring surgery. Major anatomic or physiologic alterations, such as vulvectomy, penis amputation, or impotence associated with diabetic neuropathy, require permanent changes in the patient's sexual activity. Planning for these changes should start early in the patient's hospital stay to promote coping and to facilitate home management of the problem.

This clinical plan focuses on the patient whose sexual gratification is inhibited by illness. If the patient has a temporary problem, care centers on helping the patient resume satisfactory sexual activities as soon as possible. If the problem is permanent, care centers on helping the patient explore new approaches for achieving sexual satisfaction.

Keep in mind that solutions to sexuality problems associated with illness can come only from within the patient, and that the nurse can only help the patient discover these solutions. Towards this end, the nurse should try to understand the patient's perception of the problem and encourage open and honest discussions of the patient's sexual concerns. Questions must be answered directly and solutions must address the patient's specific problems. The nurse must keep in mind that sexual behaviors that are personally satisfying for the nurse may not be appropriate for or acceptable to the patient, and vice-versa. If the nurse feels uncomfortable discussing such sexual practices as multiple sexual partners, homosexuality, bisexuality, oral sex, or anal sex, the patient should be referred to another nurse or health care provider.

■ Typical home health care length of service for a patient with a sexual problem: variable depending on the patient's primary diagnosis
■ Typical visit frequency: variable

HEALTH HISTORY FINDINGS
In a health history interview, the patient may report one of these problems (or a similar problem) that could affect sexual function:
• prostatitis
• epididymitis
• vaginitis
• mastitis
• genital cancer
• breast cancer
• recent surgery
• loss of sexual function due to spinal cord injury or other neurologic disorder
• impotence related to diabetic neuropathy or antihypertensive medication use
• altered body image related to such surgery as amputation, mastectomy, or orchidectomy

PHYSICAL FINDINGS
Physical examination findings depend on the patient's underlying medical problem, if any.

DIAGNOSTIC STUDIES
None applicable to home care

Nursing diagnosis: *Anxiety related to altered patterns of sexuality*

GOAL: To minimize the patient's anxiety about sexual concerns

Interventions

1. Encourage the patient to discuss his or her sexual concerns.

2. Use therapeutic communication techniques when discussing sexual concerns with the patient.

3. Talk to the patient about the range of sexual activities that are compatible with his or her illness. For example, a patient and partner who cannot engage in sexual intercourse may find pleasure in massage, hugging and kissing, mutual masturbation, and use of sexual aids such as vibrators.

Rationales

1. Discussing sexual concerns helps the patient define concerns and consider solutions while informing others that the concerns exist, which in turn helps decrease anxiety.

2. Therapeutic communication techniques let the patient know that you are interested and attentive. Clear communication helps reduce the patient's anxiety and helps you understand the patient's concerns.

3. An open discussion of alternatives reduces the patient's anxiety by conveying the nurse's concern, and makes the patient aware of the alternatives for existing practices. This helps the patient identify acceptable alternative behaviors.

4. As appropriate, explain that impaired sexual function or desire may result from treatments such as drug therapy, radiation therapy, or surgery.

4. Knowledge that external factors may be responsible for impaired sexual response may help reduce the patient's anxiety.

Nursing diagnosis: *Dysfunctional grieving related to loss of familiar patterns of sexuality*

GOAL: To facilitate the grieving process

Interventions

1. Accept the patient's need to grieve over the loss of familiar sexual activities, and help the patient work through the grieving process.

2. Provide emotional support while the patient grieves.

3. Assess the patient's willingness to modify customary sexual activities.

Rationales

1. Grieving, the normal period of emotional adjustment that follows a loss, helps a patient recover from emotional trauma. As the patient works through the grieving process, he or she can begin to identify acceptable alternatives for sexual expression.

2. Emotional support can facilitate the grieving process by letting the patient know that someone cares about his or her loss and is willing to listen and try to help.

3. This helps the nurse determine if the patient has completed the grieving process, has accepted his or her situation, and is ready to explore alternative sexual activities.

Nursing diagnosis: *Disturbance in self-concept: personal identity, related to loss of usual sexuality patterns*

GOAL: To help the patient develop a positive self-concept that incorporates his or her altered patterns of sexuality

Interventions

1. Convey an accepting attitude of the patient's feelings about the loss of familiar patterns of sexual behavior, and encourage the patient's partner to do so as well.

2. Help the patient understand the importance of satisfying sexual activity to a positive self-concept, and encourage the patient to explore alternative methods of sexual expression.

3. Help the patient understand that sexuality is only one of many factors that influence self-concept, and that sexual problems need not destroy self-concept.

4. Provide feedback that emphasizes the patient's unique intrinsic value. Encourage the patient's partner to do the same.

Rationales

1. Acceptance by others will help enhance the patient's self-esteem.

2. The patient must acknowledge that his or her sexual problem may be contributing to a negative self-concept, and understand that discovering new ways of attaining sexual satisfaction can help restore a positive self-concept.

3. This understanding allows the patient to begin to develop an accurate perspective, accept his or her circumstances, and redefine his or her self-concept.

4. Identifying and reinforcing the patient's desirable qualities helps the patient develop a positive self-concept.

Nursing diagnosis: *Knowledge deficit related to available and appropriate methods of achieving sexual satisfaction*

GOAL: To teach the patient ways to enhance his or her sexual satisfaction

Interventions

1. Assess the patient's understanding of the sexual

Rationales

1. Patients learn best when teaching builds on previous

problem, its anticipated duration, and possible alternative methods of sexual expression.

2. Explain to the patient the importance of achieving sexual satisfaction even when illness-imposed limitations interfere. Encourage the patient to consider alternatives to his or her pre-illness sexual practices.

3. As appropriate, teach the patient and partner about methods to enable or enhance intercourse, such as alternative positioning and use of water-soluble vaginal lubricants.

4. As necessary, teach the patient about alternatives to intercourse for achieving sexual satisfaction, such as massage, hugging and kissing, mutual masturbation, and use of sexual aids such as vibrators. Encourage the patient to investigate any activities that he or she finds appealing.

5. Explain to the patient and partner the importance of effective communication to sexual expression. Help the patient and partner identify ways to improve their communication by focusing on skills such as active listening, clarification, and restatement. Provide the patient and partner with examples of effective and ineffective communication techniques drawn from your observation of their interaction.

6. As necessary, provide the patient with a list of sex therapists or psychologists who can provide professional help with sexual problems or concerns beyond the scope of nursing practice.

knowledge. Assessing the patient's knowledge level enables the nurse to identify and correct any knowledge gaps or misconceptions.

2. Patients will be more willing to discuss sexual activity as they begin to accept their current circumstances. The patient should understand the benefits of exploring new ways of achieving sexual satisfaction within the constraints imposed by the illness.

3. Positions that place less strain on the patient, such as female-superior for a male patient or male-superior for a female patient, may enable the patient to engage in sexual intercourse. Water-soluble vaginal lubricants can make intercourse more comfortable for a female patient and her partner.

4. Such teaching may help the patient discover several acceptable alternative methods for satisfying sexual needs that he or she may not have known about or may have considered unacceptable before the onset of illness.

5. Effective communication involves open and honest discussion between partners. Sexual satisfaction improves when partners can express sexual preferences and discuss the status of the relationship openly and honestly. Using examples of communication between the patient and partner most effectively illustrates effective and ineffective communication skills.

6. Appropriate professional referrals can help the patient manage problems that require more specialized evaluation and intervention.

ASSOCIATED CARE PLANS
• Acquired Immunodeficiency Syndrome
• Acute Myocardial Infarction
• Amputation
• Breast Cancer
• Cerebrovascular Accident
• Chronic Obstructive Pulmonary Disease
• Coronary Artery Bypass Grafting
• Diabetes Mellitus
• Grief and Grieving
• Hospice Care
• Hypertension
• Ineffective Coping
• Multiple Sclerosis
• Pain
• Prostate Cancer
• Sexually Transmitted Diseases
• Spinal Cord Injuries
• Uterine Cancer

NETWORKING OF SERVICES
• mental health organizations
• sex therapy agency

CARE TEAM INVOLVED
• nurse
• doctor
• patient and family
• social worker
• sex therapist

IMPLICATIONS FOR HOME CARE
• telephone (communication)
• safe environment with adequate privacy
• sexual aids, such as vibrators and massage equipment

PATIENT EDUCATION TOOLS
• literature on human sexuality

DISCHARGE PLAN FROM HOME HEALTH CARE
Before discharge from home health care, the patient should:
• know alternative methods of achieving sexual satisfaction
• explore ways to modify customary sexual practices to satisfy both partners
• have access to resources for ongoing guidance about sexual concerns.

SELECTED REFERENCES

Anon, J. "The PLISSIT Model," *Journal of Sex Education and Therapy* 2:1, Spring-Summer 1976.

Gordon, M. *Nursing Diagnosis: Process and Application*, 2nd ed. New York: McGraw-Hill Book Co., 1987.

Lion, E., ed. *Human Sexuality in Nursing Process*. New York: John Wiley & Sons, 1982.

Luckmann, J., and Sorensen, K. *Medical-Surgical Nursing: A Psychophysiologic Approach*, 3rd ed. Philadelphia: W.B. Saunders Co., 1987.

GENERAL CARE PLANS
Intermittent I.V. Therapy

DESCRIPTION AND TIME FOCUS
Intermittent I.V. therapy is used most often in home
health care to treat patients with osteomyelitis, endocarditis, virulent respiratory disorders, or cancer. Some
home health nurses use I.V. therapy to correct electrolyte imbalances (although this is risky because the de-
hydrated patient usually requires the services of an
acute-care hospital) or to maintain a dying patient (despite recent evidence indicating that additional fluids
given to a dying patient increase adverse reactions,
such as nausea, vomiting, crackles, pulmonary edema,
pedal edema, restlessness, seizure, and insomnia). Refer to the care plan for the specific disorder to obtain
further information about applicable I.V. therapies.
   This clinical plan focuses on the patient who requires I.V. therapy because of an infectious disorder.
Services are delivered according to doctor's orders. The
nurse must choose appropriate I.V. sites, teach the patient the rationale for I.V. therapy, and obtain the patient's consent for the procedure.
   ■ Typical home health care length of service for a
patient needing I.V. therapy: usually 4 to 6 weeks, depending on the amount of treatment the patient received in the acute-care setting
   ■ Typical visit frequency: initially, according to I.V.

medication administration times (every 4 to 12 hours)
to provide patient and family teaching; gradually reducing visits to once daily to monitor the I.V. site

HEALTH HISTORY FINDINGS
In a health history interview, the patient may report
one of these findings:
• osteomyelitis
• endocarditis
• virulent respiratory disorder

PHYSICAL FINDINGS
In a physical examination, the nurse may detect infiltration, as evidenced by swelling or skin coolness at
the I.V. site or diminished flow rate.

DIAGNOSTIC STUDIES
The following studies may be performed to evaluate the
patient's health status:
• white blood cell (WBC) count—weekly; levels should
decrease during treatment
• erythrocyte sedimentation rate (ESR)—weekly; rate
should slow during treatment
• wound culture—organism should be absent at end
of therapy

Nursing diagnosis: *Potential fluid volume deficit related to infection*

GOAL: To ensure adequate fluid volume

Interventions

1. Explain the procedure to the patient. Discuss why he
needs I.V. therapy, and explain his role in treatment.
Review activity restrictions, possible adverse effects,
and fluid requirements.

2. Help the patient into the semi-Fowler's position. Have
him lie on three pillows to ensure proper positioning.
Be sure lighting is adequate.

3. Monitor and record the patient's temperature, pulse
rate, blood pressure, and respiratory rate at each visit.

4. Choose an appropriate I.V. site, and use the distal
end of the vein. Avoid the legs entirely, if possible, and
also avoid extremities with burns, surgical wounds,
casts, or splints. If the patient has undergone a mastectomy or suffered a cerebrovascular accident (CVA),
avoid the affected side.

Rationales

1. Teaching the patient about the procedure helps reduce apprehension and fear, particularly if this is his
first experience with I.V. therapy.

2. The semi-Fowler's position helps the patient relax.
Proper lighting facilitates I.V. insertion.

3. The nurse uses this information to detect changes in
the patient's condition. Abnormal findings may indicate
infection at the I.V. site or a worsening of the underlying
disease. Infection rate increases significantly after the
I.V. has been in place for 72 hours.

4. The best venipuncture sites are on the lower arm,
lower hand, upper arm, and antecubital fossa. Venipuncture in the legs increases the patient's risk for
thrombophlebitis. I.V. fluids should not be infused into
an extremity with poor circulation (for example, after
a mastectomy or CVA) because of increased risk of
phlebitis.

I.V. THERAPY GUIDELINES FOR THE PATIENT

Following proper procedures for I.V. therapy can prevent complications and help ensure consistency of care. Review these guidelines with your caregiver, and make them a part of your daily routine.

• Become thoroughly familiar with I.V. administration and care. Read all literature provided by the nurse and equipment manufacturer. Ask the nurse to repeat explanations or demonstrations until you and your caregiver can comfortably perform the procedure.

• Record the date and time you use any part of the I.V. system (bottle or bag, tubing, filter, needle, or heparin lock plug). Place a timing label on continuous I.V. bottles or bags.

• Preflush the I.V. tubing and heparin lock with 2 ml of normal saline solution before connecting them, and secure and tape all connecting points.

• Administer all I.V. fluids and medications at the proper dose, volume, and rate.

• Instill 2 ml of normal saline solution and 2 ml of heparinized solution to flush the heparin lock at least every 24 hours and after administering any medication.

• Flush the lock with 2 ml of normal saline solution before and after administering any medication, followed by 2 ml of heparin at the end of each dose.

• Keep a daily diary to monitor your status. Indicate whenever you start or stop an I.V. solution or medication. Record the date, time of day, your temperature, and a brief description of how you feel.

• Assess the I.V. site frequently. Keep the area dry, and report any redness, pain, swelling, tenderness, or leakage to the doctor.

• Take your temperature daily, preferably in late afternoon or early evening. Notify the home health agency if you develop a fever. Also report shaking, chills, light-headedness, shortness of breath, chest pain, sweating, coughing, or change in bowel or urinary patterns.

• Replace the I.V. bottle or bag, tubing, and filter every 24 hours.

• Replace the I.V. needle, dressing, and heparin lock plug every 48 hours (or more often if a problem develops).

• Never reuse an I.V. bottle or bag after taking it down nor reuse an I.V. filter, tubing, or needle.

• Place used needles in a sealed container; then discard the container.

• If you note signs of adverse reactions, air embolus, or systemic infection, stop the infusion and notify the doctor and home health agency. In an emergency, call the ambulance service immediately.

• If the I.V. solution does not flow, is plugged, or contains blood, call the home health agency for assistance.

• Develop a plan to follow in an emergency. For example, if the catheter becomes dislodged, remove the catheter and dressing, apply pressure at the site for 5 minutes or until bleeding stops, cover the site with an adhesive bandage, and notify the home health agency.

• Make sure you have 24-hour access to a professional nurse.

5. Teach the patient and caregiver to administer I.V. therapy as ordered. Explain the use of the heparin lock to start and run the I.V. infusion. Tell them to:
• wash hands thoroughly before beginning
• allow refrigerated I.V. bags or bottles to warm to room temperature before starting the I.V.
• assemble necessary items, such as the new I.V. tubing, administration set, and alcohol swab
• check the I.V. site for problems and, if any are detected, call the agency nurse for advice and assistance
• wipe the heparin lock entry port with the alcohol swab and let it dry
• flush the lock with 2 ml of normal saline solution
• call the agency nurse for advice or assistance if resistance is felt or the patient experiences pain or a severe burning sensation
• attach the I.V. tubing to the I.V. bag or bottle without touching or contaminating sterile surfaces
• hang the I.V. bag or bottle
• flush all air from the tubing; then stop the flow and attach the sterile I.V. needle
• start a flow of one or two drops through the needle to ensure that no air remains in the system
• insert the needle into the heparin lock entry port and secure with tape

5. The heparin lock is a simplified patent conduit that permits the patient and caregiver to administer intermittent I.V. therapy after they have received appropriate instruction and demonstrated their understanding. The heparin lock minimizes vein damage while facilitating adequate fluid flow.

• set the flow rate (drops/minute) as directed, and place a timing label on the bottle
• periodically check the flow rate and timing label to be sure the infusion pump is running at the proper rate
• readjust the flow rate and check the I.V. site as needed.

6. Teach the patient and caregiver how to use the infusion pump to monitor the flow rate.

6. An I.V. infusion pump provides a more accurate flow rate than conventional gravity and clamp systems, provides a steady infusion from bottles or bags, and is easy to use.

7. Explain the dangers of lying on or kinking the tubing or raising the pole height above 30″.

7. Kinked tubing can slow or stop the infusion. Raising the pole height can increase the infusion. The solution container should hang 30″ above the venipuncture site to maintain a proper flow rate.

8. Teach the patient and caregiver the importance of assessing the infusion rate every 15 minutes during intermittent infusion.

8. A faster-than-ordered rate can cause fluid overload and shock. A slower-than-ordered rate, which may indicate that the I.V. needle has changed position, can lead to unstable antibiotic blood levels.

9. Teach the patient and caregiver the proper method of completing intermittent I.V. infusion. Tell them to:
• shut off the flow when about 3 ml of I.V. solution remain
• disconnect and remove the I.V. needle from the heparin lock entry port
• place the needle in a closed container, and discard the needle, tubing, and I.V. bottle or bag
• flush the heparin lock with 2 ml of normal saline solution; then instill 2 ml of heparinized normal saline solution
• document infusion completion, observations, and questions.

9. Properly completing the I.V. infusion ensures continued patency.

10. Teach the patient and caregiver to inspect each I.V. bottle or bag for dust, debris, glass fragments, and cloudiness; to notify the pharmacy if they detect any; and to use another bottle or bag.

10. Dust, debris, glass fragments, or cloudiness may indicate I.V. solution contamination.

11. Explain that the I.V. site is changed only when the flow is impeded, the site shows signs of irritation, or the patient complains of burning or pain.

11. Changing the I.V. site causes pain and discomfort and increases the patient's risk for infection. If the I.V. is functioning, a site change is unwarranted.

Nursing diagnosis: *Potential impaired skin integrity related to I.V. therapy*

GOAL: To prevent infiltration and infection

Interventions

1. Teach the patient and caregiver to assess for infection or infiltration in an I.V. that does not include drugs. Tell them to monitor for redness, swelling, tenderness, pain, or elevated skin temperature at the site or erythema along the venipuncture vein. If infiltration occurs, tell them to disconnect the I.V.; cover the site with a warm, moist dressing; elevate the extremity; and notify the doctor and agency nurse, who will start the I.V. at a new site.

Rationales

1. Infiltration impairs absorption and threatens the patient's safety.

2. Teach the patient and caregiver how to assess for infiltration in an I.V. that includes drugs (see signs and symptoms listed in Intervention #1). If infiltration occurs, tell them to disconnect the I.V.; notify the doctor and agency nurse; administer an antidote; cover the site with a warm, moist dressing; elevate the extremity; and give the patient pain medication.

2. Infiltration involving a toxic drug can cause sloughing and extensive tissue necrosis.

I.V. THERAPY TROUBLESHOOTING GUIDE

Problem	Possible cause	Solution
I.V. solution not flowing	• No solution in the bottle or bag	• Replace the bottle or bag, prime the tubing, and start the infusion.
	• Kinked tubing	• Be sure the patient is not lying on the tube; then check for kinks.
	• Closed clamp	• Check all push clamp sites. Open any closed clamp, and set the appropriate rate.
	• I.V. infiltration	• Check the insertion site for swelling, redness, or pain. If you note any, stop the infusion and call the doctor or home health agency.
	• Bottle or bag too low	• Hang the bottle or bag 30″ above the venipuncture site.
	• Wet I.V. air filter	• Remove the filter, shake it to dislodge fluid, and reinstall. If the solution stops, use a new filter. If this fails, stop the solution, discard the old tubing, install new tubing and a new filter, invert the bottle, prime the tubing, and restart the infusion.
	• Needle pushing against the side of the vein	• Reposition the patient's arm or hand. If this fails to help, try pressing lightly on the dressing over the needle insertion site.
I.V. solution flowing too quickly	• Disconnected tubing	• Ensure that all tubing connections are intact and that the solution is flowing at the ordered rate.
I.V. solution flowing too slowly	• Clamped tubing	• Open the roller clamp slightly until the ordered drip rate is achieved.
	• Bottle or bag too low	• Hang the bottle or bag 30″ above the venipuncture site.
	• I.V. infiltration	• Check the insertion site for swelling, redness, or pain. If you note any, stop the infusion and call the doctor or home health agency.
	• Needle pushing against the side of the vein	• Reposition the patient's arm or hand. If this fails to help, try pressing lightly on the dressing over the needle insertion site.
Blood in the I.V. tubing (*Note:* A small amount of pink blood just above the needle is normal.)	• Normal blood return and pressure from venous flow, causing a small amount of red blood near the needle	• Flush the catheter with heparin solution to prevent clot formation at the needle tip.
	• Kinked tubing, leaving a large amount of blood backed up several inches into the tubing	• Straighten any kinked sections. If the I.V. solution does not flow properly, remove the I.V. line and call the nurse for reinsertion.
	• No solution in the bottle or bag	• Irrigate the heparin lock, replace the bottle or bag, prime the tubing, and start the infusion. If the tubing fails to clear, change the tubing and restart the infusion.

3. During each visit, assess the I.V. site for infection. Wash hands thoroughly, and remove the dressing. Assess for purulent drainage or odor.

4. During each visit, assess the I.V. site for signs of phlebitis, such as tenderness or redness along the vessel. If these signs exist, remove the I.V.; apply a warm, moist dressing; assess the patient for fever, pain, or fatigue; and contact the doctor.

5. If the doctor confirms phlebitis, place an ice pack over the affected insertion site.

3. Tissue around the site must remain healthy for optimum absorption of I.V. fluid. Purulent drainage and odor indicate infection.

4. To prevent emboli formation, the I.V. must be discontinued immediately if phlebitis is suspected.

5. Ice packs minimize pain and swelling.

ASSOCIATED CARE PLANS
• Brain Tumors
• Breast Cancer
• Colorectal Cancer
• Lung Cancer
• Osteomyelitis
• Pain
• Uterine Cancer

NETWORKING OF SERVICES
• home pharmaceutical agency
(See also "Networking of Services" in the care plan applicable to the patient's condition.)

IMPLICATIONS FOR HOME CARE
• 24-hour monitoring of I.V. flow rate
• refrigeration for I.V. medication and solution storage
• microwave unit, in select cases, to warm solution to room temperature
• adequate supplies to ensure the patient's safety
• clean work area with adequate lighting and ventilation
• home health agency nurse on call 24 hours a day, 7 days a week for I.V. emergencies

CARE TEAM INVOLVED
• nurse certified for I.V. therapy
• doctor
• patient and family
• pharmacist
• home health aide

PATIENT EDUCATION TOOLS
• written instructions, including patient-teaching aids, on I.V. administration and site care
• Centers for Disease Control and National Intravenous Therapy Association guidelines for I.V. care at home

DISCHARGE PLAN FROM HOME HEALTH CARE
Before discharge from home health care, the patient

should:
• post telephone numbers of the doctor and home health agency by the phone
• arrange to have I.V. equipment removed from the home when no longer in use
• know the signs and symptoms that indicate a recurrence of the underlying disease
• know safety measures to take if the disease is caused by trauma
• know the time and date of the next doctor appointment.

SELECTED REFERENCES
Hower, D. "Using Special I.V. Lines at Home," *Nursing87* 17(7):58-61, July 1987.
Moore, C.L., et al. "Nursing Care and Management of Venous Access Parts," *Oncology Nursing Forum* 13(3):35-39, March 1987.
Schakenbach, L., and Dennis, M. "And Now, a Quad-Lumen I.V. Catheter," *Nursing85* 15(11):50, November 1985.

GENERAL CARE PLANS

Malnutrition

DESCRIPTION AND TIME FOCUS

Malnutrition is a state of dietary deficiency. *Primary malnutrition* results from inadequate intake of calories and nutritional components, such as vitamins. *Secondary malnutrition* results from inadequate digestion, absorption, transportation, storage, metabolism, or elimination of nutrients. Primary and secondary malnutrition commonly occur together.

Proper nutrition is especially important for the patient subjected to the stress of illness, injury, or surgery. Maintaining a well-balanced diet can be difficult if his condition makes eating laborious, painful, or unappealing.

This clinical plan focuses on the patient at home with a diagnosis of malnutrition. Nursing care centers on helping the patient make home adaptations that ensure adequate nutrition. Interventions include helping the patient plan meals, employ measures to improve his appetite, use special utensils to make eating easier, and prepare a food budget.

■ Typical home health care length of service for uncomplicated malnutrition: 6 weeks
■ Typical visit frequency: once weekly

HEALTH HISTORY FINDINGS

In a health history interview, the patient may report many of these findings:
• history of inadequate nutritional intake
• decreased appetite
• weakness
• fatigue
• weight loss or difficulty maintaining weight

PHYSICAL FINDINGS

In a physical examination, the nurse may detect many of these findings:

Neurologic
• irritability
• confusion

Gastrointestinal
• hunger or anorexia
• nausea
• chronic vomiting or diarrhea
• abdominal pain
• difficulty in chewing or swallowing

Integumentary
• little or no subcutaneous fat
• pallor
• paresthesia
• impaired wound healing
• edema
• ascites
• brittle, ridged nails
• bleeding or recessed gums, with loose teeth or poor-fitting dentures

DIAGNOSTIC STUDIES

The following studies may be performed to evaluate the patient's health status:
• blood tests (hemoglobin; hematocrit; complete blood count; iron; protein; vitamins A, B complex, B-12, C, and E; calcium; glucose; iodine; magnesium; phosphorus; potassium; sodium; coagulation studies)—at baseline and then weekly until results are normal; to pinpoint inadequate dietary intake; abnormal digestion, absorption, or elimination; or other nutritional problems
• urine tests (acetone, glucose, protein, creatinine, blood urea nitrogen)—at baseline and then weekly until results are normal; to identify inappropriate metabolism of nutrients
• stool tests (blood, fat, ova, parasites)—at baseline and then weekly until results are normal; to identify abnormal digestion, absorption, or elimination or to detect infection
• liver function tests—at baseline and then weekly until results are normal; to identify abnormal nutrient metabolism

---

Nursing diagnosis: *Altered nutrition: less than body requirements, related to dietary deficiency*

GOAL 1: To help the patient maintain a well-balanced diet that enhances his appetite and meets his nutritional needs

Interventions

1. Encourage the patient and food preparer to consider the patient's food preferences when menu planning.

2. Teach the patient to follow a diet that includes items from the four basic food groups, with sufficient vita-

Rationales

1. Including foods the patient enjoys may stimulate his appetite and promote increased food intake.

2. A well-balanced diet that includes sufficient vitamins, minerals, protein, and calories promotes increased en-

mins, minerals, protein, calories, and fluids. Advise him to include yogurt or buttermilk unless the prescribed diet prohibits these foods.

3. Instruct the patient to limit salt, sugar, fat, and caffeine; to increase protein, calories, and fiber; and to limit or increase other additives, according to prescribed guidelines.

4. Teach the patient and food preparer alternative methods of preparing food, such as steaming instead of boiling or frying foods. Encourage him to eat fresh instead of canned foods and to use herbs, spices, lemon, garlic, or onion to vary flavor, if these items are permitted. Explain that liquid supplements can be served in frozen or pudding form or mixed with soup or fruit.

5. Encourage the patient to replace sweets and junk foods with nutritious snacks, such as raw vegetables and fruits.

6. Warn the patient not to use mineral oil laxatives.

7. Teach the patient with dysphagia how to prepare foods to minimize gagging, such as thickening liquids or pureeing solid foods in a blender.

8. Teach the patient and food preparer the importance of presenting food attractively. Encourage the family to make mealtimes pleasant, social occasions that progress at a pace comfortable for the patient.

9. Encourage the patient to eat small, frequent meals rather than one or two large meals and to drink fluids about 1 hour before or after eating.

10. Instruct the patient to brush his teeth before and after meals, and discourage him from smoking.

11. Coordinate daily activities and treatments to minimize the patient's discomfort and tiredness at mealtimes.

12. If needed, demonstrate use of special feeding devices, such as utensils with built-up handles, plate guards, mugs with weighted bases, and a universal cuff.

13. Compliment the patient when he demonstrates improved dietary habits, such as eating appropriate foods and maintaining a regular meal schedule.

GOAL 2: To help the patient maintain a desirable weight

Interventions

1. Weigh the patient weekly until he achieves the desired weight; then teach him to measure and record body weight weekly to maintain the desired weight.

2. Assess the patient's diet, cooking facilities, food shopping practices, and attitudes toward food during each visit.

ergy, activity, and tissue growth. Fluids help maintain many body functions. Yogurt and buttermilk facilitate nutrient absorption.

3. The doctor may have established dietary guidelines or restrictions to treat the patient's medical condition. Compliance with treatment increases the likelihood that the patient's condition will improve.

4. Steaming helps preserve the nutrient content of foods. Fresh food contains more nutrients than the same food does after canning. Added flavor and menu variety can enhance the patient's appetite.

5. Sweets and junk foods provide empty calories that lack essential vitamins and nutrients.

6. These medications reduce vitamin absorption in the intestines.

7. Preparing foods in this manner can make swallowing easier and may encourage the patient to eat more.

8. Visually appealing meals and a pleasant atmosphere may enhance the patient's appetite. Rushing through a meal can frustrate the patient and suppress his desire to eat.

9. These measures prevent the patient from feeling empty or bloated, either of which can lead to nausea.

10. A fresh, clean mouth may enhance the patient's appetite. Smoking suppresses appetite.

11. Exhaustion and persistent pain suppress appetite.

12. Such feeding devices help a patient with limited mobility, coordination, or range of motion to eat food more easily, thus enabling him to meet his nutritional needs.

13. Positive reinforcement encourages compliance with the prescribed diet.

Rationales

1. Regular weighings detect changes in body weight, which can indicate decreased appetite, abnormal food absorption or metabolism, or poor nutrition.

2. Assessment helps in evaluating caloric and nutrient intake and compliance with the prescribed diet.

3. Teach the patient and family to plan menus and prepare foods according to the prescribed diet. Explain how to use exchange lists and how to measure foods after cooking to ensure adequate weights.

3. Knowledge about menu planning and food preparation helps the patient comply with the prescribed diet and maintain a desirable weight.

4. Warn the patient to watch for and report any signs or symptoms of diet intolerance, such as nausea, vomiting, inadequate food intake, and abdominal distention.

4. Diet intolerance interferes with maintenance of desired weight.

5. Minimize unpleasant sensations or negative stimulation during mealtime. For example, if the patient is confined to bed, prevent unpleasant odors at mealtime by removing the bedpan or urinal. If the patient complains of an unpleasant taste in his mouth, suggest he drink plenty of water or eat sweet fruit or hard, sugarless candy. If the patient is nauseated, recommend dry crackers or toast, lemon wedges, or crushed ice.

5. Associating eating with unpleasant sensations can inhibit the patient's appetite and adversely affect nutrition.

6. Involve the patient in developing all facets of the care plan.

6. Involving the patient promotes compliance with the prescribed diet and maintenance of desired weight.

7. Help the patient develop an adequate food budget. If he requires financial assistance, refer him to appropriate community resources, such as the local food bank.

7. An adequate food budget (or the local food bank, if necessary) can help ensure that the patient gets enough nutritious food to maintain desired body weight.

ASSOCIATED CARE PLANS
- Diabetes Mellitus
- Hypoglycemia
- Ineffective Coping
- Total Parenteral Nutrition

NETWORKING OF SERVICES
- Meals On Wheels
- American Diabetes Association
- American Heart Association
- American Cancer Society
- pharmacy
- local food bank

CARE TEAM INVOLVED
- nurse
- doctor
- patient and family
- dietitian
- medical social worker
- extension service home economist

IMPLICATIONS FOR HOME CARE
- accurate bathroom scale
- blender to puree solid foods for dysphagic patient
- over-the-bed table for meals
- assistive feeding devices
- dietary restrictions
- aspiration precautions for dysphagic patient
- cultural food preferences
- degree of patient independence in feeding activities
- budgeting for food

PATIENT EDUCATION TOOLS
- literature on dietary requirements and food preparation
- literature on normal weight and intake for patient
- forms for recording dietary intake and weight
- literature on home care tips for feeding the sick
- literature and forms for planning a food budget

DISCHARGE PLAN FROM HOME HEALTH CARE
Before discharge from home health care, the patient should:
- know the causes of malnutrition and the rationale for treatment
- know the signs and symptoms of malnutrition
- know when and how to contact the doctor, nurse, or emergency department with questions on his diet or for assessment and treatment
- adhere to the prescribed diet
- understand how cultural and personal preferences affect diet
- know the goals for and record dietary intake and weight gain
- know how to contact community resources for help with meal planning, preparation, and delivery
- help plan the food budget
- assume as much responsibility for planning and performing daily dietary management as possible.

SELECTED REFERENCES

Campbell, C. *Nursing Diagnosis and Intervention in Nursing Practice,* 2nd ed. New York: John Wiley & Sons, 1984.

Dudrick, S., et al. *Tips for Feeding the Sick.* Springhouse, Pa.: Springhouse Corporation, 1986.

Hufler, D. "Helping Your Dysphagic Patient Eat," *RN* 36, September 1987.

Mezzanotte, E. J. "A Checklist for Better Discharge Planning," *Nursing87* 17(10):55, October 1987.

Stuart-Siddall, S., ed. *Home Health Care Nursing.* Rockville, Md.: Aspen Systems Corporation, 1986.

Tucker, S., et al. *Patient Care Standards,* 3rd ed. St. Louis: C.V. Mosby Co., 1984.

Total Parenteral Nutrition

DESCRIPTION AND TIME FOCUS
Total parenteral nutrition (TPN) is a nutritional support program that provides all nutrients through infusion into the central venous system. TPN is ordered to maintain nutritional status in patients who either cannot eat, cannot eat enough, should not eat, or will not eat. TPN involves a higher risk for complications than enteral nutrition and is only used when enteral nutrition is not possible. Possible complications of TPN include sepsis, fluid and electrolyte imbalances, and metabolic problems such as hyperglycemia and hypoglycemia. Medicare regulations consider the TPN infusion system a prosthetic device for a patient with a permanently inoperative body organ—the GI tract.

This clinical plan focuses on home care for a patient receiving long-term TPN. A typical regimen involves daily infusion of 2 liters of a solution containing crystalline amino acids (proteins), dextrose, and electrolytes. Vitamins, trace elements, or such medications as insulin may be added to the solution. The regimen also may include infusion of ½ liter of 10% fat emulsion twice each week.

■ Typical home health care length of service for a patient receiving TPN: variable, depending on the underlying GI problem. The patient requires ongoing supervision and monitoring throughout TPN therapy.

■ Typical visit frequency: variable; a patient typically requires one or two visits a day initially, and then one visit a day for 10 days or until the patient and family can adequately manage and monitor the infusions. The nurse then visits two or three times weekly to monitor for complications and to provide teaching and support. Visit frequency decreases as the patient's confidence and ability to recognize and manage adverse effects improve.

HEALTH HISTORY FINDINGS
During a health history interview, the patient may report many these findings:
• nausea and vomiting
• diarrhea
• excessive thirst (may point to dehydration or hyperglycemia)
• chest pain (may point to air embolism)
• muscle weakness (may point to dehydration)
• fatigue, malaise, anxiety, headache, and excessive hunger (symptoms of hypoglycemia)
• history of GI cancer with intestinal obstruction
• history of inflammatory bowel syndrome with malabsorption
• history of radiation enteritis
• history of mesenteric infarction
• history of malabsorption disorder
• history of motility disorder (pseudo-obstruction)
• history of high enterocutaneous fistula

PHYSICAL FINDINGS
In a physical examination, the nurse may detect many of these findings:

Cardiovascular
• tachycardia (may point to dehydration or hypoglycemia)
• hypertension (may point to fluid overload)
• hypotension (may point to dehydration)

Respiratory
• dyspnea (may point to air embolism or fluid overload)
• coughing (may point to air embolism)
• productive cough (may point to fluid overload)
• crackles (may point to fluid overload)

Gastrointestinal
• GI problems related to the underlying pathology

Integumentary
• poor wound healing
• alopecia
• brittle nails
• irritation or phlebitis at the I.V. insertion site
• cyanosis (may point to air embolism)
• poor skin turgor (may point to dehydration or hyperglycemia)

Renal and urinary
• decreased urine output with concentrated urine

T.P.N. AND NUTRITIONAL SUPPLEMENTS

• **Water-soluble vitamins** (B complex and vitamin C) and special preparations of vitamins A, D, and E, can be added to the TPN solution; folic acid, vitamin K, and vitamin B_{12} must be administered separately. TPN solution containing vitamins should be administered promptly after mixing, because vitamin C is lost if the solution stands for 24 hours.

• **Electrolytes,** such as sodium, potassium, chloride, calcium, magnesium, and phosphorus, also may be added to TPN solutions. Amounts depend on the patient's renal status and general condition. During infusion of a TPN solution with electrolytes, the nurse must monitor the patient's cardiac and renal status and electrolyte values closely.

• **Trace elements,** such as zinc, copper, chromium, iron, manganese, selenium, molybdenum, iodine, and fluoride, usually are added to the TPN solution for a patient receiving long-term TPN therapy to prevent the serious complications that accompany trace element deficiencies.

(may point to dehydration)
• increased urine output (may point to hyperglycemia or fluid overload)

General
• dependent edema (may point to fluid overload)
• sudden weight gain (may point to fluid overload)
• sudden weight loss (may point to dehydration)
• signs of vitamin or micronutrient deficiency

DIAGNOSTIC STUDIES
The following studies may be performed to evaluate the patient's health status:
• complete blood count (CBC) and platelet count—twice weekly, then less often after TPN is well established and the patient is stable; to help detect infection
• serum electrolytes (sodium, potassium, chloride, calcium, phosphorus, and magnesium)—twice weekly at first, then less often after TPN is well established and the patient is stable; values determine the makeup of TPN solution necessary to maintain electrolytes within normal limits
• serum glucose—twice weekly at first, then less often after TPN is well established and the patient is stable; helps evaluate the body's metabolic response to TPN
• serum total protein and albumin—twice weekly at first, then less often after TPN is well established and the patient is stable; monitors nutritional status and response to TPN
• renal function tests (blood urea nitrogen [BUN] and creatinine)—twice weekly at first, then less often after TPN is well established and the patient is stable; monitors the kidneys' ability to handle the fluid and nitrogen infused in TPN therapy
• hepatic function tests (alkaline phosphatase, aspartate aminotransferase [AST, formerly SGOT], alanine aminotransferase [ALT, formerly SGPT], bilirubin, iron content and iron-binding capacity, uric acid, and prothrombin time [PT])—twice weekly at first, then less often after TPN is well established and the patient is stable; monitors liver function as an aid to evaluating the body's response to TPN
• urine glucose and acetone—once or twice daily, to detect metabolic complications

---

Nursing diagnosis: *Potential for infection related to I.V. catheter use*

GOAL: To prevent or control infection

Interventions

1. Monitor the patient for signs and symptoms of systemic infection: fever, chills, increased pulse and respiratory rates, diaphoresis, weakness, and fatigue. Assess the catheter site for signs of local infection, such as redness, swelling, and purulent drainage.

2. If you suspect that the TPN solution may be contaminated, immediately taper the I.V. infusion rate until it stops and then convert to a heparin lock. Return the suspect solution to the laboratory for culture.

3. Follow strict sterile technique when handling I.V. tubing and equipment and when performing dressing changes.

Rationales

1. Local infection can occur at the catheter site; systemic infection can result from infusion of contaminated solution. Prompt recognition of infection facilitates timely intervention to control it.

2. TPN solution is an excellent medium for bacterial growth. Contaminated solutions must not be infused. Appropriate antibiotic therapy must start as soon as possible to prevent serious systemic infection.

3. Strict sterile technique decreases the risk of infection.

Nursing diagnosis: *Knowledge deficit related to home management of TPN*

GOAL: To teach the patient and caregiver proper TPN management techniques

Interventions

1. Teach the patient and caregiver proper techniques for administering the TPN solution, including how to record the time, amount, and infusion rate of each infusion. (See *A Personal Home TPN Record* for a form the patient and caregiver can use.)

Rationales

1. The patient and caregiver will be responsible for TPN therapy when the home health nurse is not present. They must know proper administration techniques to ensure effective therapy.

A PERSONAL HOME TPN RECORD

Week of

ROUTINE	Sun		Mon		Tues		Wed		Thurs		Fri		Sat	
Temperature time [ ]														
Urine testing result % time [ ]	am	pm	am	pm	am	pm	am	pm	am	pm	am	pm	am	pm
Handwashing ✔														
TPN solution start up [cc] at rate [cc/hr]	cc		cc		cc		cc		cc		cc		cc	
TPN infusion [cc] at rate [cc/hr]	cc		cc		cc		cc		cc		cc		cc	
TPN taper off [cc] at rate [cc/hr]	cc		cc		cc		cc		cc		cc		cc	
Catheter flush ✔														
Fat emulsion [cc] days [ ]	cc		cc		cc		cc		cc		cc		cc	
Dressing change ✔ redness ✔ discomfort ✔ drainage														
Other:														
Note how you feel today														

What questions do you have?

2. Teach the patient and caregiver how to use an infusion pump and how to troubleshoot problems with this device.

3. Teach the patient and caregiver the proper procedure for administering lipid infusions. Teach them to recognize and report adverse reactions, such as chills, fever, diaphoresis, flushing, allergic reaction, headache, dizziness, or sleepiness.

4. Teach the patient and caregiver to reduce the risk of infection by properly storing and using the TPN solution. Explain that the solution must be refrigerated to the temperature stipulated by the manufacturer and must be used before the expiration date.

2. An infusion pump is mandatory for the safe administration of TPN solution. The patient and caregiver must be thoroughly familiar with its operation to ensure safe, effective therapy.

3. Independent lipid infusion involves a separate rate and separate tubing connected to the system below the TPN filter. Prompt reporting of adverse reactions by the patient facilitates timely intervention.

4. Improperly stored solution can serve as a medium for bacterial growth.

5. Teach the patient and caregiver to use sterile technique when handling the equipment and solutions and when changing dressings.

5. Sterile technique decreases the risk of infection.

6. Teach the patient and caregiver to monitor and record daily weight, temperature, urine glucose and acetone levels, and intake and output during TPN therapy.

6. These parameters help evaluate the effectiveness of TPN therapy and detect any impending complications.

7. Teach the patient and caregiver to recognize the signs and symptoms of local and systemic infection and stress the importance of promptly reporting these signs and symptoms if they occur.

7. Early recognition of signs and symptoms enables prompt intervention to treat infection and prevent sepsis.

Nursing diagnosis: *Potential for disturbance in self-concept: self-esteem, related to TPN dependence*

GOAL: To enhance the patient's self-esteem and help him cope with life-style changes

Interventions

1. Assess the patient's and family's response to activity and life-style restrictions imposed by the infusion schedule. Consult with the doctor about the possibility of nighttime infusions to facilitate independence during the day.

2. Refer the patient to a social services agency, religious advisor, or other members of the nutritional support team when appropriate.

Rationales

1. This assessment helps the nurse identify factors that may be inhibiting the patient's ability to adapt to the life-style changes imposed by the treatment.

2. An interdisciplinary approach may be necessary to resolve complex adjustment problems.

ASSOCIATED CARE PLANS
• Colorectal Cancer
• Gastroenteritis
• Gastrointestinal Cancer
• Grief and Grieving
• Hospice
• Ineffective Coping
• I.V. Therapy
• Malnutrition
• Sex and Sexuality

NETWORKING OF SERVICES
• TPN solution supply company
• infusion pump manufacturer for pump, supplies, and service
• job placement service
• vocational rehabilitation service
• counseling service for patient or family members

CARE TEAM INVOLVED
• nurse
• doctor
• patient and family
• pharmacist
• nutritionist
• medical social worker
• religious advisor

IMPLICATIONS FOR HOME CARE
• functional features of the home (adequate refrigeration for TPN solution)
• a caregiver willing to learn to administer and monitor TPN therapy when the patient requires assistance

PATIENT EDUCATION TOOLS
• literature about infusion pump use and troubleshooting
• forms for recording results of daily infusion monitoring, temperature, weight, urine glucose test results, and catheter site care
• written instructions for storing and administering the TPN and lipid solutions, including rate changes and a list of possible complications and appropriate responses

DISCHARGE PLAN FROM HOME HEALTH CARE
Before discharge from home health care, the patient should:
• demonstrate the procedure for storing and administering TPN and lipid infusions
• demonstrate the use of the infusion pump, including changing the rate when starting and stopping the intermittent infusion
• know whom to call for assistance with catheter and site care, solutions, pump, and medical or nursing care
• organize the infusion schedule to permit a return to work and usual daily activities, unless contraindicated by the underlying disease process

• demonstrate acceptance of the inability to consume foods orally

• plan enjoyable social, recreational, and daily activities within the limits imposed by TPN therapy

• contact representatives of the company supplying the TPN solution, who will provide continuing supervision and monitoring after the patient is discharged from home health care

• know the signs and symptoms of complications which must be reported to the nurse or doctor

• demonstrate how to record the time and date of solution administration and the results of daily monitoring

• know when to seek medical assistance.

SELECTED REFERENCES

ASPEN Board of Directors. "Guidelines for Use of Total Parenteral Nutrition in the Hospitalized Adult Patient," *Journal of Parenteral and Enteral Nutrition* 10(5):441-45, September/October 1986.

Burtis, G., Davis, J., and Martin, S. *Applied Nutrition and Diet Therapy*. Philadelphia: W.B. Saunders Co., 1988.

Carr, P. "When the Patient Needs TPN at Home," *RN* 49(6):25-29, June 1986.

Howard, L., Heaphey,L., and Timchalk, M. "A Review of the Current Status of Home Parenteral and Enteral Nutrition from the Provider and Consumer Perspective," *Journal of Parenteral and Enteral Nutrition* 10(4):416-23, July/August 1986.

Kee, J. *Fluids and Electrolytes with Clinical Applications: A Programmed Approach*, 4th ed. New York: John Wiley & Sons, 1986.

Mathewson, M. *Pharmacotherapeutics: A Nursing Process Approach*. Philadelphia: F.A. Davis Co., 1986.

Metheny, N. *Fluid and Electrolyte Balance: Nursing Considerations*. Philadelphia: J.B. Lippincott Co., 1987.

Shils, M., Baker, H., and Frank, O. "Blood Vitamin Levels of Adult Long-Term Home Total Parenteral Nutrition Patients: The Efficacy of the AMA-FDA Parenteral Multivitamin Formulation," *Journal of Parenteral and Enteral Nutrition* 9(2):179-88, March/April 1985.

Section IV

Community-Based Care Plans

Sexually Transmitted Diseases

DESCRIPTION AND TIME FOCUS

Sexually transmitted diseases (STDs), comprising more than 50 diseases caused by more than 20 microorganisms, refers to diseases predominantly spread by sexual contact, although certain systemic diseases can be transmitted by direct contact with blood, urine, feces, or breast milk from an infected individual. The term has replaced *venereal disease,* which had been used primarily to denote syphilis and gonorrhea. Some STDs have short-lived effects and respond well to treatment. Others require lengthy periods of treatment and can cause serious complications, permanent physical damage requiring surgical intervention, or death.

STD can affect children, infants, and fetuses in addition to sexually active adults and adolescents. Incidence is highest among individuals from low-income, urban areas, especially Blacks and Hispanics, and in those under age 25. About two-thirds of reported cases of gonorrhea involve this age-group, and adolescents experience the highest incidence of syphilis, gonorrhea, and hospitalization for pelvic inflammatory disease (PID).

This clinical plan focuses on the patient with an STD. Nursing care centers on promoting the patient's health, providing comfort, and teaching the patient about STD and techniques for preventing future infections. Education and counseling help the patient understand the risks involved in various sexual activities.

■ A patient with an STD usually is treated in a clinic. If the patient is being treated at home for another disease, home health care length of service and visit frequency will depend on the primary disease.

HEALTH HISTORY FINDINGS

In a health history interview, the patient may report many of these findings:
• anxiety
• emotional stress
• denial
• embarrassment
• sexual intercourse before age 20
• pregnancy before age 20
• history of more than three sexual partners
• partner who has had more than three sexual partners
• partner with a high risk for STD
• risky sexual behavior (oral, anal, or genital intercourse without using a condom)
• homosexuality
• I.V. drug use
• exposure to infected blood products or blood transfusions

• diabetes
• history of travel to the tropics (particularly India or Papua, New Guinea)

PHYSICAL FINDINGS

In a physical examination, the nurse may detect many of these findings:

Respiratory
• pneumonitis

Neurologic
• headache
• lassitude
• fever
• encephalitis

Gastrointestinal
• nausea
• vomiting
• pharyngitis
• oral thrush
• oral herpes simplex
• anal herpes simplex
• abdominal pain
• enterocolitis
• enlarged liver

Integumentary
• herpes zoster
• erythema
• excoriation
• edema
• itching
• lesions
• maculae and papules
• subcutaneous nodules
• urticaria
• blisters
• vesicles
• soft, fleshy, wartlike growths, usually on genitalia
• ulcers
• chancre
• pustules

Reproductive
• discharge from vagina, anus, or urethra
• dyspareunia
• ovarian enlargement; cystic ovaries
• adnexal mass

• painful, tender pelvic organs
• genital vesicles (herpes)
• genital chancre (syphilis)
• pubic nits, crab louse on genital hairs
• abnormal menses
• labial edema and excoriation
• cervicitis
• proctitis
• abnormal vaginal bleeding
• pain with manipulation of cervix during bimanual examination
• inguinal lymphadenopathy
• buboes

Renal and urinary
• dysuria
• urethritis
• frequency
• pyuria
• hematuria

DIAGNOSTIC STUDIES
The following studies may be performed to evaluate the patient's health status:

For acute urethral syndrome or cystitis
• urine culture and sensitivity—at time of diagnosis and 2 weeks after treatment is completed
• microscopic exam of urinary sediment—at time of diagnosis and 2 weeks after treatment is completed
• gonorrhea culture—at time of diagnosis
• chlamydia culture—at time of diagnosis; if inconclusive, may want to test for other sexually transmitted infections
repeat chlamydia test 6 weeks after treatment is completed

For cervical intraepithelial neoplasia
• Pap smear—every 6 months or annually until Pap smear is normal
• colposcopy—annually to rule out papilloma virus and cervical warts

For chancroid
• dark-field microscopic examination of all lesions—at time of diagnosis and if chancroid reappears
• herpes titer (blood test)—at time of diagnosis and if chancroid reappears
• syphilis (serologic test syphilis [STS]), at time of diagnosis and if chancroid reappears
Progress evaluated 3 to 5 days after therapy begins and then biweekly until infection subsides

For cytomegalovirus (CMV) infections
• CMV titer (blood)—at time of diagnosis and during pregnancy
• tissue or excretion examination—at time of diagnosis and if reinfection is suspected

For enteric infections
• microscopic examination for ova and parasites (amebiasis, giardiasis)—at time of diagnosis
• cultures (shigellosis)—at time of diagnosis
• serologic tests (hepatitis A)—at time of diagnosis

For genital warts
• examination of external genitalia—at time of diagnosis, weekly until lesions disappear, then 6 months after lesions disappear
• Pap smear for koilocytosis—at time of diagnosis, then every 6 months until pap smear is normal
• colposcopy—at time of diagnosis, then annually until normal
• syphilis (STS) to rule out condylomata lata—at time of diagnosis
• biopsy—at time of diagnosis to rule out neoplasia

For gonorrhea
• gonorrhea culture—at time of diagnosis, then 4 to 7 days after therapy is completed and if infection recurs

For granuloma inguinale
• microscopic examination of scraping—at time of diagnosis, then 3 to 5 days after therapy is completed, then weekly or biweekly until healed

For hepatitis B
• hepatitis B surface antigen (HBsAg) for patients with infection or carriers—at time of diagnosis
• anti-HBsAg for patients with infection history and present immunity—at time of diagnosis
• anti-HBe core antigen for patients with past or current infection—at time of diagnosis
• liver chemistry, bilirubin, alkaline phosphatase, aspartate aminotransferase (AST, formerly SGOT) and alanine aminotransferase (ALT, formerly SGPT)—at time of diagnosis, then 6 weeks later; patient may have negative serology test but elevated ALT if hepatitis was contracted sexually or after transfusion.

For herpes genitalis
• herpes simplex virus (HSV) tissue culture—during initial visit and then if disease recurs
• Pap smear—at time of diagnosis, then annually
• serologic test—at time of diagnosis

For lymphogranuloma venereum (LGV)
• LGV complement fixation test—at time of diagnosis

For chlamydia trachomatis
• chlamydia culture—at time of diagnosis, then at 6 months or if disease recurs
• gonorrhea culture to rule out gonorrhea—at time of diagnosis. If negative, no need to repeat; if positive, culture repeated 4 to 7 days after therapy is completed

For molluscum contagiosum
• microscopic examination of lesion—at time of diagnosis, then 1 month after treatment is completed to remove new lesions, then 1 month later if lesions persist

For mucopurulent cervicitis
• speculum examination of cervix—at time of diagnosis, after 6 months, then at 1 year if symptoms persist
• wet-mount, saline, and potassium hydroxide (KOH) microscopic examination—at time of diagnosis, repeated if symptoms persist
• chlamydia culture—at time of diagnosis, then every 6 months if symptoms persist
• gonorrhea culture—at time of diagnosis, then every 6 months if symptoms persist

For nongonococcal urethritis
• chlamydia culture—at time of diagnosis, repeated in 3 to 6 months if symptoms recur with a new partner
• gonorrhea culture—at time of diagnosis, repeated in 3 to 6 months if symptoms recur with a new partner
• wet mount microscopic examination of urethral-cervical discharge to rule out trichomonas, candida—at time of diagnosis, repeated in 3 to 6 months, or if symptoms persist or recur
• herpes titer—at time of diagnosis, repeated if symptoms recur with new partner
• syphilis (STS)—at time of diagnosis, repeated if symptoms recur with new partner

For pediculosis pubis
• inspection of genital hair for lice or nits—at time of diagnosis, then 7 to 10 days after treatment
• microscopic examination of crab louse—at time of diagnosis

For pelvic inflammatory disease
• temperature, pulse, respiration measurements to rule out elevated temperature—at time of diagnosis, then 48 to 72 hours after therapy begins
• white blood cell (WBC) count to rule out elevated WBC count—at time of diagnosis, then 48 to 72 hours after therapy begins, again 2 to 3 days after therapy is completed if warranted by infection severity
• urine pregnancy test or serum beta subunit—if applicable
• wet-mount microscopic examination of discharge to rule out trichomonas or candida—at time of diagnosis
• pelvic ultrasound to rule out ectopic pregnancy or adnexal mass—at time of diagnosis, depending on infection severity and pelvic examination findings
• serum erythrocyte sedimentation rate (ESR) to rule out elevated ESR—at time of diagnosis, again 2 to 3 days after therapy is completed
• Gram stain of endocervical discharge to rule out gonorrhea or chlamydia—at time of diagnosis
• culdocentesis to rule out WBC or bacteria in peritoneal fluid—at time of diagnosis, depending on infection severity and pelvic examination findings

For scabies
• microscopic examination of mite, eggs, larvae, or feces in scrapings—at time of diagnosis, 1 week after treatment begins, and 1 week after treatment ends
• cutaneous biopsy—at time of diagnosis if required

For syphilis
• STS, required for all patients with genital lesions—at time of diagnosis; if positive, every 3 months for 2 years after treatment is completed

For trichomoniasis
• saline wet-mount microscopic examination of cervical, vaginal, or urethral discharge for pear-shape motile protozoan—at time of diagnosis, repeated if reinfected
• Pap smear (not diagnostic of active infection)—annually
• chlamydia culture—sometimes performed after treatment for trichomoniasis is completed if symptoms persist
• gonorrhea culture—sometimes performed after treatment for trichomoniasis is completed if symptoms persist

For bacterial vaginosis
• saline wet-mount or Gram stain microscopic examination of cervical, vaginal, or urethral discharge to identify clue cells—at time of diagnosis, repeated after treatment if reinfected
• elevated vaginal pH (above 4.5 to 5.5)—at time of diagnosis, repeated after treatment if reinfected by untreated partner
• evaluation of vaginal discharge with wet mount prepared with 10% KOH solution—at time of diagnosis, repeated after treatment if reinfected by untreated partner
• chlamydia and gonorrhea cultures—at time of diagnosis (if diagnosis is questionable) or if discharge persists after treatment

For candidiasis
• Pap smear—annually
• vaginal pH test (should be normal pH of 3.8 to 4.2)—at time of diagnosis and if disease recurs
• glucose tolerance test to rule out diabetes—if reinfection occurs more than three times per year

Nursing diagnosis: *Knowledge deficit related to STD*

GOAL: To improve the patient's knowledge of STD

Interventions	**Rationales**
1. Assess the patient's life-style, ability to learn, and current knowledge about the infection. Determine the partner's understanding and willingness to support the patient and participate in teaching sessions.	1. A baseline assessment helps in preparing appropriate teaching sessions.
2. Teach the patient and partner about the infection; discuss the cause, routes of transmission, signs and symptoms, treatment, and prevention methods. Provide appropriate literature to reinforce concepts covered in teaching sessions.	2. Teaching the patient and partner about STD reduces the likelihood of reinfection. Pamphlets, reprints, and books are powerful teaching aids and reference materials the patient can use whenever accurate information is needed.
3. Teach the patient about prescribed medications, such as oral antibiotics, topical ointments and creams, or vaginal suppositories. Explain the appropriate administration method, schedules, adverse effects, and the importance of complying with treatment.	3. Proper administration and compliance help ensure treatment effectiveness.
4. If the patient is pregnant, encourage her to talk with the obstetrician about possible risks to the fetus. Explain that the disease may cause scarring of the fallopian tubes and uterine wall and that sterility may result.	4. Pregnant patients must be informed of the disease's potential effects.
5. Explain the importance of notifying all sexual contacts of their exposure to the disease.	5. Prompt testing and treatment help prevent disease dissemination.

Nursing diagnosis: *Altered patterns of sexuality related to infection*

GOAL: To help the patient develop normal sexual patterns and avoid recurrence of the infection

Interventions	**Rationales**
1. Take the patient's sexual history; include the age at which the patient first had intercourse, number of sexual partners, pregnancies or terminations, and sexual preference. Assess his knowledge, concerns, and attitudes about sexual activity and disease transmission.	1. A baseline assessment helps in planning appropriate teaching sessions.
2. Encourage an honest discussion by developing a caring and confidential relationship with the patient. Assure him that this information will be kept confidential.	2. Many patients with STD are reluctant to discuss their sexual conduct. Conveying an honest interest in the patient's well-being and assuring confidentiality helps in overcoming this reluctance.
3. Explain to the patient the need to abstain from sexual intercourse. Discuss alternative methods of achieving sexual satisfaction, such as cuddling, kissing, massage, and mutual masturbation. Encourage the patient to express concerns and ask questions.	3. Understanding alternative methods of sexual expression helps the patient cope with the need to abstain from sexual intercourse. The patient also may need advice and emotional support before discussing with their partners the necessary changes in routine sexual practices.
4. If the patient has multiple sexual partners, stress the importance of using a latex condom when resuming sexual intercourse.	4. Using a latex condom may help prevent infection.

Nursing diagnosis: *Disturbance in self-esteem related to stigma of STD*

GOAL: To promote the patient's self-esteem

Interventions

1. Encourage the patient to express concerns and fears. Listen, convey reassurance, and avoid making judgments. Refer the patient to a support group or counseling service, if necessary.

2. Correct any misconceptions the patient may have about the disease, reiterate the importance of complying with treatments and notifying sexual partners, and suggest effective coping techniques.

3. Restate the disease's transmission routes and methods of preventing reinfection.

4. Encourage the patient to make decisions concerning the care plan whenever appropriate.

Rationales

1. Fear and embarrassment about the disease, its physical effects, and the need to talk with partners can damage the patient's self-esteem. An open discussion with the nurse or a counselor may help alleviate some of his concerns.

2. Inadequate information about the disease and the need for compliance can prompt the patient to make inaccurate value judgments (such as "Only bad people contract STD.") which can reduce self-esteem. Correcting misconceptions, explaining treatment rationales, and identifying coping strategies help the patient maintain self-esteem and cope with emotional difficulties during recovery.

3. Understanding how the disease is transmitted and how to prevent it may allay the patient's fears about resuming sexual intercourse.

4. Making personal health care decisions enhances the patient's self-esteem.

Nursing diagnosis: *Impaired skin integrity related to infection*

GOAL: To promote healing of lesions

Interventions

1. Administer topical ointments and creams and systemic medications as ordered.

2. Provide appropriate wound care, according to doctor's orders and agency protocol.

3. Assess the patient's anal and genital areas for herpes lesions, vesicles, or blisters during each visit. Teach him to discard dressings properly. Explain that he should wash his hands thoroughly, especially after touching infected areas.

Rationales

1. Many infections, such as herpes, scabies, and pediculosis, respond quickly to conventional therapy.

2. Some lesions require wound care to promote healing and reduce the risk of further infection.

3. Regular assessment ensures timely intervention to treat spreading infection or complications. Proper techniques of hand washing and dressing disposal help prevent further infection.

ASSOCIATED CARE PLANS
• Acquired Immunodeficiency Syndrome
• Hepatitis
• Ineffective Coping
• Sex and Sexuality

NETWORKING OF SERVICES
• state Public Health Association
• Centers for Disease Control
• Herpes Resource Center
• American Fertility Society
• Resolve (local chapters provide information, counseling, and emotional support to couples with fertility problems)
• STD clinic

• family planning clinic
• pharmacy
• outpatient laboratory services

CARE TEAM INVOLVED
• nurse
• doctor
• patient (and partner, if possible)
• sex counselor
• social worker

IMPLICATIONS FOR HOME CARE
• environment that affords privacy and physical and emotional comfort
• telephone (communication)

PATIENT EDUCATION TOOLS
• literature on diagnosis and treatment
• literature on the prescribed medication plan
• literature about the infection
• list of normal temperature, pulse, and respirations
• literature on sex and health education

DISCHARGE PLAN FROM HOME HEALTH CARE
Before discharge from home health care, the patient should:
• be coping with physical and emotional discomfort
• be aware of the risk of STD transmission during sexual activity and know the activities that increase the risk
• understand how diseases and infections are transmitted, methods of prevention, and STD consequences
• know the signs and symptoms of infection
• know the behaviors that increase the likelihood of infection
• understand the importance of complying with treatment
• know the method of administration, dosage, action, and adverse effects of each prescribed medication
• understand the importance of finishing the prescription, even if signs and symptoms of infection subside
• know when to resume sexual activity
• understand that latex condoms can help prevent infection
• have the telephone number of the doctor and home health agency for follow-up care, as needed
• know the dates of follow-up appointments with the doctor or clinic
• understand how STD affects pregnancy
• know that proper genital hygiene and postcoital urination prevent recurrent urethritis
• inform sexual partners about the disease and encourage them to consult a doctor
• understand that partners should discuss their sexual histories with each other when initiating a sexual relationship.

SELECTED REFERENCES
Connell, E.B., and Tatum, H.J. *Sexually Transmitted Diseases: Diseases and Treatment.* Durant, Okla.: Creative Infomatics, Inc., 1986.

Coles, R., and Stokes, G. *Sex and the American Teenager.* Harper & Row Publishers, 1985.

Hatcher, R.A., et al. *Contraceptive Technology 1988-1989,* 14th revised ed. New York: Irvington Publishers, Inc., 1988.

Hawkins, J.W., et al. *Protocols for Nurse Practitioners in Gynecologic Settings.* New York: Tiresias Press, Inc., 1987.

Hoole, A.J., et al. *Patient Care Guidelines for Nurse Practitioners,* 2nd ed. Boston: Little Brown & Co., 1982.

Withington, A.M., et al. *Teenage Sexual Health.* New York: Irvington Publishers, Inc., 1983.

COMMUNITY-BASED CARE PLANS

Acquired Immunodeficiency Syndrome (AIDS)

DESCRIPTION AND TIME FOCUS

Acquired immunodeficiency syndrome (AIDS) is caused by infection with the human immunodeficiency virus (HIV). HIV is transmitted through sexual contact (especially anal or vaginal intercourse), direct percutaneous exposure to infected blood, or from mother to child in utero, during delivery, or by breast-feeding.

The initial HIV infection may cause an acute febrile illness that resolves spontaneously. A period characterized by asymptomatic infections usually follows and may last more than 10 years. The limit of AIDS incubation is unknown. In later stages, HIV causes profound cellular immunodeficiency by destroying CD4 lymphocytes, thus increasing the patient's susceptibility to opportunistic disease. HIV also affects many organs directly.

An AIDS diagnosis indicates end-stage HIV infection and usually coincides with discovery of an opportunistic infection or cancer. Diagnosis may also reveal HIV encephalopathy, a progressive and incapacitating neurologic disease, or HIV wasting syndrome, characterized by profound weight loss and chronic fever or diarrhea.

AIDS progression is variable. Many AIDS patients experience periods of good health between acute episodes of opportunistic disease. However, most patients inevitably experience multiple, severe infections and dramatic deterioration of health. Profound dementia is common in later stages, and most patients die within 2 years of diagnosis.

This clinical plan focuses on home care of an AIDS patient with an opportunistic disease, encephalopathy, or wasting syndrome. A patient in the early stages of AIDS is usually well enough to participate in the care plan. The home is a comfortable and secure environment for a patient receiving short-term or intermittent care for specific infections. Home care also facilitates patient comfort during terminal care.

■ Typical home health care length of service for a patient with AIDS: depends on the disease's progression

■ Typical visit frequency: two or three times weekly, with daily visits as death nears. Hospice services should be offered to the dying AIDS patient.

HEALTH HISTORY FINDINGS

In a health history interview, the patient may report many of these findings:
• fatigue and malaise
• extreme distress due to diagnosis and prognosis
• anorexia
• nausea and vomiting
• weight loss of more than 10% of baseline weight
• social isolation or nontraditional family structure
• multiple losses (friends, employment, physical attractiveness, future) due to diagnosis and illness
• history of substance abuse (particularly I.V. drug use)
• deterioration of health before diagnosis
• anxiety
• depression
• recurrent fever
• malnutrition
• lymphadenopathy

PHYSICAL FINDINGS

In a physical examination, the nurse may detect many of these findings:

Respiratory
• dyspnea
• persistent cough
• crackles

Neurologic
• cognitive impairment
• memory loss
• apathy
• depression
• headache
• psychomotor retardation
• gait disturbance
• ataxia
• seizures
• global dementia

Gastrointestinal
• oral candidiasis
• dysphagia and anorexia
• oral and anal herpes simplex
• chronic watery diarrhea
• gingivitis

Integumentary
• Kaposi's sarcoma lesions
• herpes zoster
• dermatitis or eczema
• pruritus
• cyanosis
• alopecia

General
• vision loss or impairment

DIAGNOSTIC STUDIES

The following studies may be performed to evaluate the patient's health status:
• HIV antibody testing—antibody is usually detectable 4 to 12 weeks after infection but may be lost in the late phase of illness
• complete blood count (CBC)—to detect leukopenia, anemia, thrombocytopenia

• delayed hypersensitivity skin testing—to detect partial or complete anergy
• CD4 lymphocyte counts—usually less than 400 mm/cc² in seriously ill patients
• blood and urine cultures—often positive for cytomegalovirus (CMV), Epstein-Barr virus, or mycobacterium aviumns complex (MAC)

• Mantoux test—to detect tuberculosis; may be falsely negative in an immunosuppressed patient
• chest X-ray—for interstitial infiltrates
• brain imaging—to detect cortical atrophy, specific abnormalities, or ring-enhancing lesions
• stool for ova and parasites and culture—to detect amebiasis, giardiasis, salmonellosis, or cryptosporidiosis

PRECAUTIONS FOR CARING FOR A PATIENT WITH A.I.D.S.

Home health nurses and caregivers can attend to the needs of a patient with AIDS—and do so safely, without fear of contracting the disease—by observing special precautions when providing care. For example, HIV transmission from contact with infected body fluids during needle-stick or inspection of mucous membranes or open wounds is rare but possible, so caregivers should use simple barrier precautions to prevent contact with the patient's blood or other body fluids. (Because HIV is not transmitted through the air, food, water, or fomites, risk of transmission to family and friends is minimal.) Follow the guidelines listed here, and be sure to share them with the patient's caregivers.

• Take extra precautions to prevent injury from contaminated needles, lancets, razors, and certain I.V. catheters. Never recap, bend, clip, or break used needles or syringes by hand; instead, discard them immediately in a puncture-resistant container; seal and incinerate full containers.

• Wear disposable gloves when performing procedures that involve contact with the patient's blood, urine, feces, saliva, or other fluids and when handling or cleaning objects soiled with blood or secretions.

• Wash hands immediately with soap and water after accidental contact with any body fluid and after removing gloves.

• Wear a gown when performing procedures in which clothing may be soiled by the patient's body fluids.

• Wear a mask and eye protection when performing procedures that may involve splashing or spraying secretions, such as tracheotomy care or suctioning. Also wear a mask if the patient has pulmonary tuberculosis with a positive sputum culture or an undiagnosed productive cough.

• Clean blood and body waste spills with the bleach solution or other germicide; wear gloves and use paper towels or another disposable cleaning product.

• Be sure the patient has exclusive use of a thermometer and equipment used during wound care and dressing changes; stethoscopes and blood pressure cuffs require no special attention unless soiled with body fluids.

• Collect specimens in a leak-proof container, and place this container in another container (such as a sturdy plastic bag) for transport; label containers appropriately.

• Wash eating utensils in hot, soapy water or a dishwasher after meals; keeping separate utensils for the patient is unnecessary.

• Wear gloves to handle clothing and bed linens only if they are soiled with blood or other body fluids; wash the clothing in hot water; washing machines require no special treatment.

• Dispose of gloves, diapers, tissue, and dressings in a heavy-duty plastic bag, tie it shut, place it in a second plastic bag, and dispose with other household garbage.

• Use a solution of one part liquid chlorine bleach to ten parts water as an effective, inexpensive disinfectant. HIV is fragile and easily killed by commercial germicides, alcohol, Betadine, and other disinfectants.

Nursing diagnosis: Anxiety related to the stigma associated with AIDS; poor prognosis and uncertain course of disease; guilt about sexual history, drug use, or possible infection of partners or children; lack of a cure; or process of dying and death

GOAL 1: To alleviate the patient's anxiety

Interventions

1. Cultivate an honest, nonjudgmental, and accepting relationship with the patient to encourage discussion of concerns and fears.

2. Explain the rationale for using barrier precautions during physical care. Touch the patient whenever skin-to-skin contact is safe and appropriate, such as shaking hands or providing a back rub.

Rationales

1. The patient may experience rejection and discrimination because of his diagnosis, sexual orientation, or drug use. Interacting with an accepting person may reduce anxiety or anger and increase self-esteem.

2. Using barrier precautions when they are unwarranted increases the patient's feelings of isolation and anger.

3. Refer the patient for treatment of persistent anxiety or depression, if necessary.

3. Medication or psychotherapy may alleviate anxiety and depression.

GOAL 2: To establish a support system of family, friends, and community resources

Interventions

1. Involve the patient's family and friends in all facets of the patient's care.

2. Refer the patient, family members, or friends to appropriate community agencies or AIDS service organizations.

Rationales

1. Involving family and friends in planning and care helps them cope with the patient's illness and reduces the patient's feeling of isolation.

2. Community AIDS organizations provide the patient with emotional support, services, and counseling and can help reduce stress felt by the caregivers, thereby improving their ability to care for and support the patient.

Nursing diagnosis: *Potential for infection related to loss of cellular immunity from CD4 lymphocyte destruction or to neutropenia*

GOAL 1: To reduce the patient's risk for infection

Interventions

1. Teach the patient and caregiver to recognize and reduce infection hazards. Explain that:
• thorough housekeeping removes molds and other potentially infectious organisms
• the patient should not come in contact with animal feces, particularly of cats, birds, and fish
• the patient should consume pasteurized dairy products because nonpasteurized products contain bacteria that can cause serious illness
• foods from animals, including eggs, must be cooked thoroughly.

2. If the patient is sexually active, teach him precautions or refer him to an AIDS service group or to public health personnel for this important instruction.

3. Teach the patient and caregiver the importance of minimizing the patient's exposure to communicable diseases. Explain that:
• caregivers must wash their hands before providing direct care
• persons with acute communicable disease should be excluded from patient care or should exercise precautions (such as wearing a mask) if patient contact is unavoidable
• a patient caring for a young child should wash hands thoroughly after diapering or feeding the child and after attending to the child's cuts or scrapes
• a child living with the patient should receive a polio vaccine injection instead of an orally administered polio vaccine.

Rationales

1. Opportunistic diseases can originate in the patient's home (for example, *Toxoplasma gondii* in raw meat and cat feces; *Salmonella* in animal feces, raw poultry, and eggs; and nonpasteurized milk).

2. Techniques that make HIV transmission less likely include using a latex condom and a spermicide containing nonoxynol-9 during intercourse and employing methods that do not include penetration. These techniques also protect the patient from other sexually transmitted diseases and, possibly, other strains of HIV.

3. Precautions are necessary because household members and caregivers can transmit serious illnesses to the patient. A child who receives an oral polio vaccine excretes the virus in stool.

GOAL 2: To identify early signs and symptoms of opportunistic disease

Interventions	**Rationales**
1. Assess the patient for signs and symptoms of *Pneumocystis carinii* pneumonia, such as dyspnea, nonproductive cough, crackles, and rhonchi.	1. *P. carinii* pneumonia, the most common serious infection found in AIDS patients, is a major cause of death. Treatment usually succeeds if the disease is identified in its early stages.
2. Monitor the patient's temperature, and report increases to the doctor.	2. Increased temperature may indicate a new or recurring infection.
3. Frequently assess the patient's skin and mouth for infections and lesions.	3. Prompt treatment of common infections, such as oral candidiasis or anal herpes, can prevent serious and extensive infection.
4. Administer prophylactic antibiotics as ordered.	4. Infectious organisms are difficult to eradicate in the AIDS patient; prophylactic antibiotics may be ordered to prevent recurrence.
5. Administer antiviral medications such as zidovudine (Retrovir), as ordered.	5. Zidovudine, which inhibits the replication of HIV, may prevent opportunistic diseases.

Nursing diagnosis: *Altered thought processes related to HIV infection of the central nervous system, specific opportunistic infections or cancers, or medication*

GOAL 1: To recognize changes in the patient's mental status

Interventions	**Rationales**
1. Assess the patient's mental status during the first visit. Document assessment findings.	1. A baseline assessment helps the nurse recognize changes in the patient's mental status.
2. Periodically reassess the patient's mental status.	2. A sudden change in mental status can indicate an opportunistic infection (such as toxoplasmosis or cryptococcal meningitis), central nervous system neoplasm, or HIV encephalopathy. Onset of dementia may necessitate a change in the home care plan.
3. Carefully assess the patient's ability to comprehend and remember information during teaching sessions.	3. Cognitive impairment and short-term memory loss are common in AIDS patients. Teaching sessions may require reinforcement or repetition.

GOAL 2: To protect the patient from health hazards in the home

Interventions	**Rationales**
1. Assess the patient's need for supervision.	1. Continuous care may be necessary for a severely impaired patient.
2. Eliminate household hazards that can cause falls, fires, or other accidents. Encourage the family to install protective equipment, such as gates, in appropriate locations.	2. A disoriented and forgetful patient is vulnerable to household hazards.
3. Monitor self-administered medications by counting pills and encouraging the patient to use reminders, such as alarm clocks or individual dosage devices.	3. Monitoring reduces the likelihood of overdose or missed doses. A patient on zidovudine, which must be taken every 4 hours around the clock, must be particularly attentive.

Nursing diagnosis: *Altered nutrition: less than body requirements, related to anorexia, frequent oropharyngeal infections, nausea and vomiting, or chronic diarrhea*

GOAL: To ensure adequate nutrition and fluid balance

Interventions	Rationales
1. Assess the patient's current weight and recent changes, current diet, food preferences, and food intolerances.	1. This baseline information helps the nurse plan interventions.
2. Monitor the patient's weight, intake and output, caloric intake, and hydration status.	2. Sudden deterioration in the patient's nutritional status may indicate a new infection or the need for parenteral nutrition.
3. Encourage the patient to eat small, frequent meals of preferred foods. Explain that bland and soft foods may be better tolerated. Also suggest palatable nutritional supplements.	3. An anorexic patient usually tolerates small, palatable meals more easily.
4. Refer the patient for nutritional consultation as necessary.	4. Consultation may help a patient who has several nutritional problems.
5. Encourage the patient to use Meals On Wheels, homemaker services, or food stamps, when appropriate.	5. The patient may lack the financial resources, energy, or motivation to buy and prepare food.

Nursing diagnosis: *Impaired skin integrity related to infection, immobility, incontinence, or chronic diarrhea*

GOAL 1: To promote healing of skin lesions

Interventions	Rationales
1. Administer topical and systemic medications as ordered.	1. Many skin problems, such as herpes simplex lesions, respond to conventional therapy.
2. Perform wound care and decubitus care as necessary.	2. Proper wound care promotes healing and reduces the risk of further infection.

GOAL 2: To maintain skin integrity

Interventions	Rationales
1. Teach the patient and caregiver the importance of changing the patient's position frequently and protecting bony prominences. Encourage use of protective items, such as heel guards, pads, and fleeces, to promote skin integrity.	1. Frequent position changes and pressure point protection prevent skin breakdown.
2. Frequently assess the region around the patient's anus and genitals for skin irritation or breakdown. When necessary, use such devices as external catheters or diapers to protect skin.	2. Skin breakdown from chronic diarrhea or incontinence is common among AIDS patients.
3. Help the patient bathe. Apply lotions and other skin-care products as necessary.	3. The patient may be too weak or confused to maintain adequate hygiene without assistance.

Nursing diagnosis: *Sleep pattern disturbance related to the AIDS process or opportunistic disease*

GOAL: To promote adequate rest and sleep

Interventions

1. When planning patient care, consider the patient's existing sleep and rest schedule and activity tolerance. Plan to let the patient rest after bathing, wound care, or other stressful or tiring procedures.

2. If necessary, encourage the patient and caregiver to obtain homemaker services or to enlist a volunteer to help with activities of daily living (ADLs).

3. Teach the patient methods of conserving energy, such as using a shower stool or bedside commode.

4. If the patient has trouble sleeping, assess his need for pharmacologic intervention.

Rationales

1. Preventing disruptions in the patient's existing schedule and planning additional respites after procedures promote adequate rest.

2. The patient may have trouble performing ADLs independently because of chronic fatigue and weakness.

3. The need for frequent toileting and clean-up can deplete the patient's energy.

4. Appropriate medication can alleviate sleep disorders caused by anxiety or depression.

ASSOCIATED CARE PLANS
• Brain Tumors
• Esophagitis
• Gastroenteritis
• Grief and Grieving
• Hospice
• Pneumonia
• Seizure Disorders
• Sex and Sexuality
• Substance Abuse
• Total Parenteral Nutrition
• Tuberculosis

NETWORKING OF SERVICES
• AIDS service organizations
• Meals On Wheels
• hospice
• AIDS hot-line services
• homemaker service

CARE TEAM INVOLVED
• doctor
• nurse
• patient and family
• homemaker
• nutritionist
• medical social worker

PATIENT EDUCATION TOOLS
• free or low-cost materials from local or state health departments and AIDS service organizations
• American Red Cross
• materials from the San Francisco AIDS Foundations
• literature on each medication ordered

IMPLICATIONS FOR HOME CARE
• safe, clean environment
• telephone (communication)
• availability of support system

DISCHARGE PLAN FROM HOME HEALTH CARE
Before discharge from home health care, the patient and caregiver should:
• know the signs and symptoms of the most common opportunistic diseases, such as pneumonia and meningitis
• know the schedule and possible adverse effects of each medication prescribed
• contact appropriate agencies for services and support
• understand routes of HIV transmission and precautions necessary to prevent sexual and body fluid-borne transmission.

SELECTED REFERENCES
American Red Cross and U.S. Public Health Service. *Caring for the AIDS Patient at Home.* October 1986.
Bryant, J. "Home Care of the Client with AIDS," *Journal of Community Health Nursing* 3(2):69-74, 1986.
Centers for Disease Control. "Recommendations for Prevention of HIV Transmission in Health-Care Settings," *MMWR* 36 (suppl. no. 2S), 1987.
Centers for Disease Control. "Revision of the CDC Surveillance Case Definition for Acquired Immunodeficiency Syndrome," *MMWR* 36 (suppl. no. 1S), 1987.
Carr, G. and Gee, G. "AIDS and AIDS-Related Conditions: Screening for Populations at Risk," *Nurse Practitioner* 11:25-48, October 1986.
New Jersey Home Health Agency Assembly and New Jersey State Department of Health. *Home Care Guidelines for AIDS Patients.* October 1987.
Salyer, J., et al. "AIDS: Holistic Home Care," *Home Healthcare Nurse* 5(2):10-18, 1987.
San Francisco General Hospital. "Nursing Care Plan for Persons with AIDS," *Quality Review Bulletin* 12(10):361-65, October 1986.
Scheitinger, H. "A Home Care Plan for AIDS," *AJN* 86(9):1021-28, October 1986.

Teenage Pregnancy

DESCRIPTION AND TIME FOCUS

After a brief decline in the early 1980s, sexual activity among teenagers in the United States is increasing; current estimates indicate that 70% of females and 80% of males have sexual intercourse by age 20. Of sexually active women ages 15 to 19, about 65% either use no birth control method or use one inconsistently. As a result, 1 in 10 teenage women become pregnant each year, and 4 in 10 become pregnant before they reach age 20. Incidence is highest in low-income, urban areas and in areas where adequate sex education is lacking.

This clinical plan focuses on the adolescent patient during pregnancy and the postpartum period. Adolescence is a unique developmental stage with specific health care requirements; health care services must address these requirements. Teenage mothers suffer higher-than-average levels of toxemia, anemia bleeding, cervical trauma, and premature delivery and are more likely to give birth to low-birthweight infants. Nursing care centers on monitoring the patient during pregnancy and after delivery for complications, teaching health-promoting activities, assessing her relationships with her family and the father, and determining her need for social support services.

■ Typical home health care length of service for teenage pregnancy: 6 weeks

■ Typical visit frequency: twice weekly for 2 weeks, then once weekly for 4 weeks

HEALTH HISTORY FINDINGS

In a health history interview, the patient may report many of these findings:
- anemia
- preeclampsia
- pregnancy-induced hypertension
- gestational diabetes
- malnutrition or obesity
- substance abuse
- sexually transmitted disease
- low-birthweight infant
- lack of early prenatal care
- urinary tract infection
- pelvic dystocia
- emotional stress
- low self-esteem

PHYSICAL FINDINGS

In a physical examination, the nurse may detect many of these findings:

Cardiovascular
- anemia (iron deficiency, folic acid, sickle cell)
- increased heart rate
- pregnancy-induced hypertension
- preeclampsia, eclampsia
- faintness
- ankle edema
- varicose veins
- spider nevi

Respiratory
- shortness of breath
- dyspnea
- nasal congestion

Neurologic
- carpal tunnel syndrome
- Bell's palsy
- numbness or tingling in hands

Gastrointestinal
- hyperemesis gravidarum
- nausea and vomiting
- constipation
- hemorrhoids
- heartburn
- food cravings
- bleeding gums
- dental caries
- cholelithiasis, cholecystitis

Integumentary
- pruritus
- striae gravidarum
- melasma
- linea nigra

Musculoskeletal
- contracted pelvis
- leg cramps
- joint pain
- back pain

Reproductive
- genital herpes
- gonorrhea
- syphilis
- chlamydia
- vaginitis

Renal and urinary
- nephritis
- cystitis
- urinary frequency

General
- gestational diabetes
- extreme obesity
- malnutrition

• hyperthyroidism or hypothyroidism
• hypoglycemia

DIAGNOSTIC STUDIES

The following studies may be performed to evaluate the patient's health status:
• hemoglobin and hematocrit—initially, then repeated every 2 to 3 months to detect anemia
• hemoglobin electrophoresis—to detect sickle cell anemia and hemoglobinopathy
• alpha-fetoprotein—to screen for neural tube defect in fetus
• Rh typing—to identify erythroblastosis fetalis in fetuses or hyperbilirubinemia in newborns
• fasting blood glucose and 1-hour glucose tolerance—to detect diabetes mellitus or gestational diabetes
• rubella titer—to determine rubella immunity
• Venereal Disease Research Laboratories (VDRL) test—initially, then repeat at 32 weeks' gestation to detect untreated syphilis
• blood urea nitrogen (BUN), creatinine electrolytes, creatinine clearance, total protein excretion—to evaluate level of renal compromise
• urinalysis, including microscopic examination—during each prenatal visit to detect unsuspected renal disease, hypertension, or diabetes
• gonorrhea culture—to screen for asymptomatic infection
• Papanicolaou smear—to screen for intraepithelial neoplasia, herpes simplex type II
• ultrasound—during first trimester to confirm pregnancy, establish dates, identify uterine mass, confirm viability; during second trimester to verify dates and fetal size, rule out intrauterine growth retardation, and detect congenital anomalies or multiple gestation; during third trimester to verify dates and fetal size, deter-mine fetal position, ascertain cardiac activity, rule out placenta previa or abruptio placentae, and determine amniotic fluid volume
• amniocentesis—at 16 weeks' gestation to detect genetic problems (such as Down's syndrome or neural tube defects), if warranted by family history, or to detect sex-linked and metabolic disorders; in late pregnancy to ascertain fetal age
• fetal heart rate—during each visit, first heard between 8 and 12 weeks' gestation
• nonstress test—recommended in high-risk pregnancies and repeated twice weekly to ascertain accelerated fetal heart rate in response to fetal activity. A reactive test indicates a normal fetus with a good perinatal prognosis; a nonreactive test indicates a need for further tests
• nipple stimulated contraction stress test—nipple stimulation for 10 minutes should cause uterine contractions 10 minutes later with no deceleration in fetal heart rate (negative result); positive result of decelerated fetal heart rate indicates increased risk of perinatal morbidity and mortality
• daily fetal movement count—recommended for high-risk patients or when decreased fetal movement is reported; counts number of fetal movements during 1 hour. Three or more movements is the desired result; less than three movements necessitates immediate stress test
• oxytocin-stimulated contraction stress test—rarely ordered, involves I.V. drip of oxytocin; considered negative when three uterine contractions last 40 to 60 seconds without a decrease in fetal heart rate; positive result indicates increased risk to the fetus and the need for an expeditious vaginal delivery (if the patient has a successful induction) or cesarean section

---

Nursing diagnosis: *Knowledge deficit related to teenage pregnancy*

GOAL 1: To improve the patient's knowledge of pregnancy, labor, and delivery

Interventions	Rationales
1. Assess the patient's reaction to her pregnancy by establishing a therapeutic relationship.	1. Adolescents usually wait until pregnancy is advanced before seeking care. The nurse should try to minimize barriers, such as financial hardship or accessibility, that prevent the teenager from using the health care system.
2. Assess the patient for physiologic and psychological effects of pregnancy. Be alert for pregnancy-induced hypertension, intrauterine growth retardation, denial, and a delay in prenatal attachment behaviors.	2. Adolescents are prone to pregnancy complications, which can be treated if detected early.
3. Teach the patient about proper nutrition and its importance during pregnancy. Encourage proper nutrition by helping the patient establish a food budget and plan meals.	3. A proper diet promotes normal weight gain during pregnancy and delivery of a healthy infant.
4. Provide primary nursing care in a nonjudgmental manner. Work closely with the patient and obstetrician to ensure the patient's optimum health. Direct the pa-	4. People learn by various educational strategies. Education provides an excellent vehicle for optimum health care.

tient to appropriate classes, demonstrations, and literature.

Interventions	Rationales
5. Assess the educational needs of the patient, family members, and father (if present). Help the patient explore alternative methods of meeting health and educational requirements, if necessary.	5. Keeping the patient in school may be impractical. Such alternatives as night school or tutoring can help pregnant patients meet educational requirements for graduation.

GOAL 2: To help the patient develop a support system

Interventions	Rationales
1. Teach family members about the physical and psychological changes that occur during pregnancy.	1. Family members are better prepared—and often more willing—to provide support when they understand the patient's physical and emotional needs.
2. Assess the patient's need for financial assistance, infant care, and social acceptance. Refer the patient to appropriate community services, such as a Women's, Infants, and Children (WIC) program, day care center, women's center, counseling service, and religious group. Encourage participation in school programs.	2. Community resources constitute an integral part of the patient's support network and can help her develop and improve parenting and coping skills.

Nursing diagnosis: *Knowledge deficit related to parenting and infant care*

GOAL: To improve the patient's knowledge of parenting and infant care

Interventions	Rationales
1. Assess the patient and caregiver to determine knowledge deficiencies. Begin teaching the patient about infant care before delivery.	1. A baseline assessment of knowledge helps the nurse plan appropriate instruction. Learning about infant care before delivery prepares the patient for duties that will begin immediately after delivery and helps her adjust to the new role of parent.
2. Teach the patient the importance of proper self-care, including personal hygiene, exercise, rest, nutrition, and breast care.	2. Inadequate rest and poor nutrition can cause postpartum hemorrhage. Proper breast care promotes an adequate milk supply in nursing mothers.
3. Assess the patient for mood changes and feelings of inadequacy. Encourage the patient to express her concerns and needs. Develop a teaching plan that helps her adapt to her new role as parent.	3. Information about infant care and parenting helps the patient understand and adapt to the role of parent. Discussing concerns and fears alleviates anxiety.
4. Determine if adequate preparations have been made at home for infant care. Assist the patient with preparations, if necessary. (See the "Postpartum Period" care plan in this section for more information.)	4. Adequate preparation helps ensure continuity of care after delivery.
5. Teach the patient about the infant's unique abilities. Explain the importance of interaction to the parent-child bonding process. Discuss the infant's temperament and nursery activities. (See the "Postpartum Period" care plan in this section for more information.)	5. Interaction with the infant provides valuable information about the infant. Learning to recognize infant behavior promotes parent-child bonding and helps reduce the patient's tension and anxiety.

Nursing diagnosis: *Anticipatory grieving related to plans to give the infant up for adoption*

GOAL: To support the patient during the grieving process

Interventions	Rationales
1. Determine the patient's decision about adoption.	1. Preparation for the loss and the grieving process

Note that the patient may change her mind, perhaps more than once, or have serious misgivings about her decision. If appropriate, encourage her to talk with her parents, a counselor, or a religious advisor.

should begin before delivery.

2. Discuss adoption agency options with the patient. Answer any questions she may have, and once she has selected an agency, help her establish a working relationship with the agency's social worker. Provide generous emotional support during this process.

2. The patient may have many questions and concerns and need guidance when choosing an adoption agency. Continued emotional support from the nurse can be reassuring to the patient during this emotionally unsettling time.

3. Coordinate standard postpartum care for the mother and infant. Encourage the patient to see and hold the infant after birth.

3. Seeing and holding the infant helps the mother adjust to her decision.

4. Observe the patient for signs of loss and grief, such as anxiety, depression, or crying. Document the patient's reaction to the loss.

4. Documentation can verify the need for crisis intervention.

Nursing diagnosis: *Knowledge deficit related to birth control*

GOAL: To improve the patient's knowledge of birth control methods

Interventions

1. Assess the patient's knowledge of birth control methods.

2. Teach the patient about birth control and the types of contraceptive devices available. Provide her with appropriate literature on each method.

3. Stress the importance of using birth control while breast-feeding.

Rationales

1. A baseline assessment helps the nurse develop an appropriate teaching plan.

2. Most adolescents have a poor understanding of birth control and the available options. Knowledge may help prevent unwanted pregnancies in the future.

3. The patient may mistakenly believe that breast-feeding prevents conception.

ASSOCIATED CARE PLANS
• Grief and Grieving
• The Postpartum Period
• Sex and Sexuality
• Sexually Transmitted Disease

NETWORKING OF SERVICES
• Women, Infants, and Children program
• Aid to Dependent Children
• Division of Youth and Family Services
• La Leche League
• American Society for Psychoprophylaxis in Obstetrics
• Planned Parenthood
• Catholic Charities
• community services

CARE TEAM INVOLVED
• nurse
• perinatal nurse clinician
• pediatric nurse practitioner
• obstetrician
• pediatrician

• patient (and, if possible, partner and family)
• certified Lamaze instructor
• social worker
• dietitian
• home health aide
• school authorities
• lactation consultant

IMPLICATIONS FOR HOME CARE
• condition of the home, including adequacy of water supply, refrigeration, cooking facilities, plumbing, furniture, and sleeping area for all family members
• appropriate clothing for infant
• necessary equipment for preparing infant formula
• appropriate toys for infant
• adequate financial assistance

PATIENT EDUCATION TOOLS
• list of normal temperature, pulse rate, respiratory rate, and blood pressure
• appropriate dietary information
• literature on birth control methods
• list of available community resources, including

La Leche League, cesarean section support group,
March of Dimes (if infant has an anomaly)
• information on breast pump use (if mother is breast-
feeding)

DISCHARGE PLAN FROM HOME HEALTH CARE
Before discharge from home health care, the patient
should:
• understand that mood swings are common
• know the signs and symptoms of postpartum
hemorrhage
• understand that an increase in temperature may
indicate postpartum or postoperative infection
• know how to recognize and cope with breast
enlargement
• know when to resume sexual activity
• be familiar with available birth control methods
• know the community resources available to a
single mother
• understand the importance of follow-up care for
herself and the infant
• know the signs and symptoms of infant illnesses
• know the proper method of preparing formula,
if bottle-feeding
• be able to properly feed, burp, diaper, and bathe the
infant
• display confidence in her abilities as a new mother
• know how to prevent sexually transmitted diseases.

SELECTED REFERENCES
Adams, B. *Adolescent Health Care: Needs, Priorities and Services.* The Nursing Clinics of North America. Philadelphia: W.B. Saunders Co., 1983.

Aukamp, V. *Nursing Care Plans for the Childbearing Family.* East Norwalk, Conn.: Appleton-Century-Crofts, 1984.

Boback, I., and Jensen, M. *Essentials of Maternity Nursing.* St. Louis: C.V. Mosby Co., 1984.

Taylor, B., et al. "School-Based Prenatal Services: Can Similar Outcomes Be Attained in a Non-School Setting?," *Journal of School Health* 53:480-85, October 1983.

Ziegel, E., and Cranley, M. *Obstetric Nursing,* 8th ed. New York: Macmillan Publishing Co., 1985.

The Postpartum Period

DESCRIPTION AND TIME FOCUS

The postpartum period, or puerperium, begins after the third stage of labor and continues until uterus involution is completed, typically 4 to 6 weeks. During this time the woman's organs and physiology return to a normal, nonpregnant state. Psychological and behavioral changes also occur during the postpartum period as the woman adapts to her new role as parent.

Common complications during the postpartum period include abdominal diastasis, sore or cracked nipples, plugged breast ducts, poor let-down reflex, inadequate milk supply, constipation, strong afterpains, breast engorgement, and depression.

This clinical plan focuses on the patient discharged home from an acute-care hospital after giving birth. Nursing care centers on helping the patient cope with physical, emotional, and behavioral changes and adapting the home to meet the needs of mother and infant. The home is a familiar, secure setting that enhances the parent-child bonding process. The nurse promotes physical and emotional adjustments and monitors the patient's postpartum physical process.

■ Typical home health care length of service for a patient with no complications: 2 weeks

■ Typical visit frequency: three visits during the 2 week period

HEALTH HISTORY FINDINGS

In a health history interview, the patient may report many of these findings:
- abdominal diastasis
- sore or cracked nipples
- plugged breast ducts
- poor let-down reflex
- inadequate milk supply
- constipation
- strong afterpains
- breast engorgement
- depression
- hemorrhage
- puerperal infection
- uterine atony
- retained placental tissue
- cervical or vaginal lacerations
- thrombophlebitis
- mastitis
- bladder distention
- cystitis
- pyelonephritis
- subinvolution
- hematomas in connective tissue of vulva or under vaginal mucosa

PHYSICAL FINDINGS

In a physical examination, the nurse may detect many of these findings:

Cardiovascular
- vericose veins

Neurologic
- passive, dependent behavior followed by increased independence
- postpartum depression
- mood swings
- nervousness
- anxiety

Gastrointestinal
- GI organs restored to normal placement
- GI motility restored
- reduced tone of anal sphincter
- abdominal distention
- flatus
- hemorrhoids
- constipation
- hunger or thirst
- nausea or vomiting (rare)

Integumentary
- skin desquamation
- fading of spider nevi
- lightening of striae gravidarum (stretch marks)
- fading or disappearance of pregnancy-related pigment changes

Musculoskeletal
- improved abdominal muscle tone and strength
- weight loss

Reproductive
- uterine involution
- uterine contractions
- endometrium regeneration
- lochia
- vaginal healing
- cervical healing
- perineal healing
- restoration of external genitalia appearance
- lactation
- return of menstruation and ovulation

Renal and urinary
- improved tone and dilation of ureters and renal pelvis
- diuresis

• bladder edema or loss of bladder tone
• occasional reflex spasm of urethral muscle
• occasional lack of sensation to void
• bladder distention

• urine retention

DIAGNOSTIC STUDIES
None applicable

Nursing diagnosis: *Potential for infection related to perineal laceration, placental site wound, breast-feeding, changes in blood coagulability, venous stasis, or temporary loss of bladder tone*

GOAL: To prevent infection

Interventions

1. Monitor the patient for—and teach her to recognize—signs and symptoms of infection. Check the perineum for swelling, redness, warmth, tenderness, and drainage. Assess lochia for color. odor, amount, and consistency. Monitor the patient's temperature. Assess for abnormal abdominal pain. Examine the breasts for warmth, tenderness, localized ervthema, and cracked nipples. Document all findings.

2. Teach the patient the importance of thorough hand washing.

3. Teach the patient the proper technique for cleansing the perineum. Tell her to rinse the perineum with warm water from a peri bottle and to dry the area thoroughly, moving from the vaginal and perineal areas to the rectal area to prevent infection.

4. Show the patient how to fit a perineal pad so it will not slide.

5. Teach the patient proper techniques of breast and nipple care, including cleansing, drying, gentle handling, and using lubricants. Tell the breast-feeding patient to use nipple shields when nipples are sore, and suggest that she try more frequent feedings of a shorter duration.

6. If the patient is breast-feeding, teach her how to break the infant's suction on the nipple before removing the infant from the breast. Demonstrate the technique.

7. Teach the patient the importance of emptying the breasts after each feeding, using manual expression or a pump.

8. Teach the patient the importance of reporting and treating cracked nipples as soon as they occur. Tell her to feed the infant by bottle with milk expressed manually or by a pump. Explain the benefits of breast creams and nipple shields.

Rationales

1. Abnormal findings may indicate infection. Early detection helps ensure prompt treatment.

2. Thorough hand washing helps prevent bacteria from spreading, thus reducing the risk of infection.

3. Proper perineal care keeps the area clean and dry and promotes healing.

4. If the pad slides, bacteria from the rectum can contaminate the perineal-vaginal area.

5. Proper care can prevent injury and infection.

6. Removing the infant without first breaking the suction can injure the nipple and cause cracking.

7. Emptying the breast of leftover milk can prevent engorgement, in which the breasts become hard, full, and painful and the nipple disappears into the areola, so the infant cannot grasp it properly.

8. Bacteria can infect the body through cracked nipples.

Nursing diagnosis: *Altered comfort: pain, related to perineal edema, episiotomy, or hemorrhoids*

GOAL: To minimize the patient's discomfort

Interventions

1. If the patient has participated in an early discharge program, tell her to apply cold packs to the perineum during the first 24 hours after delivery.

2. Tell the patient to apply heat to the perineum (after the first 24 hours postpartum) by using a heat lamp for 20 minutes two or three times daily or by taking a sitz bath when necessary.

3. Teach the patient to apply topical anesthetics, such as benzocaine or dibucaine hydrochloride, as needed.

4. Teach the patient to inspect the perineum daily for signs and symptoms of infection, such as swelling, redness, warmth, tenderness, or drainage.

5. Teach the patient Kegel exercises and encourage their use.

6. Teach the patient to tighten buttocks muscles before sitting.

7. Obtain an inflatable plastic air ring for the patient to use when sitting. If the patient has hemorrhoids, have her use Tucks pads (witch hazel, glycerin, and water) between the perineal pad and the hemorrhoids.

Rationales

1. Cold application during the first 24 hours postpartum minimizes edema and discomfort by reducing circulation to the area.

2. Heat application after the first 24 hours postpartum reduces discomfort by relaxing tissue. Heat also promotes healing by increasing circulation.

3. Topical anesthetics reduce perineal discomfort by numbing the area. They also keep sutures soft and pliable.

4. Infection can cause edema and pain. Early detection helps ensure prompt treatment.

5. Kegel exercises promote healing by increasing circulation to the perineum.

6. Tightening buttocks muscles before sitting prevents trauma to the perineal area and minimizes discomfort.

7. An air ring reduces discomfort by relieving pressure on the perineal area when the patient is sitting. Witch hazel is an astringent that promotes comfort by reducing the swelling of hemorrhoidal tissues.

Nursing diagnosis: *Sleep pattern disturbance related to demands of infant*

GOAL: To promote adequate sleep and rest

Interventions

1. Teach the patient and family the importance of sleep and rest to the patient's physical and mental health.

2. Schedule periods of undisturbed sleep and rest for the patient. Help family members adapt their schedules to include more household tasks and infant care.

3. Evaluate the patient's and family's need for assistance, such as a home health aide.

4. If the infant is fed with a bottle, encourage family members to take turns feeding the infant during the night to allow the patient occasional nights of uninterrupted sleep.

5. If the patient is breast-feeding the infant, explain the relationship between milk secretion and adequate sleep and rest.

Rationales

1. Family members are more likely to help the patient—and the patient is less inclined to overexert herself—when they understand the rationale for adequate sleep and rest.

2. New mothers rarely receive enough sleep at night. Periods of undisturbed sleep and rest during the day ensure that the patient remains well rested.

3. A home health aide can assist with household tasks, allowing the patient to rest while the infant sleeps.

4. Adequate assistance with infant care helps the patient reestablish normal sleep and rest patterns.

5. Fatigue can inhibit milk secretion and the let-down reflex.

Nursing diagnosis: *Altered role performance related to newly acquired role of parent*

GOAL: To help the patient and partner adapt to their new roles as parents

Interventions	Rationales
1. Encourage the patient and partner to discuss their feelings and fears about parenthood. Listen attentively and remain nonjudgmental.	1. An open discussion helps the nurse evaluate the parents' emotional status and helps the parents begin to understand and accept their feelings.
2. Assess the parent-infant bonding process (touching, establishing eye contact, calling the infant by name, communicating with the infant, identifying the infant as a family member).	2. Lack of intimacy and poor communication with the infant may indicate that one or both parents do not accept their new role.
3. Assume role model responsibilities to help the patient and partner learn appropriate parenting behavior, such as patience, confidence, flexibility, and maintaining a sense of humor.	3. Watching a role model helps the new parents learn proper techniques of handling and caring for the infant.
4. Encourage the patient and partner to cultivate new skills appropriate for their role as parents, such as bathing and changing the baby and performing umbilical cord and circumcision care. Commend them when they accomplish parenting tasks.	4. Successfully performing new skills can increase the parents' confidence in their parenting abilities. Positive reinforcement encourages the patient and partner to continue improving these skills.
5. Provide the patient and partner with literature on the family and parent-infant bonding. Refer them to a new-parent support group, if necessary.	5. Teaching aids help convey the importance of parenthood. A support group provides a forum for the new parents to talk with others who share their feelings and concerns; such discussion may promote acceptance of their parental roles.

ASSOCIATED CARE PLANS
• Ineffective Coping
• Pain
• Sex and Sexuality
• Teenage Pregnancy
• Thrombophlebitis

NETWORKING OF SERVICES
• new-parent support group
• breast-feeding group, such as La Leche League
• home health aide service
• professional homemaker program
• well child clinic
• financial aid program

CARE TEAM INVOLVED
• nurse
• doctor
• patient and family
• medical social worker
• home health aide or homemaker
• childbirth educator
• lactation consultant

IMPLICATIONS FOR HOME CARE
• functional features of the home
• support person for assistance with home maintenance and infant care
• telephone (communication)
• necessary equipment and supplies—and financial assistance, if needed—to ensure proper care of mother and infant

PATIENT EDUCATION TOOLS
• literature on each medication or vitamin ordered
• current edition of infant care and development book
• current edition of breast-feeding book
• hospital discharge sheets from obstetrician and pediatrician with instructions and activity restrictions
• literature on infant bonding
• literature on contraceptive options

DISCHARGE PLAN FROM HOME HEALTH CARE
Before discharge from home health care, the patient should:
• have a firm, gradually descending uterus
• be free of signs or symptoms of infection and postpartum complications
• know the normal amount, color, odor, and consistency of lochia
• know the signs and symptoms of thrombophlebitis, cystitis, urine retention, upper urinary tract infection, mastitis, and breast complications
• have hospital discharge instruction sheets from the obstetrician and pediatrician
• demonstrate proper technique for breast-feeding or bottle feeding and for manually expressing milk
• understand that proper diet and adequate fluid intake prevent constipation
• understand the need for proper nutrition while breast-

feeding and realize that components of most foods the
mother ingests are secreted in her breast milk
• understand the need for frequent rest periods during
the day
• demonstrate proper breast and perineal care
• demonstrate proper method of fundal massage
• demonstrate proper hemorrhoid care
• perform postpartum exercises prescribed by the
obstetrician
• know and follow activity and exercise restrictions
• understand current contraceptive options
• demonstrate proper techniques for bathing and diapering the infant
• demonstrate appropriate parent-infant bonding
• demonstrate emotional adjustment to family life
• have telephone numbers for the obstetrician, pediatrician, home health agency, new-parent support group,
and breast-feeding support group (if nursing)
• know the dates of follow-up appointments with the
obstetrician and pediatrician.

SELECTED REFERENCES

Burroughs, A. *Bleier's Maternity Nursing,* 5th ed. Phila-
delphia: W.B. Saunders Co., 1986.
Campbell, C. *Nursing Diagnosis and Intervention in
Nursing Practice,* 2nd ed. New York: John Wiley &
Sons, 1984.
Carpenito, L. *Handbook of Nursing Diagnosis,* 2nd ed.
Philadelphia: J.B. Lippincott Co., 1987.
Gordon, M. *Nursing Diagnosis: Process and Application,*
2nd ed. New York: McGraw-Hill Book Co., 1987.
Moore, M.L. *Realities in Childbearing,* 2nd ed. Philadel-
phia: W.B. Saunders Co., 1983.
Ziegel, E.E., and Cranley, M.S. *Obstetric Nursing,* 8th ed.
New York: Macmillan Publishing Co., 1984.

Lyme Disease

DESCRIPTION AND TIME FOCUS
Lyme disease is a multisystemic inflammatory disorder caused by the spirochete *Borrelia burgdorferi,* which is transmitted by *Ixodes dammini* ticks. Lyme disease was first identified in a group of children living in Lyme, Connecticut. Infected ticks are found in wooded areas and suburban lawns, and the disease has been reported in 32 states and on all continents except Antarctica. The tiny *I. dammini* tick is carried by mice, birds, deer, and other mammals.

Lyme disease has three clinical stages. Stage one is characterized by flulike symptoms and an expanding skin lesion (erythema chronicum migrans). In Stage two the patient experiences neurologic and cardiac involvement. Stage three is characterized by musculoskeletal and chronic neurologic involvement. The spirochete *Borrelia* is susceptible to ceftriaxone, amoxicillin, tetracycline, and penicillin V. If the disease is diagnosed early, oral antibiotic therapy can be successful, although I.V. therapy sometimes is the treatment of choice.

This clinical plan focuses on the patient with Lyme disease. Nursing care centers on teaching the patient and family to avoid tick sites, explaining medical and nursing interventions, and helping them adapt to necessary life-style changes during treatment.

■ Typical home health care length of service and visit frequency vary according to disease stage. *Stage one*—daily to administer I.V. therapy. *Stage two*—twice weekly for 3 months to monitor the illness; daily visits if high-dose I.V. therapy is ordered. *Stage three*—twice weekly for 6 months to help the patient with rehabilitation goals; daily for I.V. therapy if penicillin treatment is ordered

HEALTH HISTORY FINDINGS
In a health history interview, the patient may report many of these findings:
• flulike signs and symptoms (headache, chills, fever)
• skin lesion (erythema chronicum migrans)
• fatigue
• arthritis
• history of cardiac disease

PHYSICAL FINDINGS
In a physical examination, the nurse may detect many of these findings:

Cardiovascular
• fatigue
• atrioventricular heart block
• anemia
• dysrhythmias
• erratic pulse

Neurologic
• malaise
• cranial neuropathy
• Bell's palsy
• headache
• meningitis
• peripheral neuropathy
• ptosis
• strabismus
• diplopia
• increased intracranial pressure
• dementia

Integumentary
• expanding skin lesions (red macule or papule)
• swollen glands
• malar rash
• urticaria

Musculoskeletal
• large joint swelling
• arthritis
• migrating pain
• bone erosion

DIAGNOSTIC STUDIES
The following studies may be performed to evaluate the patient's health status:
• hemoglobin and hematocrit—weekly until normal; hemoglobin: men, 14 to 18 g/dl; women, 12 to 16 g/dl; hematocrit: men, 42% to 54%; women: 38% to 46%
• erythrocyte sedimentation rate—weekly until normal; men: 0 to 10 mm/hour; women: 0 to 20 mm/hour
• leukocyte count—weekly until normal or until white blood cell (WBC) count is 4,100 to 10,900/mcg/l
• aspartate aminotransferase (AST, formerly SGOT)—monthly until normal (8 to 20 units/liter)
• spinal tap—once for diagnosis

Nursing diagnosis: *Altered nutrition, less than body requirements, related to fatigue or medication*

GOAL: To ensure adequate nutrition

Interventions

1. Encourage the patient to eat small, frequent meals rather than one or two larger meals.

2. Monitor and record the patient's weight each day.

3. Consult with a dietitian about the patient's diet.

4. Formulate a nutritional plan for the patient. Consider the patient's food preferences when preparing the plan.

5. Advise the patient to eat yogurt to prevent severe diarrhea.

Rationales

1. Eating and digesting small meals requires less oxygen.

2. Daily weighings help in assessing the patient's caloric intake and need for dietary supplements.

3. Early consultation may prevent complications (aseptic meningitis, encephalitis, Guillain-Barré syndrome, polyradiculitis) that can cause increased debilitation.

4. The patient is more likely to comply with a dietary regimen that includes preferred foods.

5. Antibiotics affect the normal flora in the intestinal tract. *Lactobacillus acidophilus,* found in yogurt, helps prevent severe diarrhea associated with antibiotic therapy.

Nursing diagnosis: *Activity intolerance related to fatigue, muscle weakness from lack of physical activity, or depression*

GOAL: To improve the patient's activity tolerance

Interventions

1. Teach the patient breathing techniques that conserve oxygen during activities of daily living (ADLs).

2. Develop an exercise program for the patient.

3. Monitor the patient's blood pressure, pulse rate and rhythm, skin color, and respiratory rate before, during, and after exercise. Document all findings.

4. Document episodes of shortness of breath.

Rationales

1. Breathing techniques promote full exhalation and inhalation, thus facilitating a broader range of activities.

2. Exercise improves the patient's endurance and can prevent fatigue, muscle weakness, and depression.

3. Documentation helps the nurse assess the patient's response to various forms of exercise and determine an appropriate regimen.

4. Shortness of breath may be related to cardiac complications, such as heart block or dysrhythmias. Episodes should decrease or disappear as therapy progresses.

Nursing diagnosis: *Sleep pattern disturbance related to medication, depression, or anxiety*

GOAL: To promote adequate sleep

Interventions

1. Determine the patient's normal sleep patterns before he acquired Lyme disease. Teach him about normal and abnormal sleep patterns.

2. Teach the caregiver to monitor the patient's episodes of sleeplessness.

Rationales

1. Teaching the patient about normal and abnormal sleep patterns can clear up misunderstandings he may have about insomnia and may promote more restful sleep. (See the "Sleep Disorders" care plan for more information.)

2. Observation may uncover reasons for sleeplessness and provide clues to effective prevention or treatment.

3. Teach the patient relaxation techniques, such as hypnosis, guided imagery, biofeedback, or distraction.

3. Relaxation techniques reduce the patient's oxygen demand and promote sleep.

Nursing diagnosis: *Altered patterns of sexuality related to perceived changes in relationship with spouse*

GOAL: To promote resumption of normal sexual activity

Interventions

1. Discuss sexual pattern changes with the patient and partner. Encourage them to express their concerns.

2. Help the patient identify times of the day when he feels well rested.

Rationales

1. Discussion helps clarify the issues. The patient and partner must express feelings to identify perceived changes.

2. Sexual activity expends energy. Scheduling sexual activity for times when the patient is well rested enhances the sexual satisfaction of both partners.

Nursing diagnosis: *Altered bowel elimination: constipation or diarrhea, related to inactivity, medication, or disease*

GOAL: To help the patient achieve a normal bowel pattern

Interventions

1. Assess the patient's normal bowel patterns.

2. Administer antidiarrheal medication as needed.

3. Teach the patient to alleviate constipation by consuming more dietary fiber, drinking warm fluids, and exercising.

Rationales

1. Assessment helps the nurse recognize abnormal patterns and develop an appropriate plan of care.

2. These medications slow gastric motility.

3. Vegetables, fruits, and whole grain breads provide dietary fiber and promote bowel elimination. Liquids increase peristalsis. Exercise increases abdominal muscle contraction and facilitates bowel elimination.

Nursing diagnosis: *Altered comfort: pain, related to immobility or muscle spasm secondary to arthritis*

GOAL: To alleviate pain

Interventions

1. Assess the patient for pain or discomfort; pay particular attention to joints.

2. Administer pain medications as ordered, and document adverse effects.

3. Encourage the patient to use noninvasive pain-relief methods, such as proper positioning, massage, and whirlpool baths. Tell him to place a bed board under his mattress and to lie in the prone position twice a day for 15 minutes, with his toes hanging over the foot of the bed.

4. Plan four daily rest periods for the patient, each lasting 1 to 2 hours.

5. If activity is permitted, teach the patient to use muscle groups rather than joints when lifting, standing, and moving.

Rationales

1. Pain occurs in affected joints. Some patients will not report pain unless they are asked.

2. Medications reduce pain and allow the patient to perform ADLs.

3. These methods promote the release of endorphins, opiatelike substances in the brain that help reduce pain.

4. Rest promotes healing.

5. Using muscles rather than joints prevents further trauma.

ASSOCIATED CARE PLANS
• Grief and Grieving
• Ineffective Coping
• Intermittent I.V. Therapy
• Osteoarthritis
• Pain
• Sex and Sexuality

NETWORKING OF SERVICES
• public health department
• durable medical equipment supplier
• I.V. therapy pharmacy
• Lifeline
• Arthritis Foundation
• American Heart Association

CARE TEAM INVOLVED
• nurse
• doctor
• patient and family
• physical therapist
• pharmacist
• laboratory technician

IMPLICATIONS FOR HOME CARE
• telephone for communication in emergency
• adaptation and safety of home
• storage of I.V. supplies
• durable medical equipment

PATIENT EDUCATION TOOLS
• information from the National Lyme Borreliosis
Foundation, Box 462, Tolland, Conn., 06084;
telephone 203-871-2900
• Arthritis Foundation literature
• patient booklet on I.V. therapy

DISCHARGE PLAN FROM HOME HEALTH CARE
Before discharge from home health care, the patient
should:
• state the early signs of a tick bite (redness, warmth,
itch)
• know the areas where ticks are prevalent (tall grass,
woods)
• cite personal drug allergies
• understand activity restrictions, including overexertion
• demonstrate how to use a home infusion pump for
I.V. therapy
• try to maintain a normal life-style during home
treatment
• know the adverse effects of prescribed drugs
• post the telephone numbers of the doctor and home
health agency by the phone.

SELECTED REFERENCES
Habicht, G.S., et al. "Lyme Disease," *Scientific American,* July 1987.
Melski, J., and Mitchell, P. Proceedings of Lyme Disease Conference, Marshfield, Wis., June 3, 1988.
Steere, A.C., et al. "Successful Parenteral Therapy of Established Lyme Arthritis," *New England Journal of Medicine* 312:869, April 1985.

Substance Abuse

DESCRIPTION AND TIME FOCUS

Substance abuse is an addiction to mood- or behavior-altering substances, such as alcohol or prescribed, over-the-counter, or illicit drugs. Incidence is increasing as more and more individuals use alcohol and drugs to cope with or escape from the anxiety and stress associated with daily living. Abusers exhibit various physiologic and psychological sequelae, from weight loss to mood swings. Research indicates that 5 million Americans abuse cocaine, 20 million abuse alcohol, and roughly one-third of the population smoke cigarettes. These figures do not reflect the myriad other substance addictions present in American society. Research also indicates that children of substance abusers have a higher-than-average risk for becoming substance abusers.

Substance abuse is a chronic disease that usually stems from a complex interaction of family rituals, genetic predisposition, and various environmental influences. Rehabilitation is particularly difficult because the patient must typically change friends, jobs, and methods of solving problems and managing stress while enduring the physical and psychological discomforts of withdrawal. Consequently, relapse during the first year after detoxification is common.

This clinical plan focuses on the patient with an addiction to alcohol, cocaine, or nicotine. Nursing care centers on promoting the patient's health and helping him adopt a substance-free life-style. The nurse must be compassionate, familiar with family systems theory and applicable community resources (such as Alcoholics Anonymous or Narcotics Anonymous), and aware that everyone has the ability to change unhealthy behavior. The home provides the patient with comfort and security as the nurse teaches effective coping techniques and helps alter patterns of thinking, perceiving, communicating, and problem solving.

■ Typical home health care length of service: 4 weeks

■ Typical visit frequency: twice weekly

HEALTH HISTORY FINDINGS

In a health history interview, the patient may report many of these findings:
• fatigue
• weight loss
• low tolerance for anxiety, guilt, and anger
• family history of substance abuse
• poor physical appearance and grooming
• lack of responsibility
• low self-esteem
• pattern of dysfunctional anger, manipulation, impulsiveness, avoidance, and grandiosity
• association with known abusers
• history of stealing from family or employer
• inconsistent interpersonal relationships
• lack of a philosophical or spiritual base
• inability to make decisions

PHYSICAL FINDINGS

In a physical examination, the nurse may detect many of these findings:

Cardiovascular
• tachycardia
• palpitations
• restlessness
• hypertension

Respiratory
• crackles
• shortness of breath on exertion
• history of respiratory infections

Neurologic
• tremors
• memory lag
• insomnia

Gastrointestinal
• indigestion
• nausea
• constipation or diarrhea
• irritation of mouth and gums
• anorexia

Integumentary
• diaphoresis

DIAGNOSTIC STUDIES
None applicable

Nursing diagnosis: *Activity intolerance related to metabolic disturbances resulting from substance abuse*

GOAL: To improve the patient's activity tolerance

Interventions

1. Help the patient plan adequate rest and relaxation periods during the day.

2. Assess the patient's past and current sleep patterns, and encourage him to get adequate sleep at night.

3. Explain the relationship between activity tolerance and stress. Review the signs and symptoms of stress (sighing, nausea, anorexia, sweating, apprehension, uncertainty, shakiness, restlessness, distress, glancing about, hand tremors, facial tension, self-focus) and appropriate responses.

4. Teach the caregiver to monitor and record the patient's pulse rate, respiratory rate, and blood pressure during activity, rest, and sleep and to document episodes of tachycardia and tachpnea.

5. Encourage the patient to exercise regularly.

Rationales

1. Rest and relaxation promote physical endurance.

2. Many substance abusers have poor sleep patterns. Adequate sleep may reduce the patient's stress and lower his pulse rate and blood pressure.

3. Stress can impair the patient's activity tolerance. The patient must learn to recognize signs and symptoms of stress and practice methods to reduce it.

4. Pulse rate, respiratory rate, and blood pressure are reliable indicators of activity tolerance. Increased pulse rate may indicate exertional discomfort. Tachycardia and tachypnea may result from stress.

5. Increased physical activity improves muscle tone and cardiac output.

Nursing diagnosis: *Altered nutrition: less than body requirements, related to lack of information and drug use*

GOAL: To restore nutritional balance

Interventions

1. Assess the patient's nutritional status and dietary habits. Have him keep a food diary for several days.

2. Teach the patient principles of sound nutrition. Urge him to follow a well-balanced diet high in protein and carbohydrates and low in fat, and advise him to avoid caffeine.

Rationales

1. Many substance abusers are underweight from inadequate nutrition. A food diary helps in assessing the patient's dietary habits.

2. A high-protein, high-carbohydrate, low-fat diet helps repair and maintain body tissue. Avoiding caffeine decreases central nervous system stimulation.

Nursing diagnosis: *Potential for respiratory infection related to smoking*

GOAL: To improve the patient's respiratory status

Interventions

1. Teach the patient to collect a sputum sample for culture and have it tested for sensitivity. Advise him to make an appointment to have a chest X-ray taken.

2. Monitor the patient's compliance with antibiotic therapy.

Rationales

1. These procedures can detect opportunistic infections.

2. Prophylactic antibiotic therapy is indicated in a high-risk patient, such as a substance abuser.

3. Tell the patient to drink at least 3 liters of fluid daily.

3. Adequate fluids help the patient loosen and expectorate respiratory tract secretions.

4. Explain the value of regular exercise.

4. Regular exercise promotes effective gas exchange.

5. Refer the patient to a smoking-cessation program.

5. A formal smoking-cessation program provides structure and support that can help motivate the patient to quit smoking.

Nursing diagnosis: *Potential for injury related to poor oral hygiene*

GOAL: To help the patient develop proper oral hygiene habits

Interventions

1. Teach the patient proper techniques for oral hygiene, and explain their importance. Supervise his use of these techniques.

2. Refer the patient to the dentist for necessary dental care.

3. Refer the patient to hospital outpatient classes that teach proper grooming and hygiene behaviors.

Rationales

1. Instruction increases the patient's awareness of the need for proper oral hygiene; supervision helps ensure compliance with the techniques.

2. Timely dental intervention can prevent problems and may enhance the patient's self-esteem.

3. Classroom instruction may help the patient establish more desirable grooming and hygiene habits.

Nursing diagnosis: *Altered family processes related to emotional stress associated with substance abuse*

GOAL: To promote effective communication among family members

Interventions

1. Encourage family discussions that explore each member's concerns.

2. Assess the family's communication patterns.

3. Encourage family members to explore methods of altering dysfunctional behaviors.

4. Refer the family for counseling, if necessary.

5. Refer family members to community education and self-help programs, such as Al-Anon and Nar-Anon.

Rationales

1. Discussions may help family members understand one another's concerns and needs, which are often overlooked because the family's collective energy has been focused on the substance abuser. *

2. Assessment helps the nurse identify patterns of anger, rejection, indifference, and inconsistency.

3. Focusing on dysfunctional behaviors helps family members recognize personal deficiencies and identify constructive alternative behaviors.

4. Counseling provides a reasonable, consistent, and clearly defined framework for exploring family interactions and can enhance interpersonal family relationships.

5. Support groups help family members cope with the patient's substance abuse by teaching them about the disease, explaining that they are not at fault, and providing emotional support.

Nursing diagnosis: *Disturbance in self-esteem related to a lack of philosophical or spiritual pursuits*

GOAL: To promote the patient's self-esteem

Interventions

1. Urge the patient to focus on the daily tasks he must accomplish to achieve a goal. Help him understand that mistakes are common and are not synonymous with failure.

2. Encourage the patient to think about getting a job if he has none.

3. Assess the patient's perception of the steps needed to secure a job. Discuss the tasks associated with each step.

4. Encourage the patient to apply for an appropriate job.

5. Encourage the patient to continue attending Narcotics Anonymous or Alcoholics Anonymous meetings biweekly after discharge.

6. Encourage the patient to pursue interesting hobbies and to try to establish a philosophical or spiritual belief system.

Rationales

1. A substance abuser may focus on the grand scheme while ignoring the daily tasks necessary to reach goals. He also may view mistakes as failures. These attitudes inhibit progress, cause frustration, and damage the patient's self-esteem.

2. This is the first task in a series of manageable tasks that have a specific, achievable goal.

3. These discussions help the patient focus on the specific tasks necessary to reach the specified goal and serve as a model for problem solving in the future.

4. Assuming responsibilities enhances the patient's self-esteem.

5. These meetings can help the patient avoid relapse by providing emotional, philosophical, and spiritual support.

6. Pursuing personal interests and having a spiritual base can make life more interesting and bearable and may ease the patient's desire to use drugs or alcohol.

ASSOCIATED CARE PLANS
- Acquired Immunodeficiency Syndrome
- Grief and Grieving
- Ineffective Coping
- Smoking Cessation

NETWORKING OF SERVICES
- Alcoholics Anonymous
- Al-Anon
- Narcotics Anonymous
- Nar-Anon
- American Cancer Society
- religious groups

CARE TEAM INVOLVED
- nurse
- doctor
- patient and family
- social worker
- nutritionist
- vocational counselor
- family service agency
- religious advisor

IMPLICATIONS FOR HOME CARE
- risk of relapse when patient returns to familiar environments
- risk of relapse because of anxiety or inability to find a desirable job
- marital problems because of ineffective communication or sexual dysfunction
- children at high risk for becoming substance abusers

PATIENT EDUCATION TOOLS
- literature from Alcoholics Anonymous, Al-Anon, Narcotics Anonymous, or Nar-Anon
- American Cancer Society and American Lung Association literature on smoking cessation
- nutrition information

DISCHARGE PLAN FROM HOME HEALTH CARE
Before discharge from home health care, the patient should:
- understand the importance of attending biweekly self-help group meetings
- experience less stress
- demonstrate improved sleeping and eating habits
- participate in a drug rehabilitation program or attend Alcoholics Anonymous or Narcotics Anonymous meetings
- know that *substance abuse* and *addiction* are synonymous
- know that alcoholism and drug abuse are chronic diseases that can be arrested but never cured
- know that I.V. drug users have a high risk for human immunodeficiency virus (HIV) infection (AIDS)
- know what to do in the event of relapse
- practice self-hypnosis and posthypnotic suggestions from smoking-cessation clinic to relieve nicotine craving
- have an appointment to visit the doctor in 3 weeks.

SELECTED REFERENCES

Drucker, E. "AIDS and Addiciton in New York City," *American Journal of Drug and Alcohol Abuse*, 12:165-81, 1986.

Hein, K., "AIDS in Adolescents: A Rationale for Concern," *New York State Journal of Medicine*, May 1987.

Selwyn, P.A., et al. "Knowledge About AIDS and High-Risk Behavior Among Intravenous Drug Abusers in New York City." Presented at annual meeting of APHA, Washington, D.C., November 18, 1985.

Wesson, D.R., and Smith, D.E. "Cocaine Use in America: Epidemiologic and Clinical Perspectives." National Institute on Drug Abuse Research Monograph 61. DHHS Pub. No. (ADM) 85-1414, Washington, D.C.: U.S. Government Printing Office, 1985.

Wise, R.A. "Neuralmechanisms of the Reinforcing Action of Cocaine," in *Cocaine: Pharmacology, Effects, and Treatments of Abuse.* Edited by Grabowski, J.G. National Institute on Drug Abuse Research Monograph 50. DHHS Pub. No. (ADM) 84-1326, Washington, D.C.: U.S. Government Printing Office, 1984.

Zeigler, S., et al. *Nursing Process, Nursing Diagnosis, and Nursing Knowledge.* Norwalk, Conn.: Appleton-Lange, 1986.

Smoking Cessation

DESCRIPTION AND TIME FOCUS

Tobacco use is the number-one addiction in the world and the leading avoidable cause of death in the United States. Smoking significantly increases an individual's risk for heart disease and cancer of the lungs, larynx, and oral cavity. Studies link breathing difficulties in children, such as asthma, bronchitis, and frequent upper respiratory infections, to second-hand (passive) smoking. Nonsmoking adults who live with smokers have an increased risk of lung cancer and other respiratory problems. Other effects may include eye, nose, and throat irritation, headaches, dizziness, and nausea.

This clinical plan focuses on the patient who smokes, regardless of the underlying disorder or the patient's desire to quit smoking. Nursing care centers on teaching the patient and family general principles of good health and discouraging smoking. The nurse must practice good health habits to establish credibility as a health educator. Patients wishing to quit smoking are more likely to listen to and comply with instruction presented by a nonsmoking nurse.

■ Typical home health care length of service and visit frequency depend on the underlying disease.

HEALTH HISTORY FINDINGS

In a health history interview, the patient may report many of these findings:
• reduced activity tolerance
• history of tobacco use
• family pattern of nicotine abuse
• chronic cough that is unrelated to a disease
• frequent or tenacious respiratory infections
• increased sputum production
• oral lesions
• anxiety

PHYSICAL FINDINGS

In a physical examination, the nurse may detect many of these findings:

Cardiovascular
• tachycardia
• palpitations
• increased blood pressure

Respiratory
• shortness of breath on exertion
• dyspnea
• chronic cough
• abnormal breath sounds

Gastrointestinal
• stomach irritation
• gastric ulcer

Integumentary
• cyanosis
• skin temperature decrease in fingers and toes
• yellow-orange stains on teeth, fingernails, fingertips

DIAGNOSTIC STUDIES

The following studies may be performed to evaluate the patient's health status:
• chest X-ray—before quitting, then 3 to 6 months after cessation
• pulmonary function studies—before quitting, then 3 to 6 months after cessation

---

Nursing diagnosis: *Altered health maintenance related to tobacco use*

GOAL: To help the patient quit or significantly reduce smoking

Interventions

1. Be alert for clues that the patient wants to quit smoking. Offer encouragement and emotional support, and try to remain sympathetic and nonjudgmental.

2. Encourage the patient to set a quitting date within 30 days of his decision to quit.

3. Have the patient identify and list reasons to quit smoking, and encourage review of the list several times daily.

Rationales

1. Expressing the desire to quit smoking is the first step in a smoking-cessation program. Support from the nurse may enhance the patient's commitment to quit.

2. The patient should choose a date while determination to quit is strong. Procrastination is less likely if the date is in the near future.

3. Frequently reviewing a list of his reasons for quitting helps reinforce the desire to quit.

4. Help the patient study his smoking habit to determine situations or times of day that stimulate the urge to smoke (when drinking coffee, after meals, during stress) and behaviors that support the habit (leaving ashtrays and other smoking supplies in convenient places at home, buying cigarettes by the carton, carrying tobacco products).

4. The effectiveness of a smoking-cessation program depends, in part, on how well the patient understands all facets of his smoking behavior.

5. Discuss measures that may reduce the urge to smoke, such as regular exercise and deep-breathing and relaxation techniques.

5. The patient may believe that tobacco relaxes him, perhaps unaware that nicotine is a stimulant and that muscle relaxation results from deep-inhalation that increases oxygen to body tissues. Regular exercise and deep-breathing and relaxation techniques can help reduce tension.

6. Teach the patient about emotional and physical withdrawal symptoms, such as cravings, depression, irritability, sleep disturbances, and changes in bowel patterns. (See interventions under the "Knowledge deficit" nursing diagnosis in this care plan.)

6. Knowledge helps the patient cope with unpleasant withdrawal symptoms.

7. Discuss eating habits and weight control with the patient. Remind him not to use food as a substitute for smoking.

7. If the patient is aware of his eating habits, he is more likely to use self-control.

8. Have the patient identify situations that could precipitate a relapse and methods of coping with these situations.

8. Preparing for a relapse promotes effective coping when a crisis occurs.

Nursing diagnosis: *Knowledge deficit related to withdrawal symptoms associated with smoking cessation*

GOAL: To improve the patient's knowledge of withdrawal symptoms and appropriate treatments

Interventions

Rationales

1. Inform the patient of techniques that can minimize withdrawal symptoms, such as listening to relaxation tapes, deep breathing, and exercising regularly.

1. Withdrawal symptoms are the primary reason for relapse. These activities help alleviate nervousness, irritability, and restlessness.

2. Encourage the patient to drink plenty of water and juice and to avoid caffeine and alcohol.

2. Liquids help flush nicotine out of the patient's system. Caffeine and alcohol can stimulate the urge for a cigarette.

3. Encourage the patient to exercise daily and to get sufficient sleep at night.

3. Regular exercise and undisturbed sleep help reduce fatigue and increase energy level.

4. Advise the patient to suck on sugarless hard candy or ice chips throughout the day.

4. These measures can alleviate increased coughing and mucus, indications that the lungs are cleansing themselves.

5. Teach the patient about dietary modifications that help alleviate bowel problems. Tell him to increase fluid and fiber intake to relieve constipation and scalded milk or hard cheeses for diarrhea.

5. The patient may experience constipation or diarrhea during smoking cessation.

6. Tell the patient not to start new projects while trying to quit smoking.

6. Poor concentration is a major withdrawal symptom. The patient will probably have trouble concentrating on other matters if he is focusing attention on quitting smoking.

7. Encourage the patient to discuss the withdrawal symptoms he is experiencing. Provide emotional support, and urge nonsmoking family members and friends to voice their encouragement.

7. The patient needs support as he copes with withdrawal symptoms and with the sense of loss he may feel at relinquishing a familiar habit.

8. Explain to the patient that withdrawal symptoms usually abate after 1 or 2 weeks and that mild analgesics and extra sleep can alleviate physical symptoms. Refer him to the doctor if his discomfort lasts longer than 2 weeks.

9. Assess the patient's need for a formal smoking cessation program. If necessary, refer him to the local chapter of the American Lung Association or American Cancer Society for further information.

8. Headaches, muscle aches, and other complaints of physical discomfort are common in the first 2 weeks after smoking cessation. If discomfort persists, the patient should consult the doctor to determine whether an underlying problem exists.

9. The patient may respond more positively to a formal program that can offer regular direction and emotional support from peers.

ASSOCIATED CARE PLANS
• Angina Pectoris
• Bronchitis
• Chronic Congestive Heart Failure
• Chronic Obstructive Pulmonary Disease
• Hypertension
• Substance Abuse

NETWORKING OF SERVICES
• American Lung Association
• American Cancer Society
• American Heart Association
• smoking-cessation programs

CARE TEAM INVOLVED
• nurse
• doctor
• patient, family, and friends
• smoking-cessation program leader

IMPLICATIONS FOR HOME CARE
• telephone numbers of the doctor and nonsmoking support persons posted by the phone
• smoke detectors

PATIENT EDUCATION TOOLS
• American Lung Association literature
• relaxation tapes

DISCHARGE PLAN FROM HOME HEALTH CARE
Before discharge from home health care, the patient should:
• understand the detrimental health effects of smoking
• know the positive health effects of quitting smoking
• know typical withdrawal symptoms and methods to alleviate them
• identify personal coping strategies
• quit smoking by the designated date or be enrolled in a smoking-cessation program.

SELECTED REFERENCES
Aucoin, R.A. "Smoking Behavior and the Efficacy of Nurses as Role Models," *Health Values,* 10(4):25-29, July/August 1986.
Carpenito, L. *Nursing Diagnosis: Application to Clinical Practice.* Philadelphia: J.B. Lippincott Co., 1987.
Dalton, J.A., and Swenson, I. "Nurses and Smoking: Role Modeling and Counseling Behaviors," *Oncology Nursing Forum,* 13(2):45-48, March/April 1986.
Ferguson, T. "Helping Smokers Quit the Habit," *Medical Self-Care,* 40-45, May/June 1987.
McKool, K. "Facilitating Smoking Cessation," *Journal of Cardiovascular Nursing* 1(4):28-41, August 1987.
Papier, C.M., and Stellman, S. *Health Risks of Passive Smoking.* New York: Haworth Press, Inc., 1987.

Hospice Care

DEFINITION AND TIME FOCUS

Set in patients' homes, nursing homes, or inpatient settings, a hospice program aims to provide coordinated physical, psychological, social, and spiritual care for dying persons and their families. It recognizes dying as part of the normal process of living and focuses on maintaining the quality of the patient's remaining life. The hospice approach is interdisciplinary in nature, centered around patients' and families' needs. This focus on the family is a major aspect of hospice care and contrasts with the usual focus of hospital care, which is almost solely on the patient.

Although hospice care is commonly perceived as applying only to patients with terminal cancer, patients enter hospice programs in the terminal stages of many different illnesses.

This clinical plan provides information applicable to most hospice patients, with nursing diagnoses covering physiologic, psychosocial, and spiritual needs of the dying patient and bereaved family. When applying this plan to a particular patient, the nurse also should refer to other care plans covering the patient's specific medical problems.

■ Typical length of service for a patient in a hospice program: varies depending on the nature and stage of the patient's terminal illness and on the amount of support needed to supplement family care

■ Typical visit frequency: also varies; may range from as many as three visits daily to as few as one visit weekly

HEALTH HISTORY FINDINGS

Health history findings will be based on the patient's specific terminal illness and the stage of the dying process. Findings that patients in hospice care commonly report include:
• diagnosis of terminal illness, typically with a prognosis of less than 6 months to live
• fear and anxiety over impending death
• feelings of powerlessness and hopelessness
• chronic pain
• anorexia
• altered taste sensation
• decreased fluid intake
• constipation
• urinary incontinence
• muscle weakness
• decreased range of motion
• difficulty breathing
• alteration in sleep and activity patterns

PHYSICAL FINDINGS

Physical examination will reveal findings associated with the patient's terminal illness; common findings for patients in hospice care include:

Cardiovascular
• tachycardia or bradycardia
• hypotension or hypertension
• dependent edema

Respiratory
• dyspnea
• shallow respirations
• crackles and rhonchi

Neurologic
• altered level of consciousness

Gastrointestinal
• nausea and vomiting
• diarrhea or constipation
• hiccoughing and belching

Integumentary
• decubiti
• dryness and pruritus
• pallor
• cyanosis
• mottling
• diaphoresis

Musculoskeletal
• weakness
• muscle atrophy
• limited range of motion, perhaps immobility
• contractures

Renal and urinary
• signs of urinary tract infection
• urinary incontinence or retention

DIAGNOSTIC STUDIES

None applicable to hospice care

Nursing diagnosis: *Altered comfort: pain, related to effects of terminal illness*

GOAL: To control pain and make the patient as comfortable as possible in the last stages of life

Interventions

1. See the "Pain" care plan, page 254.

2. Assess the patient's level of pain frequently; encourage use of prescribed pain medication before pain becomes severe.

3. As appropriate, intervene to relieve conditions that may be causing or contributing to pain or interfering with pain relief; for example, administering enemas if pain is related to abdominal distention, and positioning the patient for optimum comfort.

4. When possible, control pain with oral medications, such as Brompton's cocktail or an equivalent narcotic mixture, rather than with intramuscular injections.

5. Keep in mind that usual "safe dose" levels may not apply for the terminally ill patient, and consult the doctor if the ordered dose no longer seems effective.

6. As appropriate, teach the patient and family about alternative pain control measures, such as relaxation techniques, massage, guided imagery, hypnosis, and biofeedback.

Rationales

1. This care plan provides interventions applicable to any patient in pain.

2. A patient's level of pain significantly affects his emotional adjustment to terminal illness and impending death; patients with poorly controlled pain tend to have more difficulty with adjustment. Pain medication is most effective when administered early in the pain cycle.

3. Many factors can contribute to pain or interfere with pain relief. Correcting such problems allows optimum pain control.

4. Repeated intramuscular injections, particularly in the debilitated patient, traumatize skin and gradually become less effective as areas of scarring develop and inhibit absorption. Also, use of oral medication can help increase the patient's sense of control over the pain.

5. A patient maintained on narcotic analgesics for an extended period may develop tolerance and require larger-than-usual doses to achieve adequate pain control. The risk of narcotic addiction is not an issue for terminally ill patients.

6. Non-medicinal pain control methods may help relieve pain and increase the patient's sense of control over the pain.

Nursing diagnosis: *Altered bowel elimination: constipation, related to poor nutrition, inactivity, or medication use*

GOAL: To prevent or control constipation

Interventions

1. Determine the patient's usual bowel elimination routine. Encourage him to use the toilet if able; if he's unable, provide a bedside commode or bedpan. Assist as necessary to maintain elimination schedule.

2. As the patient's condition allows, help him increase dietary fiber intake, maintain adequate fluid intake, and engage in regular physical activity. Instruct family members in these care measures.

3. Administer enemas, stool-softeners, or laxatives, as needed. Avoid overuse.

4. Check for fecal impaction if the patient has not had a bowel movement in 3 days. Manually remove any impaction.

Rationales

1. Regular elimination is essential to physical and emotional well-being. Sitting on the toilet places the body in a position that promotes defecation.

2. These measures will promote normal bowel elimination patterns and help prevent constipation.

3. A patient who cannot assume a normal position on the toilet may require enemas or medications to aid elimination. Overuse of enemas, stool-softeners, or laxatives can lead to dependence for elimination, which can interfere with establishment of a normal bowel elimination pattern.

4. Impaction removal can relieve constipation and allow return to normal bowel function.

Nursing diagnosis: *Potential fluid volume deficit, related to anorexia and dehydration associated with terminal illness and the dying process*

GOAL: To compensate for fluid volume deficit and enhance patient comfort during the dying process

Interventions

1. Assess the patient's hydration status by monitoring intake and output, evaluating skin turgor and mucous membrane moistness, and assessing for other signs and symptoms of fluid volume deficit.

2. As appropriate for the patient's condition, encourage adequate oral fluid intake.

3. Avoid aggressive I.V. fluid replacement therapy as death becomes imminent.

4. Provide frequent mouth care and offer the patient sips of fluid (using an eyedropper or syringe if necessary), ice chips, hard candy, or artificial saliva, as appropriate.

Rationales

1. Determining the patient's hydration status helps guide appropriate interventions.

2. Adequate fluid intake is essential to proper hydration of body tissues.

3. Dehydration normally occurs during the dying process in terminal illness. Fluid replacement therapy may inappropriately prolong life in a terminally ill patient.

4. These measures can help reduce discomfort from mouth dryness due to fluid volume deficit.

Nursing diagnosis: *Altered nutrition: less than body requirements, related to anorexia associated with terminal illness and the dying process*

GOAL: To ensure adequate nutrition to promote patient comfort during the dying process

Interventions

1. See the "Malnutrition" care plan, page 277.

2. As appropriate, institute measures to enhance the patient's appetite and promote increased food intake, such as:
• eating small, frequent meals rather than fewer large ones
• cutting foods into small pieces or pureeing solid foods in a blender
• maintaining a pleasant, relaxed atmosphere during meals
• providing oral care before meals.

Rationales

1. This care plan provides interventions applicable to any patient with inadequate nutrition.

2. Various nursing interventions can help the patient meet his nutritional requirements.

• Small frequent meals are easier to eat and digest.

• This can ease chewing and swallowing and help prevent choking.
• Relaxation may enhance appetite.

• A fresh, clean mouth may enhance appetite.

Nursing diagnosis: *Potential impaired skin integrity, related to circulatory impairment or prolonged immobility associated with terminal illness*

GOAL: To maintain skin integrity and promote patient comfort during the dying process

Interventions

1. On each visit, inspect the patient's skin—especially over bony prominences—for signs of breakdown.

2. Turn the patient and massage bony prominences three or four times a day. Turn carefully to prevent shearing. Apply a skin moisturizing lotion regularly; use

Rationales

1. Dehydration and debilitation contribute to poor skin turgor and increased risk of skin breakdown. Early detection of skin breakdown enables prompt intervention to minimize damage.

2. Turning and massage stimulate circulation to the skin and help prevent breakdown. Applying moisturizing lotion helps prevent skin drying and cracking and pro-

soap sparingly. Instruct the family or other caregivers to perform these measures on the days that you do not visit.

3. Ensure the use of soft bedlinens, and pad bony prominences as necessary.

motes comfort. Soap dries skin, increasing irritation.

3. Rough linens cause friction, which can lead to skin breakdown. Padding bony prominences decreases pressure and promotes comfort.

Nursing diagnosis: *Ineffective breathing pattern, related to effects of terminal illness and prolonged immobility*

GOAL: To promote adequate respiratory function and prevent respiratory complications

Interventions

1. Each visit, assess the patient's respiratory rate and rhythm and auscultate lung sounds. Report any abnormalities.

2. Place the patient in a semi- to high-Fowler's position, as tolerated.

3. Instruct the patient to deep breathe, cough, and change position at least every 2 hours.

4. Increase the patient's fluid intake to 2 to 3 liters/day, as tolerated.

Rationales

1. Normal respirations are essential to adequate gas exchange and tissue oxygenation. Decreased elasticity of lung tissue, as often develops in terminal illness, can interfere with normal respirations and also can place the patient at risk for serious respiratory complications, such as pneumonia.

2. This position facilitates adequate lung expansion, which optimizes gas exchange.

3. These measures promote adequate lung expansion and help remove secretions from the airways.

4. Adequate hydration helps liquify secretions, which allows the patient to remove them from the airways through coughing.

Nursing diagnosis: *Impaired physical mobility, related to effects of terminal illness*

GOAL: To help the patient achieve maximum physical mobility within the limitations imposed by the terminal illness

Interventions

1. Encourage the patient to remain as physically active as possible within the limitations of his illness.

2. Assist the patient with active or passive range-of-motion exercises, as his condition allows. As appropriate, teach the family how to assist with these exercises.

3. Maintain the patient in a functional position with the body properly aligned and the extremities supported.

4. As necessary and appropriate, instruct the patient and family in the use of mobility aids, such as a cane, walker, or wheelchair, and safety devices, such as grab bars in the bathrroom and elevated toilet seats.

Rationales

1. Regular physical activity can help reduce pulmonary congestion, stimulate circulation, and promote comfort and independence.

2. Range-of-motion exercise increases blood flow to muscles and bones, strengthens muscles, and helps prevent muscle atony and contractures.

3. This helps prevent contractures and promotes circulation and comfort.

4. Such devices can improve the patient's mobility and help prevent injury.

Nursing diagnosis: *Anxiety related to the dying process*

GOAL: To reduce the patient's anxiety level and improve acceptance of terminal illness and impending death

Interventions

1. Encourage the patient to express feelings of anxiety and fear.

2. Encourage open communication and sharing of feelings between the patient and family.

3. Discuss the process of dying with the patient and family.

4. As necessary, help the patient formulate plans to complete unfinished business, such as updating a will or reconciling with estranged family members or friends.

5. If the patient or family desires, arrange for visits by clergy.

Rationales

1. Expressing anxiety and fear may help reduce these feelings.

2. Open communication can help alleviate anxiety for both the patient and family.

3. Increased understanding of the dying process can give the patient a greater sense of control over the process, which may help decrease anxiety.

4. This assistance may help the patient gain a sense of control over the last stage of life, which can help reduce anxiety.

5. A sense of spiritual peace and understanding can decrease anxiety.

Nursing diagnosis: *Disturbed self-concept: personal identity, related to imminent threat of loss of self*

GOAL: To help the patient maintain and enrich personal identity throughout the remainder of life

Interventions

1. Use active listening skills, paying special attention to nonverbal or symbolic communication. Use reflective statements and open-ended observations to offer opportunity for discussion of difficult issues. Accept and respect the patient's right to use denial or avoidance behavior. Whatever the patient's response, try to communicate the attempt to understand.

2. Be honest with the patient in answering questions, without forcing discussion of issues the patient has not introduced or chosen to respond to in discussion.

3. Encourage the patient's reminiscence and review of life experiences.

4. Promote creative expression. Encourage family and friends to provide materials for drawing, painting, writing, music, or other creative pursuits the patient enjoys.

5. Explore the option of preparing audio- or videotaped messages or mementos for family and friends to share after the patient's death (or earlier, if the patient wishes).

Rationales

1. Patients facing imminent death often use nonverbal or symbolic communication to describe their experience and to test others' willingness to talk about it. Rushed or distracted behavior from caregivers may distance the patient and contribute to feelings of alienation. Active listening and sharing show concern and respect for the patient as a unique individual. Some patients choose denial or avoidance to the end, and their right to make this choice should be respected as a reflection of their unique selfhood.

2. Honesty, even when truths are painful, shows respect for the individual.

3. Life experiences have helped to shape the patient's unique identity. Reminiscence helps the patient remain connected to important "core" experiences, and provides the caregiver with more information that may aid in understanding and responding to the patient's behavior.

4. Creative activity gives voice to individual expression, helping the patient maintain a sense of uniqueness. Moreover, drawings, paintings, or other original work by the patient may provide clues to his or her state of acceptance.

5. Some patients may feel more comfortable expressing feelings in this way. The recording process itself may help a patient achieve acceptance of impending death. Such mementos may offer the patient comfort in

the thought that some part of his or her individual identity will endure. These records may also be valued by family and friends for preserving their memories of the patient.

Nursing diagnosis: *Potential spiritual distress (distress of the human spirit) related to confrontation with the unknown*

GOAL: To help the patient achieve spiritual calm as death approaches

Interventions

1. Support the patient's personal spiritual beliefs, even if they seem unusual or unfamiliar. Keep in mind that for some people religion provides a strong, positive support system, but for others it may be a source of anger and frustration.

2. Recognize that facing death and dealing with separation and loss are developmental tasks for all persons.

3. Acknowledge what dying patients have to teach others, and express this to the patient and family as appropriate.

4. Provide privacy, as the patient desires.

5. Offer to call a spiritual advisor of the patient's choice: priest, rabbi, minister, counselor, or friend. Obtain and provide religious texts or other inspirational readings, if requested.

6. Talk with the patient while providing care, even if the patient has apparently become unresponsive or comatose. Encourage family members to continue talking to the patient.

7. Worry less about saying the "wrong thing" than about being afraid to communicate caring, and set an example that family members may follow. Avoid clichés and telling family and patient that really don't mean what they are saying.

8. Maintain a positive attitude. Promote activities that provide enjoyment, no matter how small. Avoid pat gen-

Rationales

1. Spiritual beliefs are extremely varied and usually provide comfort based on specific personal meaningfulness to the patient. Attempting to alter such beliefs or supplant them with others shows a lack of respect for the patient and may precipitate undue conflict and distress.

2. Because our culture places such emphasis on youth, we lack the societal integration of death as part of life that many primitive cultures take for granted. In order to help patients accept impending death, caregivers must acknowledge it as a stage of development and validate its importance through specific, nondisease-related interventions.

3. Nurses can learn much from a dying patient that may help them care for others who follow. In such ways, patients may touch the lives of others they will never meet. Recognition of the lessons a dying person may pass on to others in this way can help patients find meaningfulness in death and a sense of connectedness with life.

4. A patient struggling with spiritual issues may need uninterrupted periods for prayer or meditation.

5. A spiritual advisor may provide guidance or perform rituals viewed as essential by the patient. Religious readings may be satisfying to many patients with traditional religious orientation; others may find comfort in poetry or literature that has special personal significance.

6. Survivors of near-death experiences and persons who recover from deep and prolonged coma often report remembering conversation around them while they were apparently unconscious.

7. Nurses, because of prolonged close contact with dying patients and interaction with their families, are uniquely suited to help facilitate dialogue about dying between the patient and family. Often patients and families are fearful to raise the subject with each other directly, concerned they may cause pain or upset the other. There are no cultural prescriptions to guide families, but the nurse may be able to act as a liaison to help communication, thereby reducing guilt and anxiety and further preparing both the patient and family for separation.

8. A positive attitude may help the patient maintain hope and find pleasure in living, even while facing

eralizations as attempts to provide an explanation for suffering.

death. Small gestures may be extremely meaningful when the patient's worldview is narrowed by illness. Generalizations or attempts to provide an explanation ("It may be a blessing," or the like) indicate shallow appreciation for the patient's situation and may be interpreted as dismissal of real concerns.

Nursing diagnosis: *Altered family processes related to impending death of a family member*

GOAL: To minimize disruption of family dynamics by facilitating healthy coping, mutual support, and open communication

Interventions

1. Assess the family's level of acceptance and coping behaviors by observing interactions between the patient and family and by meeting with individual family members, if appropriate.

2. Encourage family members to express their feelings about the patient's imminent death to each other. If necessary, offer to introduce topics for discussion among the family.

3. Promote open communication between family members and the patient. Encourage each family member to spend time alone with the patient; as necessary, provide time for these private visits. During these visits, encourage family members to talk with, laugh with, and touch the patient and to participate in care, as appropriate.

4. Instruct family members not to neglect their own physical and emotional health. Emphasize the importance of adequate rest, good nutrition, and outside activities. Encourage them to take turns caring for the patient, if possible—or, if not possible, to take regular breaks when appropriate.

5. Encourage the family to maintain their normal family routines as much as possible, including leisure activities.

6. Help the family identify and draw on external support systems, such as friends, clergy, counselors, and social service agencies. Provide referrals as needed.

Rationales

1. Effective interventions must be based on the family's level of acceptance and coping behaviors. Each family member may be responding to the patient's imminent death in different ways.

2. Open discussion of feelings can bring sensitive issues out in the open, which may help family members resolve conflicts, explore new roles necessitated by the patient's illness and imminent death, and develop mutually supportive coping behaviors.

3. Open communication with the patient can help family members accept the patient's condition and prepare themselves for the loss of a loved one.

4. Family members' physical and emotional health is essential to continued support of the patient and each other. Breaks from caring for the patient help family members maintain their own lives and reduce the emotional stress associated with caring for a dying person.

5. Engaging in usual routines and activities can help maintain family integrity and stability and facilitate mutual support and other positive coping behaviors.

6. A family facing death often needs additional support to cope with emotional and financial burdens, especially if the dying process is prolonged.

Nursing diagnosis: *Powerlessness related to inevitability of death, lack of control over body functions, or dependence on others for care*

GOAL: To increase the patient's sense of personal power while promoting acceptance of terminal illness and impending death

Interventions

1. Encourage personal decision making whenever possible. Allow maximum flexibility for scheduling of activities, treatments, or visitors. Include the patient as a participant in decision making related to care, as appropriate.

Rationales

1. A terminally ill patient relinquishes many freedoms. Allowing as many choices as possible promotes a sense of control and increases the patient's coping ability. "Taking over" by caregivers has a devaluing effect on the patient's self-esteem and should be avoided unless absolutely necessary.

2. Recognize and support courageous attitudes.

2. Regardless of external circumstances, individuals maintain the freedom to choose their attitude and approach to life (and death). The conscious, courageous exercise of this choice decreases powerlessness.

3. Accept your own powerlessness to alter the patient's basic circumstances.

3. Health care professionals often find it difficult to be unable to "make it better" for their patients. Realistic self-assessment is essential to prevent caregiver "burnout" and maintain the ability to intervene effectively in areas that can be altered.

4. Help the patient identify inner strengths. Ask the patient to recall past losses, how he or she dealt with them, and what was learned from such experiences.

4. Recalling other losses may help the patient build on previously learned coping skills. Each person's losses throughout life may have uniquely prepared that individual with qualities that can be used in facing death.

5. Encourage the patient to establish realistic goals for the remainder of life.

5. Establishing goals provides a focus for energy and reduces the sense of helplessness. Realistic evaluation of capabilities helps in the process of acceptance.

6. Help the patient, as needed, to put affairs in order, including funeral or memorial planning, wills, settling economic affairs, and making arrangements for survivors.

6. Putting affairs in order increases the sense of control and may help soften anitcipated effects of death on loved ones.

Nursing diagnosis: *Family coping: potential for growth, related to bereavement and mourning*

GOAL: To facilitate initiation of healthy grieving after death occurs and continue to support the family during bereavement

Interventions

1. See the "Grief and Grieving" care plan, page 262.

2. Stay with the family during the dying process.

3. Allow family members to stay and hold or touch the body. Ensure that the body is respectfully covered but not inaccessible.

4. Use direct, simple sentences, avoiding use of euphemisms to describe death. Provide comforting observations, when possible; for example: "He died quietly and appeared to have no pain" or "She told me about the good times you used to have."

5. Acknowledge the family's loss by gently reorienting them to the reality of death: "It must be hard to realize he's really dead." Avoid oversentimental responses, especially if unfamiliar with the family.

6. Avoid recommending or encouraging sedation with medication, unless severely dysfunctional behavior is present.

7. Offer to call a friend, clergy, or counselor of choice to help with immediate arrangements. If the family does

Rationales

1. This care plan contains general interventions helpful in caring for bereaved families.

2. Such an intervention serves to reassure them that the patient died with the concerned caregivers at hand.

3. Seeing and touching the body of the loved one helps the family accept the reality of death. Gross blood or other secretions should be cleaned up immediately, but putting away all supplies and cleaning the room before calling the undertaker is not necessary.

4. Most family members are too anxious at this time to comprehend complex explanations. Euphemisms such as "passed on" may offend some family members and can potentially interfere with reality orientation. Sharing selected, specific observations with family members may help minimize guilt and promote healthy grieving.

5. Shock and disbelief are normal initial responses to sudden death and, to a certain degree, even to expected death. Gentle reorientation aids in the process of integrating death into reality. Oversentimental responses may be inappropriate to the family's actual relationship with the deceased.

6. Sedation may delay initiation of normal grieving process.

7. During initial stages of the grieving process, decision making becomes difficult and disorganization and dis-

not already have such a person, offer the services of a hospital chaplain or liaison nurse, or other in-house professional skilled in dealing with grief.

8. Prepare the family for the work of grieving. Emphasize the normalcy of a wide range of emotional responses (anger, guilt, sadness, frustration, resentment, fear, depression) in response to the loss of a loved one.

9. Re-emphasize the need for health-promoting self-care behavior during the grieving period.

10. Ensure that someone will be available to be with the dead patient's partner during the initial mourning period.

11. Reassure the family that feelings of loss, grief, disorientation, and isolation are valid and expected, and that grieving normally may persist for a long time.

orientation are common. Providing an advocacy person helps reduce family distress while making arrangements for disposition of the body and other arrangements.

8. Family members are sometimes unprepared for the variety of feelings experienced in the grieving process, and may feel they're "going crazy" when these occur. Understanding that such emotional disorganization is a normal (and healthy) response to loss can help families deal with these feelings.

9. Grief places additional stress on survivors, who are at increased risk for developing a physical illness during mourning. Health-promoting behavior, such as exercise, can help release emotional energy and reduce the effects of stress.

10. The grieving process is facilitated by sharing feelings with others. Few lonelinesses are as profound as that of a bereaved person, newly alone.

11. Although the grieving process varies for each person, 1 to 2 years is considered normal.

ASSOCIATED CARE PLANS
• Grief and Grieving
• Ineffective Coping
• Malnutrition
• Pain
• Sex and Sexuality
• Total Parenteral Nutrition

NETWORKING OF SERVICES
• community support groups
• durable medical equipment supplier
• Meals On Wheels
• organizations appropriate to the patient's terminal illness, such as the American Cancer Society

CARE TEAM INVOLVED
• nurse
• patient and family
• doctor
• social worker
• clergy
• hospice volunteers

IMPLICATIONS FOR HOME CARE
• telephone (communication)
• safe, accessible environment

PATIENT EDUCATION TOOLS
• information on wills and estate planning
• information on funeral planning
• information on living wills and organ donation
• instructions for pain control, including information on narcotics and nonmedicinal pain control techniques

DISCHARGE PLAN FROM HOME HEALTH CARE
A discharge plan is not applicable to hospice care because of the patient's terminal status.

SELECTED REFERENCES
Dolan, M.B. "If Your Patient Wants to Die at Home," Nursing83 13(4):50-55, April 1983.

Hoff, L.A. *People in Crisis: Understanding and Helping*, 2nd ed. Menlo Park, Calif.: Addison-Wesley Publishing Co., 1986.

Holloway, N. *Medical-Surgical Care Plans*. Springhouse, Pa.: Springhouse Corporation, 1988.

Kneisl, C., and Ames, S. *Adult Health Nursing: A Biopsychosocial Approach*. Menlo Park, Calif.: Addison-Wesley Publishing Co., 1986.

Kübler-Ross, Elisabeth. *Living With Death And Dying*. New York: Macmillan Publishing Co., 1984.

Appendices

NANDA Taxonomy of Nursing Diagnoses

This list presents the approved diagnostic labels of the North American Nursing Diagnosis Association (NANDA), as of summer 1988.

A
Activity intolerance
Activity intolerance: Potential
Adjustment, impaired
Airway clearance, ineffective
Anxiety
Aspiration, potential for

B
Body temperature, altered: Potential
Bowel elimination, altered: Colonic constipation
Bowel elimination, altered: Constipation
Bowel elimination, altered: Diarrhea
Bowel elimination, altered: Incontinence
Bowel elimination, altered: Perceived constipation
Breast-feeding, ineffective
Breathing pattern, ineffective

C
Cardiac output, altered: Decreased
Comfort, altered: Pain
Comfort, altered: Chronic pain
Communication, impaired: Verbal
Coping, family: Potential for growth
Coping, ineffective: Defensive
Coping, ineffective: Denial
Coping, ineffective family: Compromised
Coping, ineffective family: Disabled
Coping, ineffective individual

D-E
Decisional conflict (specify)
Disuse syndrome, potential for
Diversional activity, deficit
Dysreflexia

F
Family processes, altered
Fatigue
Fear
Fluid volume excess
Fluid volume deficit: Actual (1)
Fluid volume deficit: Actual (2)
Fluid volume deficit: Potential

G
Gas exchange, impaired
Grieving, anticipatory
Grieving, dysfunctional
Growth and development, altered

H
Health maintenance, altered
Health seeking behaviors (specify)
Home maintenance management, impaired
Hopelessness
Hyperthermia
Hypothermia

I-J
Incontinence, functional
Incontinence, reflex
Incontinence, stress
Incontinence, total
Incontinence, urge
Infection, potential for
Injury, potential for
Injury, potential for: Poisioning
Injury, potential for: Suffocating
Injury, potential for: Trauma

K-L
Knowledge deficit (specify)

M
Mobility, impaired physical

N-O
Noncompliance (specify)
Nutrition, altered: Less than body requirements
Nutrition, altered: More than body requirements
Nutrition, altered: Potential for more than body requirements

P-Q
Parental role, conflict
Parenting, altered: Actual
Parenting, altered: Potential
Post-trauma response
Powerlessness

R
Rape-trauma syndrome
Rape-trauma syndrome: Compound reaction
Rape-trauma syndrome: Silent reaction
Role performance, altered

S
Self-care deficit: Bathing and hygiene
Self-care deficit: Dressing and grooming
Self-care deficit: Feeding
Self-care deficit: Toileting
Self-concept, disturbance in: Body image
Self-concept, disturbance in: Personal identity
Self-esteem, chronic low
Self-esteem, disturbance in
Self-esteem, situational low
Sensory-perceptual alteration: Visual, auditory, kinesthetic, gustatory, tactile, olfactory
Sexual dysfunction
Sexuality, altered patterns
Skin integrity, impaired: Actual
Skin integrity, impaired: Potential
Sleep pattern disturbance
Social interaction, impaired
Social isolation
Spiritual distress (distress of the human spirit)
Swallowing, impaired

(continued)

NANDA Taxonomy of Nursing Diagnoses (continued)

T
Thermoregulation, ineffective
Thought processes, altered
Tissue integrity, impaired
Tissue integrity, impaired: Oral mucous membrane
Tissue perfusion, altered: Renal, cerebral,
    cardiopulmonary, gastrointestinal, peripheral

U
Unilateral neglect
Urinary elimination, altered patterns
Urinary retention

V-Z
Violence, potential for: Self-directed or directed at
    others

APPENDIX 2
Glossary

Accreditation: Means for evaluating home health care institutions for recognized approval. This evaluation includes both quantity and quality of services as well as compliance with acceptable standards of health care.

Acute care (emergency care): Treatment of a patient who is in a life-threatening situation involving physical or emotional distress.

Ambulatory (outpatient) care: Treatment provided to a patient in a doctor's office, outpatient department, or health center.

Average daily census: Number of patients receiving care during an average day; calculated by counting the number of patients on the home health roster each day.

Caregiver: Significant other (usually a family member, friend, or neighbor) who provides day-to-day home care of a patient.

Case mix: Measure of the patients (cases) handled by a health care provider reflecting their individual needs for resources.

Catastrophic care: Health care provided during the final stages of an illness.

Chronic health care: Health services provided for a patient with an incurable disease, such as hypertension or diabetes. The focus of treatment is on managing the patient's illness to prevent further debilitating effects.

Clinic (health center): Facility that provides preventive, diagnostic, and treatment services to ambulatory patients. Health services are supervised by a clinician licensed to practice in the area where the facility is located.

Community health nurse: Nurse who functions in the home and community setting to provide preventive, curative, and rehabilitative nursing services to patients and families. The main focus of the nurse's functions is teaching and assisting patients and families to achieve greater independence and self-sufficiency within the limitations of existing health problems and family capabilities.

Community resources: Health and welfare services in a community to assist individuals and families with health-related problems.

Comprehensive health care: System of health care providing a wide variety of coordinated health services to patients and families, including nursing care, social services, and nutritional planning.

Conditions of participation: Health care agency's adherence to specified standards and practices in order to receive reimbursement for services rendered, such as Medicare reimbursement for home health services.

Continuity of care: Health services that are provided without interrupting the quality and timing of needed care.

Contractual services: Written agreement whereby a health care provider or agency agrees to provide necessary health services to a patient for a set fee.

Copayment (coinsurance): Method of payment whereby a patient assumes responsibility for sharing the cost of a health care product or treatment with a health insurance agency.

Cost:benefit ratio: Ratio that assesses the cost of a service or product versus the benefits received from the service or product.

Cost control: Monitoring of health services to avoid unnecessary provision and use of services.

Cost-effectiveness analysis: Analytical technique comparing the cost of a technology or alternative technologies to the resultant benefits, with cost and benefits (effectiveness) not expressed by the same measure.

Coverage: Services or benefits provided, arranged, or paid for under a given health plan.

Deductible: Portion of covered health care costs that the insured patient must pay before benefits begin.

Diagnosis-related groups (DRGs): Classification system for reimbursement based on the principal diagnosis, secondary diagnosis, surgical procedure, and age and discharge status of patients treated in hospitals.

Discharge planning: Process of planning future care of a patient after he leaves the services of a hospital, nursing home, or home health agency.

Durable medical equipment (DME): Medical equipment prescribed by a doctor that can be rented or purchased by a patient for home use, such as oxygen tanks, hospital beds, commodes, shower chairs, hoyer lifts, wheelchairs, and walkers.

Durable power of attorney: Legal document designating an individual of choice to be responsible for a patient's health care decisions in the event the patient is incapable of making his own decisions.

Environment: Formal or informal setting (internal, external, natural, or artificial) in which a person works or resides on either a temporary or permanent basis. Usually expressed in relation to a hospital or home environment.

Fee for service: Direct purchase of health services by a patient for a specific treatment or service rendered.

Fixed costs: Costs that do not change with fluctuations in enrollment or use of services.

Follow-up: Process of continued contact with a patient or family to see whether treatment has been carried out and whether the patient's condition has improved. May refer to the initial visit after treatment or an ongoing evaluation.

Goal: Desired result to be achieved within a specified period of time.

Health care team: Various professional and nonprofessional personnel in an organization who work together in a cooperative effort to achieve successful health care.

Health maintenance: Practices involved in preventing, improving, or maintaining the current health status of a patient or family through continuity of health services.

Health maintenance organization (HMO): Health plan that combines the provision of health services in return for prospective per capita payments. The organization acts as both the insurer and provider of services.

(continued)

Glossary (continued)

Health promotion: Reinforcement of or motivation efforts stressing the improved health practices and behavior of patients, families, and communities through health education.

Holistic: Viewing the patient as a total human being rather than as fragmented parts.

Homebound: Unable to leave the home without the assistance of another person or use of an assistive device.

Home health care (home health agency, home care program, home nursing): Health services that are provided in the home setting of patients and families. Registered nurses, therapists (physical, occupational, and speech), social workers, and home health aides usually provide such health care in the home.

Home health care program: Agency-operated home health service. May be hospital-based (operated from a hospital), proprietary (operated as a private business), or public (operated as a municipal government service).

Hospice: System of family-centered care for terminally ill patients focusing on maintaining comfort and a satisfactory life-style throughout the dying process; care is multidisciplinary and may be provided in a hospice center or the home.

Hyperalimentation: Infusion of nutrient-rich formula into a central vein.

Intensive care: Medical and skilled nursing services for severely ill patients who require extensive nursing care and close supervision. Services are provided in specially equipped hospital units.

Intermediary: Agency that issues payment after intensive review of the need for skilled services; for example, an insurance company that handles Medicare claims.

Intermediate care: Health care for moderately ill patients.

Intermittent skilled care: Home care services (by a registered nurse, physical therapist, nurse's aide, occupational therapist, speech therapist, or social worker) provided in a patient's home on a part-time basis, usually not exceeding 4 hours daily.

Length of service (LOS): Anticipated time that a home health agency projects a patient will require services.

Level of care: Measure of the quality and quantity of health care services required by or rendered to a patient, family, or community.

Licensure: Process whereby an offical board grants permission to persons meeting predetermined qualifications to engage in a given occupation with use of a particular title.

Living will: Document containing the expressed wish of a terminally ill patient that no life-sustaining procedures be used on him when he is dying and can no longer actively participate in the decision-making process. Living wills are legally binding in some states.

Medicaid (Title 19): Voluntary Medicare program that aids all persons eligible for federally aided public assistance programs, such as the aged, blind, and disabled and families participating in Aid to Dependent Children (ADC).

Medicare (Title 18): Government legislation passed in 1965 as an extension of Social Security benefits to provide for basic hospital coverage with an optional plan of supplementary medical benefits for all persons age 65 or over.

Nurse clinician (nurse associate, nurse practitioner, family nurse practitioner): Registered nurse who has undergone special training to assume an expanded role in the health care of adults and children.

Ombudsman: Person who investigates patients' complaints against health care personnel or agencies.

Outpatient (ambulatory, primary) care: Facility or department where patients not requiring hospital services may receive health care.

Outreach: Process of extending personnel and services to isolated or rural areas having no access to the services of an urban or developed community.

Patient days: Total number of days of care given in a specified time period.

Patient profile: Pharmacy record system of tracking all drugs a patient is taking (or is allergic to) to prevent drug errors and misuse of drugs.

Physician assistant (PA, physician extender): Specially trained person who performs a variety of routine patient care services under the supervision or direction of a doctor. Training usually consists of 9 months of formal instruction and 15 months of clinical rotations.

Prepayment: Advance payment of a single monthly fee to cover health services received under a health insurance plan.

Preventive health care: Health services aimed at preventing illness or the further progression of disease. Preventive health care services include nutrition, family planning, immunizations, physical examinations, and screenings.

Primary health care: Continued responsibility for the care of patients and families. Also refers to the first contact between the health care provider and patient.

Prospective payment: Payment for medical care based on rates set in advance of the time period for which they apply.

Quality control: Mechanisms for setting basic minimal standards to be followed by public and private agencies to ensure protection of the public; for example, licensure, accreditation, and certification of health care facilities and personnel.

Rehabilitation: Restoration of a disabled or handicapped patient to the fullest physical, mental, social, vocational, or economic usefulness of which he is reasonably capable.

Reimbursement: Payment agreement between providers of health care and third-party payers (such as Medicare or Blue Cross) regarding which services will be paid for and at what cost.

Skilled nursing care: Nursing services provided by registered nurses to patients who need skilled care beyond the scope of lesser trained personnel.

Sliding fee scale: Method for charging various fees for health services based on a patient's individual income. With this method, patients with lower incomes pay less than patients with higher incomes for the same health services.

Specialist: Doctor or nurse who has had from 2 to 5 years of additional education and practice in a particular field of medicine. (Not to be confused with a doctor or nurse who has limited his or her practice to a particular field without the additional training).

Standards of care: Guidelines that define the level of health care acceptable to a program or organization.

Support services: Services, such as patient transportation and health education, that aid in the provision of personal health care.

Target population (service area): Specially designated group of persons who are eligible to receive health care services from a particular program or project. Designation can be by specific factors, such as geographic area, age, or sex.

Third-party payer: Agency or organization (such as Blue Cross or Medicare) responsible for the payment of a patient's health care and services.

Triage: Process of sorting out or screening patients to prioritize which individuals need immediate care and what type of care is needed.

Utilization review: Process of formal activity related to the control of health care costs in the use of health services.

Voluntary health agency: Nonprofit, nongovernmental agency governed by legislation or a professional organization created to motivate public awareness of specific health problems, to support community health services, and to assist in aiding research for specific disease categories.

Index

Page numbers with a "t" indicate tables

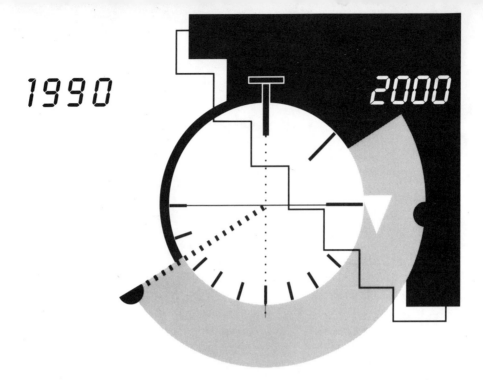

1990 · 2000

Nursing Magazine

In the future as in the past...

You can rely on *Nursing* magazine to keep your skills sharp and your practice current—with award-winning nursing journalism.

Each monthly issue is packed with expert advice on the legal, ethical, and personal issues in nursing, plus up-to-the-minute...

- Drug information—warnings, new uses, and approvals

- Assessment tips
- Emergency and acute care advice
- New treatments, equipment, and disease findings
- Photostories and skill sharpeners
- AIDS updates
- Career tracks and trends

SAVE 38%
Enter your subscription today.
